'*Clinical Handbook of Chinese Herbs* is a unique desk reference for practitioners using Chinese herbs. In a concise and easy-to-read format, Will Maclean presents a large amount of clinically useful information about individual medicinal substances. The use of tables to summarize common applications of the medicinals allows one to see what symptoms a specific substance is particularly effective at addressing. Furthermore, the text contains information about the way that processing the medicinals changes their functions. This reference text is a valuable addition to the library of books that practitioners of Chinese herbal medicine will want to have on their office shelves.'

– *Craig Mitchell, EAMP, PhD, President of the Seattle Institute of Oriental Medicine*

# CLINICAL HANDBOOK
## OF CHINESE HERBS

*of related interest*

**Discussion of Cold Damage (Shang Han Lun)**
**Commentaries and Clinical Applications**
*Guohui Liu, M.Med. L.Ac.*
*Foreword by Dr. Henry McCann*
ISBN 978 1 84819 254 6
eISBN 978 0 85701 200 5

**The Fundamentals of Acupuncture**
*Nigel Ching*
*Foreword by Charles Buck*
ISBN 978 1 84819 313 0
eISBN 978 0 85701 266 1

# CLINICAL HANDBOOK
## OF CHINESE HERBS

DESK REFERENCE, REVISED EDITION

**WILL MACLEAN**

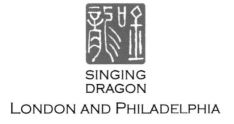

SINGING
DRAGON
LONDON AND PHILADELPHIA

First published in 2017
by Singing Dragon
an imprint of Jessica Kingsley Publishers
73 Collier Street
London N1 9BE, UK
and
400 Market Street, Suite 400
Philadelphia, PA 19106, USA

*www.singingdragon.com*

**Library of Congress Cataloging in Publication Data**
Names: Maclean, Will (Acupuncturist), author.
Title: Clinical handbook of Chinese herbs : desk reference / Will Maclean.
Description: Revised edition. | London ; Philadelphia : Jessica Kingsley
Publishers, 2017. | Includes bibliographical references and indexes.
Identifiers: LCCN 2016043864 (print) | LCCN 2016045531 (ebook) | ISBN
9781848193420 (alk. paper) | ISBN 9780857012982 (ebook)
Subjects: | MESH: Medicine, Chinese Traditional | Drugs, Chinese Herbal |
Handbooks
Classification: LCC RS180.C5 (print) | LCC RS180.C5 (ebook) | NLM WB 39 | DDC
615.3/210951--dc23

**British Library Cataloguing in Publication Data**
A CIP catalogue record for this book is available from the British Library

ISBN 978 1 84819 342 0
eISBN 978 0 85701 298 2

Printed and bound in Great Britain

# CONTENTS

# HOW TO USE THIS BOOK

The material in this book is a consensus compilation of six authoritative text books, with major guidance from the Chinese texts, *Zhong Yao Xue* (2000) and *Zhong Yao Xue* (1997). The texts consulted (see bibliography) usually agree on the major points, but sometimes vary on certain issues such as specific functions, the domain, flavour, nature, dosage and contraindications. I have adopted the consensus viewpoint for most attributes. I have retained old and less relevant indications, such as snakebite, for the sake of historical consistency.

## Indications [△ used for; ▲ strongly indicated for]

Indications, read from left to right, are the specific symptoms or disorders a herb treats. Indications are graded from average to strong on the basis of emphasis in the texts consulted, and on the basis of clinical experience with the more common items. Some obscure indications may be omitted where space is limited. When two or more items are listed in an indications box and one item is particularly indicated, it is highlighted in bold.

Abbreviations:       bld. = blood

const. = constraint

def. = deficiency

def., cold = deficiency and/or cold (yang deficiency, or excess cold)

dysenteric dis. = dysenteric disorder

mm. = muscles

painful obst. = painful obstruction (syndrome)

Sp. = Spleen; Kid. = Kidney; Lu. = Lung; Liv. = Liver; Ht. = Heart; St. = Stomach

stag. = stagnation

synd. = syndrome

↑ Ascendant, high, elevated; ↓ Decreased; → Invading, or transforming into; →ı *Not communicating*

## Functions [○ average; ● strong]

Functions are read from right to left. The functions of a herb are a summary of its general therapeutic characteristics. The original Chinese terms and their definitions, where necessary, can be found in the glossary.

## Domain

This term is usually rendered as channels entered (*gui jing* 归经). Domain is used here because it conveys the target of the herb more precisely – ingested herbs act on the organ system, which incorporates not only the channel but the organ along with associated tissues and structures. The organs listed are ordered following the five phases – metal, water, wood, fire, earth.

## Dosages

The standard dosage range given is of dried herbs, in decoction, for an average adult. Variations are noted in the accompanying text. The issue of dosage is complex and depends on factors such as the age and weight of the patient, the nature and severity of the condition being treated, and the quality of the herbs themselves. Different texts may give quite different dosage ranges. This book stays with the consensus in most cases, with a few exceptions in which clinical experience is the guide. Doses are given in multiples of three, which ties the doses to the original *qian* 钱 measurement of the classic texts. One *qian* is equivalent to 3 grams.

## Preparation and usage

If a herbs' action changes when it is processed, or if a particular cooking method is required, this is noted in the accompanying text. When no notes on preparation are included, the herb is used in the unprocessed dried state, in the dosage range noted in the text, and is decocted in the standard fashion.

## Symbols in the text

❀ Plant or ☗ animal species listed by the Convention on International Trade in Endangered Species (CITES).

† Formulae that traditionally contain items from endangered species and/or obsolete substances.

## Contraindications

Contraindications are given first. If only a caution is given, this is prefaced accordingly. The consensus contraindications and cautions are given, with the exception of those during pregnancy, in which case a conservative approach is adopted and a contraindication is noted even if only one of the source texts asserts it.

## Formulas

A selection of formulae representative of the herbs' therapeutic action are given to provide context to its clinical usage and a sense of how frequently a herb is employed. The ingredients of formulae noted can be found in Appendix 7. Most of the formulae noted are common, and detailed descriptions can be found in Formulas and Strategies (2009).

**Legend:**
△ Indication
▲ Strong Indication
E External Use
**E** Strong External Indication

○ Function
● Strong Function
❖ Domain
♦ Flavour, nature

| INDICATIONS | Shan Zhu Yu 山茱萸 | Fu Pen Zi 覆盆子 | Sang Piao Xiao 桑螵蛸 | Hai Piao Xiao 海螵蛸 | Jin Ying Zi 金樱子 | Qian Shi 芡实 | Lian Zi 莲子 | Chun Pi 椿皮 | Ji Guan Hua 鸡冠花 | Ma Huang Gen 麻黄根 | Fu Xiao Mai 浮小麦 | Nuo Dao Gen Xu 糯稻根须 | FUNCTIONS |
|---|---|---|---|---|---|---|---|---|---|---|---|---|---|
| acid reflux, heartburn | | | | ▲○ | | | | | | | | | alleviates gastric acidity |
| appetite – loss of | | | | | ○ | | △ | ○ | ○ | | | | binds the Intestines |
| bleeding – hematemesis | | ○ | | △ | | | | | | | | | brightens the eyes |
| bleeding – hemoptysis | | | | △ | | | ○ | | | | | | calms the shen |
| bleeding – hemorrhoids | | | | | | | | ○ | △ | | | | clears damp heat |
| bleeding – rectal; def., cold | | | | △ | | | | | △ | | ○ | ○ | clears deficient heat |
| bleeding – rectal, from heat# | | | | | | | | ▲○ | △ | | | | kills parasites |
| bleeding – traumatic | | | | E○ | | | | | | | | | promotes healing |
| bleeding – uterine, from heat# | ○ | ○ | ● | | | | | △ | ▲ | | | | restrains urine |
| bleeding – uterine, deficient | △○ | ○ | ○ | △ | △○ | ○ | △○ | | ▲ | | | | secures essence |
| diabetes (xiao ke) | △○ | ○ | ○ | | | ○ | ○ | ○ | | | | | stabilizes the Kidneys |
| diarrhea – Spleen def., chronic | ○ | | | △○ | △ | ▲ | △ | ○ | ○ | | | | stops bleeding |
| dizziness – Kidney deficiency | △ | | | | ○ | ○ | ○ | ○ | ○ | | | | stops diarrhea |
| dysenteric dis. – chronic; def., cold | | | | ● | △ | △ | △ | | △○ | | | | stops leukorrhea |
| dysenteric dis. – chronic; heat# | ○ | | | △ | | | | ▲ | △ | ● | ○ | ○ | stops sweating |
| ears – tinnitus, ↓hearing – Kid def. | △ | | | | | | ○ | ○ | | | | | strengthens the Spleen |
| eyes – corneal opacity, cataract | ● | ○ | ○ | △ E | | | | | | | | | tonifies the Kidneys |
| eyes – weakness of vision | | △ | | | | | | | | | | | |
| fever – bone steaming, yin def. | | | | | | | | | | | △ | △ | |
| gastritis – hyperacidity | | | | ▲ | | | | | | | | | |
| impotence – Kidney deficiency | △ | △ | △ | | | | △ | | | | | | |
| insomnia, anxiety – Ht. ↛ Kid. | | | | | | | ▲ | | | | | | |
| leukorrhea – Sp. & Kid. def. | | | △ | ▲ | △ | ▲ | △ | | △ | | | | **Domain (❖)** |
| leukorrhea – damp heat# | | | | | | △ | | ▲ | △ | ❖ | | | Lung |
| pain – abdominal, worms | | | | | ❖ | | | △ ❖ | ❖ | | | | Large Intestine |
| pain – epigastric, & hyperacidity | ❖ | ❖ | ❖ | △ ❖ | | ❖ | | | | | | | Kidney |
| pain – lower back, leg, knee | △ | △ | | | ❖ | | | | | | | | Bladder |
| palpitations – Ht. ↛ Kid. | △ ❖ | ❖ | ❖ | ❖ | | | ▲ | ❖ | ❖ | | | ❖ | Liver |
| parasites – roundworms | | | | | | ❖ | | △ | | | ❖ | ❖ | Heart |
| prolapse – rectal | | | | | △ | ❖ | ❖ | E | | | | | Spleen |
| prolapse – uterine | | | | ❖ | △ | | | ❖ | | | | | Stomach |
| skin – eczema, dermatitis | | | | E | | | | E | | | | | |
| skin – scabies, ringworm, tinea | | | | | | | | E | | | | | |
| sperm – poor motility, ↓ count | | △ | | | | | | | | | | | |
| sperm – involuntary loss of | △ | △ | △ | △ | ▲ | △ | △ | | | | | | |
| sweating – night; yin def. | △ | | | | | | | ♦ | | ▲ | △ | △ | **Flavour, nature (♦)** |
| sweating – profuse in shock | ▲ | | ♦ | ♦ | | | | | | | | | bitter |
| sweating – spontaneous; qi def. | △ ♦ | ♦ | | | ♦ | | | | | ▲ | △ | △ | salty |
| ulcers – skin, chronic | | ♦ | ♦ | E | | ♦ | ♦ | | ♦ | ♦ | ♦ | ♦ | sour |
| ulcers – gastric | | | | △ | | | | ♦ | | | | | sweet |
| urination – enuresis, nocturia | △ | △ | ▲ | | △ | △ | | | | ♦ | | | cold |
| urine – frequency, incontinence | △ | ▲ | △ ♦ | | △ ♦ | △ ♦ | ♦ | | | | ♦ | | cool |
| urination – turbid | ♦ | ♦ | | ♦ | | | △ | △ | | | | ♦ | neutral |
| **Standard dosage range (g)** | 6–12 | 6–9 | 3–9 | 6–12 | 6–18 | 9–15 | 6–15 | 6–9 | 6–15 | 3–9 | 15–30 | 15–30 | slightly warm |

Astringent herbs tone tissues, prevent passive leakage of fluids, and are used to arrest excessive sweat, urine, diarrhea and bleeding. They also enhance the tone of lax tissues and treat prolapse. They are primarily symptomatic, that is, they treat the manifestation of a disorder and not the cause. They are usually combined with appropriate tonic or heat clearing herbs. They are primarily used in cases of deficiency, and are generally contraindicated when there is any pathogen that needs clearing or venting. Some, however, may be used judiciously in combination with other appropriate herbs, when a chronic pathogen remains (damp heat in the Intestines, for example).

Astringent herbs can be divided into five broad groups, based on the main area of influence. These are not precise divisions, however, as there is considerable overlap in therapeutic action.

| Bladder, Kidneys (excessive urination, leakage of semen) | shan zhu yu, fu pen zi, sang piao xiao, jin ying zi, chun gen pi |
|---|---|
| Uterus (bleeding, leukorrhea) | hai piao xiao, ji guan hua |
| Sweat | ma huang gen, fu xiao mai, nuo dao gen xu |
| Lungs (chronic cough) | wu wei zi, wu mei, he zi, ying su ke, wu bei zi |
| Intestines (chronic diarrhea) | chi shi zhi, yu yu liang, shi liu pi, rou dou kou, lian zi, qian shi |

## Shān Zhū Yú (Corni Fructus) cornelian cherry fruit

**Preparation and usage** Up to 30 grams can be used for severe sweating or profuse urination.

**Contraindications** Damp heat and dysuria patterns.

**Formulae** *Gu Chong Tang* (uterine bleeding from Spleen qi and chōng mài / rèn mài deficiency); *Jia Wei Si Wu Tang* (menorrhagia from Liver and Kidney deficiency); *Lai Fu Tang* (severe sweating from collapse of yang qi); *Liu Wei Di Huang Wan* (Kidney yin deficiency); *You Gui Wan* (Kidney yang deficiency)

## Fù Pén Zǐ (Rubi Fructus) Chinese raspberry

**Contraindications** Kidney yin deficiency and blood deficiency patterns with heat, and in painful or difficult urination cases.

**Formulae** *Wu Zi Yan Zong Wan* (sperm disorders from Kidney deficiency)

## Sāng Piāo Xiāo (Mantidis Ootheca) praying mantis egg case

**Preparation and usage** Mostly used in pill or powders, but can be decocted.

**Contraindications** Kidney yin deficiency patterns with heat, and dysuria due to heat or damp heat.

**Formulae** *Sang Piao Xiao San* (enuresis and nocturia from Heart and Kidney deficiency); *Gu Chong Tang* (uterine bleeding from Spleen qi and chōng mài / rèn mài deficiency)

## Hǎi Piāo Xiāo (Sepiae Endoconcha) cuttlefish bone

Also known as wū zéi gǔ 乌贼骨.

**Preparation and usage** Can be stir fried (*chao hai piao xiao* 炒海螵蛸) to enhance its astringency and ability to counteract gastric hyperacidity. When used in powder form and taken directly to combat gastric acidity and epigastric pain, the dose is 1.5–3 grams.

**Contraindications** Caution in bleeding disorders from yin deficiency with heat. Prolonged use may cause constipation.

**Formulae** *Wu Bei San* (epigastric pain and acid reflux); *Bai Zhi San* (thin watery or bloody leukorrhea); *Sheng Ji Gan Nong San*† (chronic superficial suppuration)

## Jīn Yīng Zǐ (Rosae laevigatae Fructus) cherokee rosehip

**Preparation and usage** Can be cooked into a syrup with honey, which moderates it sourness with sweetness, and makes it more effective for chronic diarrhea and prolapse from Spleen deficiency. When used in this way the daily dose is up to 30 grams.

**Contraindications** Excess patterns, especially those with heat.

**Formulae** *Shui Lu Er Xian Dan* (frequent urination and leukorrhea from Kidney yang qi deficiency)

## Qiàn Shí (Euryales Semen) euryale seed

**Preparation and usage** Can be used for both deficient and damp heat types of leukorrhea, depending on the herbs with which it is combined. May be stir fried (*chao qian shi* 炒芡实) to enhance its warmth and improve its ability to treat leakage from yang deficiency.

**Contraindications** Patients with difficulty passing urine or stools.

**Formulae** *Yi Huang Tang* (chronic leukorrhea from Spleen deficiency and damp heat); *Shui Lu Er Xian Dan* (frequent urination and leukorrhea from Kidney yang qi deficiency); *Jin Suo Gu Jing Wan* (frequent urination and loss of essence from Kidney deficiency); *Gao Lin Tang* (turbid urination from Kidney deficiency)

## Lián Zǐ (Nelumbinis Semen) lotus seed

Old lotus seeds that have been harvested after frost turn black on the outside, and are known as shí lián zǐ 石莲子. They are bitter and cold, and cool the Heart and clear damp heat. The stamen of the lotus flower (lián xū 莲须, Nelumbinis Stamen) is very similar in action to the young seeds and can be used interchangeably.

**Contraindications** Patients with constipation and dry stools.

**Formulae** *Shen Ling Bai Zhu San* (Spleen qi deficiency diarrhea); *Pi Shen Shuang Bu Wan* (chronic diarrhea from Spleen and Kidney deficiency); *Jin Suo Gu Jing Wan* (frequent urination and loss of essence from Kidney deficiency); *Qing Xin Lian Zi Yin* (persistent or recurrent dysuria from Heart fire and qi and yin deficiency); *Fu Tu Dan* (leukorrhea and seminal emission from Kidney deficiency); *Kai Jin San* (anorectic dysenteric disorder)

## Chūn Pí (Ailanthi Cortex) ailanthus root bark

**Preparation and usage** This herb can be prepared as a decoction and delivered as an enema for chronic damp heat dysenteric disorder. For external use, a standard strained decoction can be used, or the herb can be powdered and mixed with a suitable carrier such as sorbolene.

**Contraindications** Caution in middle burner yang deficiency, and alone in yin deficiency patterns.

**Formulae** *Yu Dai Wan* (chronic damp heat leukorrhea with underlying qi and blood deficiency); *Gu Jing Wan* (uterine bleeding from yin deficiency with heat)

## Jī Guān Huā (Celosiae cristatae Flos) coxcomb flower

This herb is classified in the hemostatic group in some texts.

**Contraindications** Uterine bleeding from blood stasis, acute dysenteric disorder and when there is any exterior heat or cold pathogen.

## Má Huáng Gēn (Ephedrae Radix) ephedra root

**Contraindications** Sweating associated with acute external invasion, acute common cold, and lingering pathogens.

**Formulae** *Mu Li San* (sweating from deficiency)

## Fú Xiǎo Mài (Tritici Fructus levis) light wheat grain

**Contraindications** Sweating associated with acute external invasion, acute common cold, and lingering pathogens.

**Formulae** *Mu Li San* (sweating from deficiency)

## Nuò Dào Gēn Xū (Oryzae glutinosae Radix) glutinous rice root

**Contraindications** Sweating associated with acute external invasion, acute common cold, and lingering pathogens.

## Substances from other groups

Herbs from other groups with astringent properties include chao pu huang (p.12), ce bai ye (p.12) bai ji (p.14), xian he cao (p.14), zi zhu (p.14), zong lu pi (p.14), ou jie (p.14), tie xian cai (p.14), ji hua (p.14), mu li (p.48), bai guo (p.68) and long gu (p.72).

## Endnotes

\# Chronic damp heat or heat in the blood with underlying deficiency. The deficiency component is the dominant pathology.

† These formulae traditionally contain items from endangered animal species and/or obsolete toxic substances, and are unavailable in their original form.

# 1. ASTRINGENTS

| | Wu Wei Zi 五味子 | Wu Mei 乌梅 | Wu Bei Zi 五倍子 | He Zi 诃子 | Shi Liu Pi 石榴皮 | Rou Dou Kou 肉豆蔻 | Chi Shi Zhi 赤石脂 | Yu Yu Liang 禹余粮 | Ying Su Ke 罂粟壳 | FUNCTIONS |
|---|---|---|---|---|---|---|---|---|---|---|
| **△ Indication** <br> **▲ Strong Indication** <br> **E External Use** <br> **E Strong External Indication** | | | | | | | | | | ○ *Function* <br> ● *Strong Function* |
| **INDICATIONS** | | | | | | | | | | |
| appetite – loss of | ● | ○ | ○ | ○ | | △ | | | ○ | astringes the Lungs |
| bleeding – epistaxis, gums | ○ | ○ | E○ | ○ | ○ | ○ | ● | ○ | ○ | binds the Intestines |
| bleeding – hematuria | ○ | △ | △ | | | | | | | calms the shen |
| bleeding – hemoptysis | | | △ | ● | | | | | | eases the throat |
| bleeding – rectal | ○ | △○ | △ | △ | △ | | ▲ | △ | | generates fluids |
| bleeding – traumatic | | E | | | E○ | | E | | | kills parasites |
| bleeding – uterine, def. | | △ | △ | | △ | | △○ | △ | | promotes healing |
| cough – Lung def., chronic | ▲○ | △ | △○ | △ | | | | △ | | secures essence |
| diabetes (*xiao ke*) | △○ | △ | ○ | | | | | | | stabilizes the Kidneys |
| diarrhea – cockcrow | ▲ | ○ | ○ | | | ▲ | ○ | ○ | | stops bleeding |
| diarrhea – Spleen def., chronic | △● | △○ | △○ | △○ | △ | ▲ | ▲ | △ | △○ | stops cough |
| dysenteric dis. – chronic; def., cold | ○ | ▲○ | △○ | △○ | △○ | ● | ▲● | △○ | △○ | stops diarrhea |
| dysenteric dis. – chronic; heat# | | △ | | | △ | | | | ● | stops pain |
| eyes – weakness of vision | △○ | | ○ | | | | | | | stops sweating |
| insomnia – yin, blood def. | △○ | | | | | | | | | tonifies the Kidneys |
| leukorrhea – Sp. & Kid. def. | | | | | △ | ○ | △ | △ | | warms the middle burner |
| liver enzymes ↑ (AST, ALT) | △ | | | | | | | | | |
| memory – poor | △ | | | | | | | | | |
| pain – abdominal; worms | | △ | | | △ | | | | | |
| pain – abdominal; def., cold | | | | | | △ | | △ | | |
| pain – cancer | | | | | | | | ▲ | | |
| pain – sinew & bone | | | | | | | | ▲ | | |
| palpitations – yin, blood def. | △ | | | | | | | | | |
| parasites – roundworms | | | | | △ | | | | | **Domain (✣)** |
| parasites – tapeworms | ✣ | ✣ | ✣ | ✣ | △ | | | ✣ | | Lung |
| prolapse – rectal | | △✣ | △E✣ | △✣ | △✣ | △✣ | △✣ | ✣ | △✣ | Large Intestine |
| prolapse – uterine | ✣ | | E✣ | | | | | ✣ | | Kidney |
| skin – eczema | | ✣ | | E | | | | | | Liver |
| skin – tinea, ringworm | ✣ | | | E | | | | | | Heart |
| sperm – poor motility, ↓ count | ▲ | ✣ | | | | ✣ | | | | Spleen |
| sperm – involuntary loss of | △ | | △ | | ✣ | ✣ | ✣ | ✣ | | Stomach |
| sweating – night; yin def. | △ | | △ | | | | | | | |
| sweating – spontaneous; qi def. | △ | | △ | | | | | | | |
| ulcers – skin, chronic | | | E | | | | E | | | **Flavour, nature (♦)** |
| urination – enuresis | △ | | △ | | | | | ♦ | | toxic |
| urination – frequent | △ | | △♦ | | ♦ | ♦ | | | | slightly toxic |
| urination – turbid | | | △ | | | ♦ | | | | acrid |
| voice – loss of, hoarse | | | | ▲♦ | | | | | | bitter |
| vomiting, nausea – Spleen def. | ♦ | ♦ | ♦ | | ♦ | △ | ♦ | ♦ | | sour |
| warts & corns | | E | | | | | ♦ | ♦ | | sweet |
| wheezing – Lung deficiency | ▲ | | ♦ | △ | | | | | | cold |
| | | ♦ | | ♦ | | | | ♦ | ♦ | neutral |
| | ♦ | | | | ♦ | ♦ | ♦ | | | warm |
| **Standard dosage range (g)** | 1.5–6 | 9–30 | 3–9 | 3–9 | 3–9 | 3–9 | 9–18 | 9–18 | 3–9 | |

### Wǔ Wèi Zǐ (Schisandrae Fructus) schisandra fruit

**Preparation and usage** Used to restrain leakage of fluids and stop cough, either the unprocessed or vinegar processed herb (*cu wu wei zi* 醋五味子) is preferred; when used to tonify the Kidneys, the wine processed herb (*jiu wu wei zi* 酒五味子) is used. To highlight the astringent qualities, a small dose, 1.5–3 grams, is used; to tonify yin and generate fluids, a larger dose, 3–6 grams is required. When taken directly as powder the dose is 1–3 grams per day.

**Contraindications** Acute and heat type wheezing and cough, externally contracted cough, internal excess heat conditions, and the early stages of measles or other infectious rashes.

**Formulae** *Wu Wei Zi San* (chronic cough from Lung qi deficiency); *Mai Wei Di Huang Wan* (chronic cough from Lung yin deficiency); *Du Qi Wan* (chronic wheezing from Kidney not grasping qi); *Xiao Qing Long Tang* (wind cold with copious thin phlegm in the Lungs); *Sheng Mai San* (post febrile qi and yin deficiency); *Yu Ye Tang* (diabetes from yin deficiency); *Si Shen Wan* (chronic diarrhea from Spleen and Kidney yang deficiency); *Tian Wang Bu Xin Dan* (insomnia and *shén* disturbance from Heart and Kidney yin deficiency); *Wu Zi Yan Zong Wan* (sperm disorders from Kidney deficiency); *Fu Tu Dan* (leukorrhea and seminal emission from Kidney deficiency)

### Wū Méi (Mume Fructus) mume plum

**Preparation and usage** To stop bleeding, diarrhea and dysenteric disorder, the charred fruit (*wu mei tan* 乌梅炭) is used. When applied externally to warts and corns, the fruit is softened in hot water, mashed, and applied on a sterile gauze to the debrided lesion. Change the dressing every day. When applied to wounds to stop bleeding, the charred and powdered herb is applied topically.

**Contraindications** Acute common cold patterns, acute diarrhea and in internal excess heat and stagnation patterns.

**Formulae** *Wu Mei Wan* (*jué yīn* syndrome; chronic diarrhea; abdominal pain from roundworms); *Gu Chang Wan*† (chronic diarrhea from Spleen and Kidney yang deficiency); *Di Yu Wan* (incessant bloody dysentery from heat); *Yu Quan Wan* (diabetes from yin deficiency); *Yi Fu San*† (chronic cough from Lung deficiency); *Ru Sheng San* (uterine bleeding from yang deficiency); *Qin Jiao Bie Jia Tang* (bone steaming fever and night sweats from yin deficiency)

### Wǔ Bèi Zǐ (Galla Chinensis) gallnut of Chinese sumac

**Preparation and usage** When taken directly in pills and powders, the dose is 1–1.5 grams.

**Contraindications** Acute common cold patterns, externally contracted cough, and in acute, or predominantly excess patterns of damp heat diarrhea and dysenteric disorder.

**Formulae** *Yu Guan Wan* (chronic diarrhea with bleeding); *Gu Chong Tang* (uterine bleeding from Spleen qi deficiency); *Han Hua Wan* (phlegm type benign thyroid nodules and cervical lymphadenopathy); *Sheng Ji Gan Nong San*† (chronic superficial suppuration)

### Hē Zǐ (Chebulae Fructus) terminalia fruit

**Preparation and usage** To bind the Intestines and stop diarrhea, use roasted he zi (*wei he zi* 煨诃子); for chronic cough and to ease the throat and voice, unprocessed he zi is preferred.

**Contraindications** Acute damp heat patterns, and when there is any pathogen on the surface. Caution should be used in patients with significant qi deficiency, as the bitter descending component of the herb is quite strong relative to its astringency, and prolonged or excessive use can damage qi.

**Formulae** *He Zi Pi San*† (chronic diarrhea and rectal prolapse from Spleen yang deficiency); *He Zi San* (chronic dysenteric disorder from damp heat); *He Zi Qing Yin Tang* (chronic wheezing and loss of voice from Lung deficiency); *Qing Yin Wan*† (hoarse voice, loss of voice and sore throat from Lung fire); *Ke Xue Fang* (hemoptysis from fire)

### Shí Liú Pí (Granati Pericarpium) pomegranate husk

**Preparation and usage** When used in decoction for diarrhea and parasites, the unprocessed herb is used; when used for diarrhea with bleeding the charred form (*shi liu tan* 石榴炭) is preferred; when used in pills or powders, the stir fried form (*chao liu pi* 炒榴皮) is used.

**Contraindications** Acute damp heat diarrhea patterns, and in the early stages of any pattern of diarrhea and dysenteric disorder.

**Formulae** *Huang Lian Tang* (chronic diarrhea and dysenteric disorder)

### Ròu Dòu Kòu (Myristicae Semen) nutmeg

**Preparation and usage** When taken directly as powder or in pills, the daily dose is 1.5–3 grams. In general, the roasted form (*wei rou dou kou* 煨肉豆蔻) is used therapeutically, as roasting reduces its mild toxicity, and enhances its ability to warm the middle burner and stop diarrhea and vomiting.

**Contraindications** Damp heat or chronic yin deficiency type diarrhea, and Stomach heat patterns. The unprocessed herb is mildly toxic. This herb should not be used in therapeutic doses during pregnancy (the culinary use of small quantities as spice is safe), or in patients with liver damage.

**Formulae** *Si Shen Wan* (chronic diarrhea from Spleen and Kidney yang deficiency); *Yang Zang Tang*† (chronic dysenteric disorder from Spleen and Kidney yang deficiency)

### Chì Shí Zhī (Halloysitum rubrum) kaolin, a mineral clay with the chemical composition $Al_4(Si_4O_{10})(OH)_8 \cdot (4H_2O)$

**Preparation and usage** When used internally, the calcined form (*duan chi shi zhi* 煅赤石脂) is used. When decocted it should be cooked in a cloth bag[1]. When used externally, the unprocessed mineral is finely ground and applied topically.

**Contraindications** Acute damp heat or other excess patterns of diarrhea and dysenteric disorder, and when any pathogen remains in chronic cases. Caution during pregnancy. Antagonistic[2] to rou gui (p.88).

**Formulae** *Tao Hua Tang* (chronic dysenteric disorder from Spleen and Kidney yang deficiency); *Chi Shi Zhi Yu Yu Liang Tang* (chronic dysenteric disorder, fecal incontinence and rectal prolapse from yang deficiency); *Zhen Ling Dan*† (persistent uterine bleeding from yang deficiency and blood stasis); *Sheng Ji San*† (chronic non healing ulcers and sores)

### Yǔ Yú Liáng (Limonitum) limonite, an iron containing compound with the chemical composition $FeO \cdot (OH)$

**Preparation and usage** Calcining with vinegar (*cu duan yu yu liang* 醋煅禹余粮) enhances its ability to stop diarrhea and bleeding, and is the form most commonly prescribed.

**Contraindications** Acute damp heat or other excess patterns of diarrhea and dysenteric disorder, and when any pathogen remains in chronic cases. Caution during pregnancy.

**Formulae** *Chi Shi Zhi Yu Yu Liang Tang* (chronic dysenteric disorder, fecal incontinence and rectal prolapse from yang deficiency); *Zhen Ling Dan*† (persistent uterine bleeding from yang deficiency and blood stasis)

### Yīng Sù Ké (Papaveris Pericarpium) opium poppy husk

This substance is addictive when abused. It is the raw material for morphine and heroin production, and is illegal in most countries and therefore obsolete[3].

**Preparation and usage** When processed with honey (*zhi ying su ke* 炙罂粟壳) its ability to stop cough is enhanced; when processed with vinegar (*cu ying su ke* 醋罂粟壳) its ability to stop diarrhea and pain is enhanced.

**Contraindications** Pregnancy, lactation, in small children, acute diarrhea or dysenteric disorder and acute cough.

**Formulae** *Jiu Xian San*† (chronic cough); *Yang Zang Tang*† (chronic dysenteric disorder from Spleen and Kidney yang deficiency)

### Endnotes

# Chronic damp heat or heat in the blood with underlying deficiency. The deficiency component is the dominant pathology.

† These formulae traditionally contain items from endangered animal species and/or obsolete toxic substances, and are unavailable in their original form.

---

1 Appendix 6, p.109
2 Appendix 2, p.100
3 Appendix 5, p.107

**Legend:**
△ Indication
▲ Strong Indication
E External Use
**E** Strong External Indication
○ Function
● Strong Function

| INDICATIONS | Chuan Xiong 川芎 | Dan Shen 丹参 | Ji Xue Teng 鸡血藤 | Huai Niu Xi 怀牛膝 | Yi Mu Cao 益母草 | Ze Lan 泽兰 | Tao Ren 桃仁 | Hong Hua 红花 | Yan Hu Suo 延胡索 | Wu Ling Zhi 五灵脂 | Ru Xiang 乳香 | Mo Yao 没药 | FUNCTIONS |
|---|---|---|---|---|---|---|---|---|---|---|---|---|---|
| abscess – breast, mastitis | | △○ | | | △E | △E | | | | | | | calms the shen |
| abscess – Lung & Intestine | | | | | ○ | | ▲ | | | | △ | △ | clears toxic heat |
| abscesses & sores – skin | | △○ | | | △E | △ | | △ | | | △ | △ | cools the blood |
| amenorrhea | △ | △ | △ | ▲○ | △ | △ | △ | ▲ | | △ | △ | △ | directs blood & fire down |
| bleeding – hematemesis, nose | ● | | | △ | | | | | | | | | dispels wind |
| bleeding – uterine; blood stasis | | | | | △ | | ● | ● | ○ | △○ | ○ | ○ | disperses blood stasis |
| bleeding – hematuria | ● | ● | ○ | △○ | △○ | ○ | | | | | | | invigorates blood |
| cardiovascular disease | ▲ | ▲ | | | | | ○ | △ | △ | | | | moistens the intestines |
| cirrhosis of the liver – early | ● | ▲ | | | | | | | ○ | | | | moves qi |
| constipation – dryness | | | | | | | △ | | | | ○ | ○ | promotes healing |
| depression | | △ | | ○ | | | | ○ | | | | | promotes menstruation |
| dysmenorrhea | ▲ | △ | △ | △ | ▲○ | △○ | ▲ | △ | ▲ | ▲ | △ | △ | promotes urination |
| dysuria – damp heat, bld. | ● | | | △ | ● | | | | | | | | regulates menstruation |
| edema – menstrual, nephritic | ○ | ○ | | △ | △ | | | | ● | ○ | ○ | ○ | stops pain |
| headache – qi & bld. st.; cold, wind | ▲ | ○ | ○ | △ | | | | | △ | | | | tonifies blood |
| headache – Liver fire; yang↑ | △ | | | ▲○ | | | | | △ | | | | tonifies Liver & Kidney |
| hemiplegia | △ | △ | ▲○ | △ | | | △ | △ | | | | | unblocks collaterals |
| hepatitis – chronic | | △ | | | | | | | | | | | |
| hypertension – ascendant yang | | | | ▲ | | | | | | | | | |
| insomnia – heat, blood stasis | | ▲ | | | | | | | | | | | |
| labour – difficult | △ | | | △ | △ | | | | | | | | |
| leukopenia after radiotherapy | | ▲ | | | | | | | | | | | **Domain (❖)** |
| masses – abdominal | | △ | | △ | △ | △ | ▲❖ | △ | | | | △ | Lung |
| menstruation – irregular | ▲ | △ | △ | △ | ▲ | △ | △❖ | | | | | | Large Intestine |
| muscle weakness & atrophy | △ | △ | △ | ▲❖ | | | | | | | | | Kidney |
| numbness – extremities | | | ▲ | | ❖ | | | | | | | | Bladder |
| oral cavity – inflammation of | ❖ | ❖ | ❖ | ▲❖ | ❖ | ❖ | ❖ | ❖ | ❖ | ❖ | E❖ | ❖ | Liver |
| pain – & injury, trauma | △❖ | ▲ | | △ | △E | △E | △ | △E | △ | △ | ▲E | ▲E | Gallbladder |
| pain – abdominal, blood stasis | △ | △❖ | △❖ | △ | △❖ | △ | ▲❖ | △❖ | ▲❖ | △ | △❖ | △❖ | Heart |
| pain – abdominal, qi stagnation | △❖ | ❖ | | | | | | | ▲ | | | | Pericardium |
| pain – chest, angina | ▲ | ▲ | ❖ | | ❖ | | | △ | ▲❖ | △ | ▲❖ | ▲❖ | Spleen |
| pain – epigastric | | ▲ | | | | | | | ▲ | ▲ | △ | △ | |
| pain – hypochondriac | △ | △ | | | | △ | △ | △ | ▲ | △ | △ | △ | |
| pain – lower back, leg, knee | | △ | | ▲ | | | | | | | | | **Flavour, nature (♦)** |
| pain – postpartum abdominal | ▲ | △ | | △ | ▲ | △ | ▲♦ | △ | △ | △ | | | slightly toxic |
| pain – testicular | ♦ | ♦ | | | ♦ | ♦ | | ♦ | △♦ | △ | ♦ | | acrid |
| painful obst. – blood stasis | △ | △♦ | ▲♦ | △♦ | ♦ | ♦ | ♦ | | ▲♦ | ♦ | ▲♦ | ▲♦ | bitter |
| painful obst. – damp heat | | △ | | △♦ | | | | | | | | | sour |
| painful obst. – wind damp | △ | | ▲♦ | △ | | △♦ | | | ▲ | ♦ | ▲ | ▲ | sweet |
| palpitations – heat, blood stasis | | △ | | ♦ | | | ♦ | | | | | ♦ | neutral |
| placenta, lochia – retention of | △ | △♦ | | △ | ▲♦ | | ▲ | △ | | △ | | | cool |
| skin – rash, heat & bld. stasis | ♦ | | ♦ | | | | | △♦ | ♦ | ♦ | ♦ | | warm |
| ulcers, wounds – non-healing | | | | | | ♦ | | | | | ▲E | ▲E | slightly warm |
| **Standard dosage range (g)** | 3–9 | 6–15 | 9–15 | 9–15 | 9–15 | 9–15 | 6–9 | 1–9 | 3–9 | 3–9 | 3–9 | 3–9 | |

The degrees of strength in moving blood and eliminating static blood are denoted by different technical terms in Chinese medicine. Herbs that invigorate blood (*huo xue* 活血) are the mildest, with a moderate yet reliable blood stasis resolving action and some mild tonic effects. Generally well tolerated, they can be used for prolonged periods without damaging normal qi and blood. The mid range group are those that disperse stagnant blood (*qu yu* 祛血). These are stronger than the invigorating group, with little or no tonic action. They can be used for relatively long periods as long as the patient is monitored. They may disperse normal qi and blood in some patients. The strongest, those that break up static blood (*po xue* 破血), are powerful substances with the potential to damage normal qi and blood. They are used for short periods in cases of stubborn or severe blood stasis, and should be phased out in favor of dispersing or invigorating herbs as stasis resolves. Grades of strength also occur within the blood breaking group, the insect drugs being the strongest. The herbs are roughly arranged here in ascending order of strength.

The classification of strength varies between texts. Different sources emphasise different aspects of a herb's activity. The rating used here is based on the consensus of several sources and clinical experience.

### Chuān Xiōng (Chuanxiong Rhizoma) Sichuan lovage root

**Preparation and usage** When decocted, cook no longer than 5–15 minutes[1]. When taken directly as a powder the dose is 1–1.5 grams. For severe, recalcitrant and migrainous headaches, up to 50 grams in decoction may be used for a few days. Stir frying (*chao chuan xiong* 炒川芎) moderates its dispersing nature and makes it more suitable for weak and deficient patients; processing with wine (*jiu chuan xiong* 酒川芎) enhances its analgesic effect.

**Contraindications** Yin deficiency with internal heat, excessive sweating from qi deficiency, vomiting due to counterflow qi, menorrhagia and bleeding disorders. Caution during pregnancy, and alone in headache from ascendant Liver yang or blood deficiency.

**Formulae** *Chuan Xiong Cha Tiao San* (wind cold headache); *Qiang Huo Sheng Shi Tang* (wind damp headache); *Tong Qiao Huo Xue Tang*† (headache, tinnitus and hearing loss from blood stasis); *Bu Yang Huan Wu Tang* (hemiplegia from qi deficiency with blood stasis); *Wen Jing Tang* (infertility and dysmenorrhea from cold and deficient *chōng mài / rèn mài*); *Sheng Hua Tang* (postpartum pain from blood stasis); *Xue Fu Zhu Yu Tang* (qi and blood stasis); *Juan Bi Tang* (wind damp joint pain)

### Dān Shēn (Salviae miltiorrhizae Radix) salvia root

**Preparation and usage** Processing with wine (*jiu dan shen* 酒丹参) enhances its ability to invigorate blood; stir frying (*chao dan shen* 炒丹参) warms it up a little and makes it more suitable for blood stasis patterns without heat. For severe heat in the blood and damp heat painful obstruction, up to 30 grams of dan shen may be used for a few weeks. Large doses must not be used where there is bleeding.

**Contraindications** Pregnancy[2]. Caution in yang deficiency, and in the absence of stagnant blood. Incompatible[3] with li lu (p.22). Avoid concurrent use with the anticoagulant drug Warfarin.

**Formulae** *Dan Shen Yin* (chest and epigastric pain from blood stasis); *Huo Luo Xiao Ling Dan* (acute and chronic pain from blood stasis); *Tian Wang Bu Xin Dan* (insomnia and shen disturbance from Heart and Kidney yin deficiency); *Xiao Ru Tang*† (early stage of breast abscess and mastitis)

### Jī Xuè Téng (Spatholobi Caulis) chicken blood vine

**Preparation and usage** In severe cases up to 30 grams may be used.

**Contraindications** Pregnancy[4], menorrhagia, bleeding disorders.

**Formulae** *Gu Zhi Zeng Sheng Wan* (bony proliferation, osteophytes); *Lao Guan Cao Gao* (syrup for wind damp painful obstruction)

### Huái Niú Xī (Achyranthis bidentatae Radix) achyranthes root

**Preparation and usage** The downwards directing action is strongest in the unprocessed herb, used for amenorrhea, retained placenta and postpartum pain, painful urination and oral pathology from fire. Processing with wine (*jiu niu xi* 酒牛膝) enhances its ability to invigorate blood, stop pain and treat abdominal masses and joint pain; processing with salt (*yan niu xi* 盐牛膝) enhances its ability to tonify the Liver and Kidneys, strengthen sinews and bones and treat lower back and leg weakness and pain.

**Contraindications** Pregnancy, menorrhagia and bleeding disorders. The unprocessed form should be used cautiously in patients with sinking Spleen qi, diarrhea, leukorrhea, and involuntary seminal emission.

**Formulae** *Shen Tong Zhu Yu Tang* (chronic musculoskeletal pain from blood stasis); *Zhen Gan Xi Feng Tang* (headache and hypertension from ascendant Liver yang); *Shou Wu He Ji* (dizziness and numb extremities from Liver blood deficiency with ascendant yang); *Si Miao Wan* (weakness and numbness in the legs from damp heat); *Yu Nü Jian* (toothache and oral pathology from Stomach heat and yin deficiency); *Ji Sheng Shen Qi Wan* (edema from Kidney yang deficiency); *Du Huo Ji Sheng Tang* (wind damp painful obstruction with Liver and Kidney deficiency)

### Yì Mǔ Cǎo (Leonurus Herba) Chinese motherwort

**Preparation and usage** In severe cases up to 30 grams may be used. Commonly prepared as a syrup with honey (*yi mu cao gao* 益母草膏) for postpartum blood stasis. The fresh herb, or the dregs left from decoction, can be applied topically for trauma, skin lesions and mastitis.

**Contraindications** Pregnancy, and in patients with yin and blood deficiency without blood stasis.

**Formulae** *Yi Mu Sheng Jin Dan* (irregular menses and dysmenorrhea from blood deficiency with blood stasis); *Tian Ma Gou Teng Yin* (dizziness and headache from ascendant Liver yang)

### Zé Lán (Lycopi Herba) bugleweed

**Preparation and usage** The fresh herb, or the dregs left from decoction, can be applied topically for traumatic injuries and mastitis.

**Contraindications** Caution during pregnancy, and in patients with blood deficiency without blood stasis.

**Formulae** *Ze Lan Tang* (amenorrhea, dysmenorrhea, gynecological masses and postpartum pain from blood stasis)

### Táo Rén (Persicae Semen) peach seed

**Preparation and usage** Unprocessed seeds are better for dispersing blood stasis; stir frying (*chao tao ren* 炒桃仁) enhances their ability to moisten the Intestines and treat constipation. Should be pulverized before decoction. When used in pills or powder the skin around the seed should be removed by blanching. Peeled seeds are less toxic than unpeeled seeds, and decoction is safer than direct ingestion. The dosage range should not be exceeded to avoid possible toxicity[5].

**Contraindications** Pregnancy, and when used alone in blood deficiency. Caution in patients with loose stools and diarrhea.

**Formulae** *Tao Hong Si Wu Tang* (blood deficiency with mild blood stasis); *Tao He Cheng Qi Tang* (heat and blood stasis in the lower burner); *Sheng Hua Tang* (postpartum blood stasis); *Gui Zhi Fu Ling Wan* (blood stasis masses in the lower burner); *Da Huang Mu Dan Tang* (Intestinal abscess); *Wei Jing Tang* (Lung abscess); *Run Chang Wan* (chronic constipation from blood dryness); *Wa Leng Zi Wan* (abdominal masses from blood and phlegm stasis)

### Hóng Huā (Carthami Flos) safflower

**Preparation and usage** Large doses (6–9 grams) invigorate blood and disperse blood stasis; small doses (1–3 grams) are used to tonify and harmonize the blood.

**Contraindications** Pregnancy, menorrhagia and bleeding disorders.

**Formulae** *Tao Hong Si Wu Tang* (blood deficiency with mild blood stasis); *Fu Yuan Huo Xue Tang*† (blood stasis from trauma); *Xue Fu Zhu Yu Tang* (qi and blood stasis); *Dang Gui Hong Hua Yin* (skin rash from heat and blood stasis); *Jing Wan Hong* (ointment for burns and non healing sores)

---

1 Appendix 6, p.108
2 Bensky et al (2004) 3rd ed. is the only source to assert a contraindication during pregnancy. None of the Chinese sources consulted make any statement regarding usage during pregnancy. See Appendix 1.1, p.98.
3 Appendix 2, p.100
4 Chen (2004) is the only source to assert a contraindication during pregnancy. None of the Chinese sources consulted make any statement regarding pregnancy usage. See Appendix 1.1, p.98.

---

5 Appendix 3.2, p.104

| INDICATIONS | Pu Huang 蒲黄 | Yu Jin 郁金 | Hu Zhang 虎杖 | Luo De Da 落得大 | Lu Lu Tong 路路通 | Mao Dong Qing 毛冬青 | Jiang Xiang 降香 | Chuan Niu Xi 川牛膝 | Jiang Huang 姜黄 | Wang Bu Liu Xing 王不留行 | Liu Ji Nu 刘寄奴 | Su Mu 苏木 | FUNCTIONS |
|---|---|---|---|---|---|---|---|---|---|---|---|---|---|
| abscess – breast | | ○ | △ | | | | | | | ▲ | | | aids Gallbladder function |
| abscesses & sores – skin | | | ▲E | △ | | | | | △ | | ○ | | breaks up blood stasis |
| amenorrhea | | ○ | △○ | | | | | ▲ | △ | ▲ | ▲ | △ | clears damp heat |
| bleeding – hematemesis, nose | | △ | ● | ○ | | | | △ | | | | | clears toxic heat |
| bleeding – hematuria | △ | △ | | | | | | ▲○ | | | △ | | directs blood & fire down |
| breast – distension & pain | | | ○ | | △ | | | | | △ | | | dispels wind damp |
| burns & scalds | ● | ○ | E○ | ○ | ○ | E○ | ○ | ● | ○ | ○ | E | ○ | disperses blood stasis |
| cardiovascular disease | | ○ | | | | ▲ | △ | | | | | | dredges the Liver |
| cirrhosis of the liver – early | | △○ | | | ○ | | | | ○ | | | | moves qi |
| cough – Lung heat | | | △ | | | △ | | | | ○ | | | promotes lactation |
| delirium – in high fever | | △ | | | | | | | | ○ | ○ | | promotes menstruation |
| depression – phlegm, qi const. | ○ | ▲ | ○ | ○ | ○ | | | ○ | | | | | promotes urination |
| dysmenorrhea | ▲○ | △ | | | | | ○ | ▲ | △ | △ | △ | △ | stops bleeding |
| dysuria – blood | △ | ○ | ○ | | | | | ▲ | ○ | | △○ | ○ | stops pain |
| dysuria – damp heat | △ | | △ | △ | | | | ○ | | | △ | | strengthens sinew, bone |
| edema | | ○ | ○ | | △ | | | | | | | | transforms phlegm heat |
| fallopian tubes – blockage of | | | | △○ | ○ | | | | | ○ | | | unblocks collaterals |
| gallstones, cholecystitis | | ▲ | △ | | | | | | | | | | |
| hemiplegia | | | | | | △ | | △ | | | | | |
| hypertension | | | | | | △ | | ▲ | | | | | |
| jaundice – damp heat, bld. stasis | | ▲ | △ | | | | | | | | △ | | |
| lactation – insufficient | | | | | | | | | | ▲ | | | **Domain (❖)** |
| leukorrhea – damp heat | | ❖ | △❖ | | | | | | | | | | Lung |
| masses – abdominal | | △ | | ❖ | | | | ❖ | △ | | △ | | Kidney |
| menstruation – irregular | ❖ | △❖ | ❖ | ❖ | △❖ | | ❖ | △❖ | ❖ | ❖ | | ❖ | Liver |
| muscle weakness & atrophy | | ❖ | ❖ | | △ | △ | | ▲ | | | | | Gallbladder |
| nasosinusitis | | ❖ | | | △ | ❖ | ❖ | | | | ❖ | ❖ | Heart |
| numbness – extremities | ❖ | | | | △ | △ | | △ | | | | | Pericardium |
| pain – & injury, trauma | △ | △ | △ | ▲❖ | | ▲❖ | | △ | △❖ | | ▲❖ | △❖ | Spleen |
| pain – abdominal, blood stasis | ▲ | △ | | | ❖ | | | △ | △ | ❖ | △ | △ | Stomach |
| pain – abdominal, qi stagnation | | △ | | | | | △ | | △ | | | | |
| pain – arm & shoulder | | | | | | | | | ▲ | | | | |
| pain – chest, angina | △ | △ | | | | ▲ | △ | | △ | | | | **Flavour, nature (♦)** |
| pain – epigastric | ▲ | △♦ | | ♦ | △ | | ♦ | | △♦ | | | ♦ | acrid |
| pain – hypochondriac | | ▲ | | | | ♦ | △ | | △ | | | | astringent |
| pain – lower back, leg, knee | | ♦ | ♦ | ♦ | △♦ | ♦ | | ▲♦ | ♦ | ♦ | ♦ | | bitter |
| pain – postpartum abdominal | △ | | △ | | | | | △ | △ | | △ | △♦ | salty |
| pain – testicular | | | | | | | | | ♦ | △ | | | sour |
| painful obst. – damp, bld. stasis | ♦ | | △ | | △ | | | ▲ | ▲ | | | ♦ | sweet |
| placenta, lochia – retention of | ▲ | ♦ | ♦ | | | | | △ | | | △ | | cold |
| seizures, epilepsy – phlegm heat | | △ | | ♦ | | ♦ | | | | | | | cool |
| thrombophlebitis, Buerger's dis. | ♦ | | | ♦ | | ▲ | | | | ♦ | | ♦ | neutral |
| withdrawal mania (*dian kuang*) | | ▲ | | | | | ♦ | | ♦ | | ♦ | | warm |
| **Standard dosage range (g)** | 3–9 | 6–12 | 9–30 | 9–30 | 3–9 | 30–60 | 3–6 | 9–15 | 3–9 | 6–9 | 3–9 | 3–9 | |

△ Indication
▲ Strong Indication
E External Use
**E** Strong External Indication

○ Function
● Strong Function

**Yán Hú Suǒ (Corydalis Rhizoma) corydalis rhizome**

**Preparation and usage** Processing with vinegar (*cu yan hu suo* 醋延胡索) enhances its analgesic action. Can be taken alone as powder in doses of 1.5–3 grams.

**Contraindications** Pregnancy. Caution in pain from deficiency.

**Formulae** *Jin Ling Zi San* (abdominal pain from qi and blood stasis); *An Zhong San* (epigastric pain from cold); *Jiang Huang San* (chest and abdominal pain from qi and blood stasis); *Ju He Wan* (testicular swelling and pain from cold damp)

**Wǔ Líng Zhī (Trogopterori Faeces) flying squirrel feces ~ p.6**

**Preparation and usage** Decocted in a cloth bag[1], or preferably used in powder or pill form. Processing with vinegar (*cu wu ling zhi* 醋五灵脂) enhances its analgesic effect; charred wu ling zhi (*wu ling zhi tan* 五灵脂炭) is used to stop bleeding.

**Contraindications** Pregnancy, and pain from deficiency. Has a rather unpleasant and often nauseating smell and taste when decocted, and should be used cautiously in patients with Stomach qi deficiency patterns. Antagonistic[2] to ren shen (p.74) and dang shen (p.74).

**Formulae** *Shi Xiao San* (chest and epigastric pain from blood stasis); *Shou Nian San* (abdominal pain from qi and blood stasis)

**Rǔ Xiāng (Olibanum) frankincense, mastic ~ p.6**

**Preparation and usage** The raw resin can irritate the stomach and cause nausea and vomiting; processing with vinegar (*cu ru xiang* 醋乳香, also written as *zhi ru xiang* 炙乳香) alleviates this tendency, and is the preferred form for internal use. The processed resin is often used in alcohol extract. Not suitable for long term use.

**Contraindications** Pregnancy, and in the absence of blood stasis. Caution in patients with sensitive digestion and Spleen qi deficiency.

**Formulae** *Huo Luo Xiao Ling Dan* (acute and chronic pain from blood stasis); *Juan Bi Tang* (wind damp bi pain); *Qi Li San*† (traumatic injury); *Xian Fang Huo Ming Yin*† (toxic heat boils and sores); *Jing Wan Hong* (ointment for burns and non–healing sores); *Hong Teng Jian* (Intestinal abscess); *Jie Gu Dan* (slow healing broken bones)

**Mò Yaò (Myrrha) myrrh ~ p.6**

**Preparation and usage** The raw resin can irritate the stomach and cause nausea and vomiting; processing with vinegar (*cu mo yao* 醋没药, also written as *zhi mo yao* 炙没药) alleviates this tendency, and is the preferred form for internal use. The processed resin is often used in alcohol extract. Not suitable for long term use.

**Contraindications** Pregnancy, and in the absence of blood stasis. Caution in patients with sensitive digestion and Spleen qi deficiency.

**Formulae** *Huo Luo Xiao Ling Dan* (acute and chronic pain from blood stasis); *Shou Nian San* (abdominal pain from qi and blood stasis); *Shao Fu Zhu Yu Tang* (dysmenorrhea from cold and blood stasis in the lower burner); *Zi Ran Tong San* (slow healing broken bones); *Xiao Huo Luo Dan* (stubborn painful obstruction, loss of function and numbness from cold, phlegm and blood stasis); *Sheng Ji San*† (chronic non healing ulcers)

**Pú Huáng (Typhae Pollen) raw bulrush pollen**

Raw pu huang is quite different in action from the stir fried product (p.12) and is thus distinguished here.

**Preparation and usage** Should be decocted in a cloth bag[3] to prevent the tiny spores from irritating the throat.

**Contraindications** Pregnancy, and in the absence of blood stasis.

**Formulae** *Shi Xiao San* (chest and epigastric pain from blood stasis); *Hei Shen San* (postpartum blood stasis); *Shao Fu Zhu Yu Tang* (dysmenorrhea from cold and blood stasis in the lower burner)

**Yù Jīn (Curcumae Radix) curcuma root tuber**

**Preparation and usage** When taken directly as powder, the dose is 2–5 grams per day.

**Contraindications** Pregnancy[4]. Antagonistic[5] to ding xiang (p.88).

**Formulae** *Xuan Yu Tong Jing Tang* (premenstrual fever, short cycle and dysmenorrhea from qi constraint with heat in the blood); *Chang Pu Yu Jin Tang* (disturbance of consciousness in a damp warm febrile disease); *Bai Jin Wan* (seizures or mania from phlegm blocking the Heart); *Dan Dao Pai Shi Tang* (gallstones from damp heat)

**Hǔ Zhàng (Polygoni cuspidati Rhizoma) bushy knotweed**

Other texts place this herb in the damp draining[6] or wind damp dispelling group[7].

**Preparation and usage** For topical use fresh or powdered hu zhang is steeped in sesame oil for a week or so, the strained oil is then applied to the affected area.

**Contraindications** Pregnancy.

**Formulae** *Sang Zhi Hu Zhang Tang* (wind damp painful obstruction)

**Luò De Dà (Centella asiatica Herba) gotu kola**

**Contraindications** Yang deficiency.

**Lù Lù Tōng (Liquidambaris Fructus) liquidamber fruit**

Other texts place this in the wind damp dispelling[8] or qi regulating group[9].

**Contraindications** Pregnancy and in menorrhagia.

**Máo Dōng Qīng (Ilicis pubescentis Radix) hairy holly root**

**Contraindications** Yang deficiency.

**Jiàng Xiāng (Dalbergiae odoriferae Lignum) rosewood**

**Preparation and usage** Shaved or powdered before decoction. When taken directly as powder, the dose is 1–2 grams. Can be applied topically as a powder mixed with lanoline or sorbolene for injuries, fractures and sprains, or as a powder alone for traumatic bleeding.

**Contraindications** Bleeding from heat in the blood, and in the absence of blood stasis.

**Chuān Niú Xī (Cyathulae Radix) cyathula root**

**Preparation and usage** This type of niu xi is used instead of huai niu xi (p.6) when greater blood stasis dispersing action is desired.

**Contraindications** Pregnancy, menorrhagia and bleeding disorders.

**Formulae** *Shu Jin Huo Xue Tang* (hemiplegia and wind damp painful obstruction with blood stasis); *Tong Jing Wan* (amenorrhea and dysmenorrhea from blood stasis); *Xue Fu Zhu Yu Tang* (qi and blood stasis); *San Leng Wan* (abdominal masses); *Bai Ling Tiao Gan Tang* (infertility from blocked fallopian tubes or endometriosis)

**Jiāng Huáng (Curcumae longae Rhizoma) turmeric**

**Contraindications** Pregnancy, and pain from deficiency.

**Formulae** *Jiang Huang San* (chest and abdominal pain from qi and blood stasis); *Juan Bi Tang* (wind damp joint pain); *Shu Jin Tang* (arm and shoulder pain from wind damp)

**Wáng Bù Liú Xíng (Vaccariae Semen) vaccaria seeds**

**Preparation and usage** Can be stir fried (*chao liu xing zi* 炒留行子) to enhance its ability to invigorate blood and promote menstruation. Alternative to the scales of the endangered pangolin[10] (chuan shan jia 穿山甲) for blood stasis and lactation problems.

**Contraindications** Pregnancy.

**Formulae** *Bai Ling Tiao Gan Tang* (infertility from blocked fallopian tubes or endometriosis)

**Liú Jì Nú (Artemesiae anomalae Herba) anomalous artemesia**

**Preparation and usage** Can be powdered and applied topically to bleeding wounds.

**Contraindications** Pregnancy.

**Formulae** *Bi Huo Dan* (topical ointment for burns and scalds)

**Sū Mù (Sappan Lignum) sappan wood**

**Contraindications** Pregnancy, and in cases of menorrhagia.

**Formulae** *Tong Jing Wan* (amenorrhea and dysmenorrhea from blood stasis); *Ba Li San* (pain and injury from trauma)

---

1 Appendix 6, p.109
2 Appendix 2, p.100
3 Appendix 6, p.109
4 Xu & Wang (2002) is the only source asserting a contraindication. See p.99.
5 Appendix 2, p.100

6 *Zhong Yao Xue* (2000)
7 *Shi Yong Zhong Yao Xue* (1985)
8 *Zhong Yao Xue* (2000)
9 *Shi Yong Zhong Yao Xue* (1985)
10 Appendix 5, p.106

| Indication<br>△ Indication<br>▲ Strong Indication<br>E External Use<br>E Strong External Indication<br>**INDICATIONS** | Zi Ran Tong 自然铜 | Jiu Cai 韭菜 | Ji Xing Zi 急性子 | Ma Bian Cao 马鞭草 | Gan Qi 干漆 | Wa Leng Zi 瓦楞子 | Shui Hong Hua Zi 水红花子 | San Leng 三棱 | E Zhu 莪术 | Shui Zhi 水蛭 | Di Bie Chong 地鳖虫 | Meng Chong 虻虫 | ○ Function / ● Strong Function<br>**FUNCTIONS** |
|---|---|---|---|---|---|---|---|---|---|---|---|---|---|
| abscesses & sores – skin | | | | △ E | | | ○ | ○ | ○ | | | | alleviates food stagnation |
| abscess – breast, mastitis | | | | △ E | | ○ | | | | | | | alleviates gastric acidity |
| acid reflux, heartburn | | | ○ | ○ | ○ | ▲○ | ○ | △● | △● | ● | ● | ● | breaks up blood stasis |
| amenorrhea | | | △ | △○ | △ | | | △ | △ | △ | △ | △ | checks malarial disorder |
| ascites – from cirrhosis | | | | △○ | | | | | | | | | clears toxic heat |
| bones – poor healing of broken | ▲ E | | ○ | | | ○ | ○ | ● | ● | ○ | ▲E○ | ○ | dissipates masses |
| cancer – cervical | ○ | ○ | | | | | | | △ | | | | disperses blood stasis |
| cancer – esophagus, digestive tract | | | △ | | ○ | △ | | △ | △ | | | | kills parasites |
| cancer – tumours in general | | | | | | △ | | ▲○ | ▲○ | △ | △ | | moves qi |
| cancer – liver | ○ | | | | | △ | △ | | △ | | ● | | promotes healing of |
| cervical lymphadenitis (*luo li*) | | | ○ | ○ | ○ | ▲ | | | | | | | bones |
| cirrhosis of the liver – early | | | | △○ | | △ | △ | △ | | | △ | | promotes menstruation |
| cough – stubborn phlegm | | | | | | △● | | | | | | | promotes urination |
| dysenteric disorder – damp heat | ○ | | | △ | | ○ | ○ | ○ | ○ | | | | softens hardness |
| dysmenorrhea | | | | △ | | △○ | | △ | △ | | | | stops pain |
| dysphagia (esophageal mass) | | ▲ | | | | △ | | | | △ | | | transforms phlegm |
| dysuria – damp heat | | | | △ | | | | | | | | | |
| ears – insects in | | E | | | | | | | | | | | |
| edema | | | | △ | | | | | | | | | |
| fibroids, endometriosis | | | | | | △ | | ▲ | ▲ | △ | △ | | |
| food stagnation | | | | | | | | △ | △ | | | | |
| gingivitis | | | | △ E | | | | | | | | | |
| hemorrhoids | | E | | | | | | | | | | | |
| hepatitis – chronic | | | | △ | | | | | | | △ | | |
| hepatosplenomegaly | | | △ | △ | | △ | △ | ▲ | ▲ | | ▲ | | |
| malarial disorder | | | | ▲ | | | | | | | △ | | **Domain (✤)** |
| masses – abdominal, uterine | | | △ | △ | △ | △✤ | △ E | ▲ | ▲ | △ | △ | △ | Lung |
| masses – tumours, cancer | ✤ | ✤ | ✤ | ✤ | ✤ | ✤ | △✤ | △✤ | ▲✤ | △✤ | △✤ | ✤ | Liver |
| pain – & injury, trauma | △ E | E | ✤ | | | | | | | △ | △ | △ | Heart |
| pain – abdominal, blood stasis | | | | ✤ | | | | △✤ | △✤ | △ | △ | | Spleen |
| pain – abdominal, food stag. | | ✤ | | | ✤ | ✤ | △✤ | △ | △ | | | | Stomach |
| pain – abdominal, from worms | | | | | △ | | | | | | | | |
| pain – abdominal, qi stag. | | | | | | | | △ | △ | | | | **Flavour, nature (◆)** |
| pain – chest, angina | | △ | △◆ | | ◆ | | | | | ◆ | ◆ | ◆ | slightly toxic |
| pain – epigastric | ◆ | △◆ | | | ◆ | | | △ | △◆ | | | | acrid |
| pain – epigastric, & hyperacidity | | ◆ | | | | △ | | | | | | | astringent |
| pain – postpartum abdominal | | | ◆ | ◆ | ◆ | | | △◆ | △◆ | ◆ | △ | △◆ | bitter |
| pregnancy – ectopic | | | | | | ◆ | | △ | ◆ | ◆ | △◆ | | salty |
| throat – sore, acute | | ◆ | | △ E | | | | | | | | | sour |
| thyroid – benign nodules, goitre | | | | | | ▲ | △ | | | | ◆ | | cold |
| tongue – numbness of | | | | ◆ | | | ◆ | | | | E | ◆ | cool |
| ulcers – gastric | ◆ | | | | | △◆ | | | ◆ | | ◆ | | neutral |
| | | ◆ | ◆ | | ◆ | | | | ◆ | | | | warm |
| **Standard dosage range (g)** | 9–15 | 30–60 | 3–9 | 10–30 | *see* p.11 | 9–30 | 15–30 | 3–9 | 3–9 | 3–6 | 3–9 | 1–1.5 | |

### Zì Rán Tóng (Pyritum) pyrite, ferrous disulphide FeS₂

**Preparation and usage** Calcined (*duan zi ran tong* 煅自然铜) when used in decoction, in doses of 9–15 grams. In pills and powder (the preferred option) the dose is 0.3–1 grams of the calcined and pulverized substance, once or twice daily.

**Contraindications** Not suitable in the absence of blood stasis and for prolonged use. Caution in patients with heat from yin and blood deficiency.

**Formulae** *Zi Ran Tong San* (slow healing broken bones); *Ba Li San* (pain and injury from trauma)

### Jiǔ Cài (Allium tuberosum Stamen) fragrant flowered garlic

**Preparation and usage** The fresh juice is acrid, sour, astringent and very warm, disperses blood stasis in the upper digestive tract, and is an important herb for regurgitation and dysphagia caused by blood stasis in the esophagus. When cooked, it becomes sweet and warm, and is used to warm Spleen and Stomach yang, and restore the qi dynamic. To treat insects in the ear, fresh juice is dripped into the ear. For hemorrhoids, a brief decoction can be used to wash the rectal area.

**Contraindications** Patients with indeterminate gnawing hunger.

**Formulae** Wu Zhi An Zhong Yin (dysphagia from qi and blood stasis); San Zhi Yin (regurgitation from Spleen and Stomach yang deficiency)

### Jí Xìng Zǐ (Impatiens balsamina Semen) garden balsam seed

**Contraindications** Pregnancy; blood deficiency without blood stasis.

### Mǎ Biān Cǎo (Verbenae Herba) verbena

**Preparation and usage** For abscesses the fresh herb can be applied topically; for sore throat and gingivitis the extracted juice can be used as a gargle. Decoction of ma bian cao (alone or with other suitable herbs) can be given 2–3 hours before the expected onset of a malarial fever. Large doses (up to 30 grams) are required for masses and ascites.

**Contraindications** Caution during pregnancy.

**Formulae** *Zi Xue Tang* (blood stasis type amenorrhea and dysmenorrhea)

### Gān Qī (Toxicodendri Resina) Japanese lacquer tree resin

**Preparation and usage** Not suitable for decoction; only used in powder or pill form in doses of 0.06–0.1 grams. Always processed, usually stir fried or calcined.

**Contraindications** Pregnancy, in the absence of blood stasis or in patients with Spleen qi deficiency.

**Formulae** Da Huang Zhe Chong Wan (lower abdominal masses and amenorrhea from blood stasis)

### Wǎ Léng Zǐ (Arcae Concha) cockle shell

Placed in the phlegm heat clearing group in some texts[1].

**Preparation and usage** When decocted, the dose is 9–30 grams and it should be cooked for 30–60 minutes[2] before the other herbs. When taken directly in powder or in pills, the dose is 1–3 grams per day. To break up blood stasis, transform phlegm and dissipate masses, wa leng zi is untreated or processed with vinegar (*cu wa leng zi* 醋瓦楞子); to alleviate gastric hyperacidity and stop epigastric pain, it should be calcined (*duan wa leng zi* 煅瓦楞子).

**Contraindications** None noted.

**Formulae** *Wa Leng Zi Wan* (abdominal masses from blood and phlegm stasis); *Han Hua Wan* (phlegm type benign thyroid nodules and cervical lymphadenopathy); *Bie Jia Wan* (abdominal masses)

### Shuǐ Hóng Huā Zǐ (Polygonum orientale Fructus) princes feather fruit

**Contraindications** Absence of blood stasis and middle burner yang deficiency.

### Sān Léng (Sparganii Rhizoma) burr reed rhizome

**Preparation and usage** Processing with wine (*jiu san leng* 酒三棱) enhances its ability to break up blood stasis and dissipate masses; processing with vinegar (*cu san leng* 醋三棱) enhances its analgesic action; stir frying (*chao san leng* 炒三棱) enhances its ability to alleviate food stagnation.

**Contraindications** Pregnancy, women with menorrhagia or patients with bleeding disorders. Caution in weak patients with mild to moderate blood stasis.

**Formulae** *San Leng Wan* (abdominal masses)

### É Zhú (Curcumae Rhizoma) curcuma rhizome

**Preparation and usage** Unprocessed for food stagnation; processing with vinegar (*cu e zhu* 醋莪术) enhances its ability to disperse blood stasis and stop pain.

**Contraindications** Pregnancy, women with menorrhagia or patients with bleeding disorders. Caution in weak patients with mild to moderate blood stasis.

**Formulae** *Bie Jia Wan* (abdominal masses); *E Wei Hua Pi Gao*† (topical plaster for masses); *Jiang Huang San* (chest and abdominal pain from qi and blood stasis)

### Shuǐ Zhì (Hirudo) leech

**Preparation and usage** In decoction the dose is 3–6 grams; when taken separately as powder (the preferred option) the dose is 0.3–0.6 grams once or twice daily. When destined for pills or powder, the leech should be processed with talcum powder (*hua shi chao shi zhi* 滑石炒水蛭), as this makes it crispy and more easily powdered.

**Contraindications** Pregnancy, in the absence of blood stasis, in women with menorrhagia or patients with bleeding disorders.

**Formulae** *Di Dang Tang* (severe blood stasis); *Da Huang Zhe Chong Wan* (lower abdominal masses and amenorrhea from blood stasis)

### Dì Biē Chóng (Eupolyphaga/Steleophaga) wingless cockroach

Also known as zhè chóng 䗪虫 and tǔ biē chóng 土鳖虫.

**Preparation and usage** In decoction the dose is 3–9 grams, crushed; when taken separately as powder or in pills (the preferred option) the dose is 1–1.5 grams once or twice daily.

**Contraindications** Pregnancy, in the absence of blood stasis, in women with menorrhagia or in patients with bleeding disorders.

**Formulae** *Da Huang Zhe Chong Wan* (lower abdominal masses and amenorrhea from blood stasis); *Xia Yu Xue Tang* (severe dysmenorrhea from blood stasis); *Bie Jia Wan* (abdominal masses); *Can She Tang* (stubborn wind damp painful obstruction)

### Méng Chóng (Tabanus) horse fly

**Preparation and usage** In decoction the dose is 1–1.5 grams, crushed; when taken separately as powder or in pills (the preferred option) the dose is 0.3 grams once or twice daily.

**Contraindications** Pregnancy, in the absence of blood stasis, in women with menorrhagia or patients with bleeding disorders.

**Formulae** *Da Huang Zhe Chong Wan* (lower abdominal masses and amenorrhea from blood stasis); *Di Dang Tang* (severe blood stasis)

### Substances from other groups

Substances from different categories with some blood stasis dispersing action include pu huang (p.8), qian cao gen (p.12), san qi (p.12), xue yu tan (p.14), xue jie (p.24), shan zha (p.30), chi shao (p.40), mu dan pi (p.40), da huang (p.60), dang gui (p.78) and gu sui bu (p.84).

### Endnotes

† These formulae traditionally contain items from endangered animal species and/or obsolete toxic substances, and are unavailable in their original form.

---

1 *Zhong Yao Xue* (2000), *Shi Yong Zhong Yao Xue* (1985)
2 Appendix 6, p.108

| △ Indication / ▲ Strong Indication / E External Use / E Strong External Indication — **INDICATIONS** | Chao Pu Huang 炒蒲黄 | San Qi 三七 | Qian Cao Gen 茜草根 | Hua Rui Shi 花蕊石 | Xiao Ji 小蓟 | Da Ji 大蓟 | Di Yu 地榆 | Huai Hua Mi 槐花米 | Ce Bai Ye 侧柏叶 | Bai Mao Gen 白茅根 | Zhu Ma Gen 苎麻根 | Yang Ti Gen 羊蹄根 | ○ Function / ● Strong Function — **FUNCTIONS** |
|---|---|---|---|---|---|---|---|---|---|---|---|---|---|
| abscess – breast, mastitis | ○ | | | | | △ | | | ○ | | △ E | | astringes bleeding |
| abscess – Intestinal | | | | | | △ | ○ | ○ | | | | | clears damp heat |
| abscess – Lung | | | | ○ | | △● | | | | ○ | | | clears toxic heat |
| abscesses & sores – skin | | △ | ● | | △EO | ▲EO | EO | ○ | ○ | ○ | △EO | ○ | cools the blood |
| alopecia – bld. def.; heat in bld. | | | | | ○ | ○ | | ○ | ▲E | | | | cools the Liver |
| amenorrhea – blood stasis | | △ | △ | | | | | | | ● | | | cools the Lung & Stomach |
| bleeding – epistaxis | △EO | △● | ▲○ | △○ | △ | △ | △ | △ | △E | ▲ | △ | △ | disperses blood stasis |
| bleeding – gums | △E | △ | | | | △ | △ | | △ | ▲ | | ○ | kills parasites |
| bleeding – hematemesis | △ | △ | △ | △ | △ | ▲ | △ | | △○ | ▲ | △ | △ | promotes hair growth |
| bleeding – hematuria | ▲ | △ | △ | | ▲ | △ | △● | △ | △ | ▲ | △ | | promotes healing |
| bleeding – hemoptysis | △○ | △ | △ | △ | △ | ▲ | △ | △ | △ | ▲○ | △○ | △ | promotes urination |
| bleeding – hemorrhoids | △● | △● | ○ | ○ | EO | | ▲○ | ▲○ | ● | ○ | ○ | △○ | stops bleeding |
| bleeding – postpartum | ▲ | ▲ | △ | | | | | | ○ | | | | stops cough |
| bleeding – pregnancy; heat | | ○ | | | | | | | | | ▲ | | stops pain |
| bleeding – rectal; blood stasis | △ | △ | △ | | | | | | | | | | |
| bleeding – rectal; damp heat | | | △ | | △ | △ | ▲ | ▲ | △ | △ | △ | △ | |
| bleeding – skin, purpura | △ | △ | △ | | | | | | | | △ | ▲ | |
| bleeding – traumatic | E | ▲E | △ | E | | E | | | △ | | | | |
| bleeding – uterine | ▲ | ▲ | ▲ | | △ | △ | △ | △ | ▲ | | △ | △ | |
| burns & scalds | | | | | | | E | | E | | | | |
| cough – Lung heat | | | △ | | | | | | △ | ▲ | | | |
| dysenteric dis. – damp heat | | | △ | | | | ▲ | ▲ | △ | | | | |
| dysmenorrhea – blood stasis | △ | △ | △ | | | | | | | | | | |
| dysuria – blood | ▲ | △ | △ | | ▲ | △ | △ | △ | △ | △ | △ | | |
| dysuria – damp heat | △ | | | | | | | | ❖ | ▲❖ | △ | | **Domain (❖)** |
| edema – nephritic, acute; heat | | | | | | | ❖ | ❖ | | △ | | ❖ | Lung |
| headache, dizziness – Liver fire | | | | | | | | △ | | ❖ | | | Large Intestine |
| hypercholesterolemia | ❖ | △❖ | ❖ | ❖ | ❖ | ❖ | ❖ | ❖ | ❖ | | ❖ | ❖ | Bladder |
| hypertension – Liver fire | | | | | △❖ | ▲❖ | | ▲ | | | ❖ | ❖ | Liver |
| jaundice – damp heat | ❖ | | | | △ | ▲ | | | | △ | | | Heart |
| leukorrhea – damp heat | | ❖ | | | | | △❖ | | △ | ❖ | | | Pericardium |
| miscarriage – threatened; heat | | | | | | | | | | | ▲ | | Stomach |
| nausea, vomiting – St. heat | | | | | | | | | | ▲ | | | |
| pain – & injury, trauma | △ | ▲ | △ | | | | | | | | | | **Flavour, nature (♦)** |
| pain – chest, angina; bld. stasis | ♦ | ▲ | △ | ♦ | | | | | ♦ | | | ♦ | astringent |
| pain – epigastric, blood stasis | △ | △ | ♦ | | | ♦ | | ♦ | ♦ | | | ♦ | bitter |
| pain – postpartum abdominal | △ | ▲♦ | | | | | | | | | | | slightly bitter |
| painful obst. – wind damp | | | △ | ♦ | | | ♦ | | | | | | sour |
| placenta, lochia – retention of | △♦ | ▲♦ | △ | △ | | ♦ | ♦ | | | ♦ | ♦ | | sweet |
| skin – eczema, psoriasis | | | | | ♦ | ♦ | E♦ | ♦ | ♦ | | | △E | cool |
| skin – tinea, ringworm; scabies | | | ♦ | | | | | | | ♦ | ♦ | E♦ | cold |
| thrombocytopenia | ♦ | | | ♦ | | | | | | | | △ | neutral |
| ulcers, wounds – non healing | | ▲E♦ | | | | | | | E | | | | warm |
| **Standard dosage range (g)** | 3–9 | 1–3 | 9–15 | 9–15 | 9–30 | 9–15 | 9–15 | 9–15 | 9–15 | 15–30 | 9–30 | 9–15 | |

Hemostatic herbs stop bleeding. In chronic mild to moderate bleeding using hemostatic herbs alone is insufficient and the underlying pathology must also be addressed. When bleeding is acute or severe however, the main principle is to quickly staunch bleeding, and herbs that focus solely on that can be employed until the bleeding is controlled.

These herbs have specific characteristics that enable them to stop different types of bleeding. The tables are laid out according to the following four groups. These are not precise distinctions, however, as some herbs possess more than one characteristic.

| | |
|---|---|
| Blood stasis dispersing – for bleeding from blood stasis | chao pu huang, san qi, qian cao gen, hua rui shi |
| Blood cooling – for bleeding due to heat in the blood or organs. | xiao ji, da ji, di yu, huai hua mi, ce bai ye, bai mao gen, zhu ma gen, yang ti gen |
| Astringents – broad acting hemostatics for blood that leaks out (as opposed to being forced out) from causes including trauma and deficiency | bai ji, xian he cao, zi zhu, zong lu pi, xue yu tan, ou jie, tie xian cai, ji mu |
| Warming – for bleeding from yang deficiency and cold | ai ye, pao jiang, zao xin tu |

### Chǎo Pú Huáng (Typhae Pollen preparata) stir fried bulrush pollen

**Preparation and usage** Should be decocted in a cloth bag[1] to prevent the tiny spores from irritating the throat. Pu huang has contrasting actions depending on how it is processed, so the correct specification is critical. To stop bleeding, pu huang is always stir fried (*chao pu huang* 炒蒲黄). Even when stir fried, however, pu huang retains some blood invigorating action. When bleeding occurs as a result of blood stasis, a mixture of unprocessed and fried pu huang can be used.

**Contraindications** Pregnancy.

**Formulae** *Xiao Ji Yin Zi* (urinary bleeding from heat); *Dai Ge San* (cough and hemoptysis from Lung heat or Liver fire invading the Lungs); *Gu Jing Wan* (uterine bleeding from yin deficiency with heat)

### Sān Qī (Notoginseng Radix) pseudoginseng root

**Preparation and usage** Taken directly[2] as powder or pills in doses of 1–3 grams, several times daily for bleeding. In severe cases the dose or frequency can be doubled. Can be decocted with a dosage range of 3–9 grams, however prolonged decoction diminishes its hemostatic effects. Commonly available as pills packaged in blister packs.

**Contraindications** Pregnancy.

**Formulae** *Sheng Tian Qi Pian* (prepared medicine for bleeding and cardiovascular disease); *Yun Nan Bai Yao* (well known prepared medicine for traumatic bleeding); *Hua Xue Dan* (bleeding with blood stasis)

### Qiàn Cǎo Gēn (Rubiae Radix) madder root

**Preparation and usage** In severe cases, up to 30 grams may be used. When used to stop bleeding, the charred herb (*qian cao tan* 茜草炭) is used; when used to disperse static blood, qian cao gen can be used unprocessed, or processed with wine (*jiu qian cao* 酒茜草).

**Contraindications** Caution in patients with middle burner yang deficiency, or blood and yin deficiency with heat. The unprocessed form should not be used in patients without blood stasis.

**Formulae** *Gu Chong Tang* (uterine bleeding from Spleen qi deficiency); *Qian Gen San* (hematemesis from Stomach heat); *Qian Gen Wan†* (rectal bleeding from damp heat); *Shi Hui San* (bleeding from heat in the blood)

### Huā Ruǐ Shí (Ophicalcitum) ophicalcite, a form of limestone

**Preparation and usage** For internal use, hua rui shi is calcined (*duan hua rui shi* 煅花蕊石). When calcined its astringency and ability to stop bleeding, as well as digestibility, are enhanced. When taken directly in pills or powder, the dose is 1–1.5 grams, two or three times daily. Should be broken up into small pieces or powdered before decoction and cooked in a cloth bag for 30 minutes[3] prior to the other herbs in the prescription. For topical application grind to a fine powder.

1 Appendix 6, p.109
2 Ibid.
3 Ibid.

**Contraindications** Pregnancy, and the absence of blood stasis.

**Formulae** *Hua Rui Shi San* (bleeding from trauma); *Hua Rui Shi Bai Ji San* (hemoptysis with blood stasis); *Hua Xue Dan* (bleeding with an element of blood stasis)

### Xiǎo Jì (Cirsii Herba) small thistle

**Preparation and usage** Do not cook longer than 15 minutes[4]. When the fresh herb is available, 30–60 grams per packet of herbs can be used. The fresh herb can also be juiced, with the juice taken internally or applied topically to suppurative sores and hemorrhoids. To treat bleeding from heat in the blood, hypertension or sores, the unprocessed herb is used; to stop bleeding from causes other than heat, the charred form (*xiao ji tan* 小蓟炭) is preferred.

**Contraindications** Caution in patients with Spleen qi deficiency, diarrhea and loss of appetite.

**Formulae** *Xiao Ji Yin Zi* (urinary bleeding from heat); *San Xian Yin* (hemoptysis from Lung yin deficiency); *Shi Hui San* (bleeding from heat in the blood)

### Dà Jì (Cirsii japonici Herba sive Radix) Japanese thistle

**Preparation and usage** When the fresh herb is available, 30–60 grams per packet of herbs can be used. The fresh herb can also be juiced, with the juice taken internally or applied topically to suppurative lesions. When charred (*da ji tan* 大蓟炭), its cooling action is reduced and it can be used for bleeding from causes other that heat.

**Contraindications** Middle burner yang qi deficiency.

**Formulae** *Shi Hui San* (bleeding from heat in the blood)

### Dì Yú (Sanguisorbae Radix) bloodwort root

**Preparation and usage** In severe cases, up to 30 grams per dose may be used. When taken directly as powder or in pills, the dose is 1.5–3 grams, several times daily. Usually charred to stop bleeding (*di yu tan* 地榆炭). When used topically for skin lesions, burns and chronic ulceration, unprocessed di yu is ground into a fine powder and mixed with a suitable carrier, such as sesame oil (traditional), sorbolene or honey.

**Contraindications** Bleeding or dysenteric disorder from cold and deficiency, or when there is substantial blood stasis. Not suitable for widespread burns, as excessive topical coverage and absorption may be associated with induction of liver damage and hepatitis. Not suitable alone in the early stages of heat type dysenteric disorder due to its sourness.

**Formulae** *Di Yu Gan Cao Tang* (rectal bleeding with abdominal pain); *Di Yu Wan* (incessant bloody dysentery from heat); *Huai Jiao Wan* (bleeding hemorrhoids); *Jing Wan Hong* (ointment for burns and non healing sores); *An Tai Yin* (threatened miscarriage from qi deficiency with heat); *Qin Jiao Bai Zhu Wan* (chronic constipation with bleeding, itchy hemorrhoids)

### Huái Huā Mǐ (Sophorae Flos immaturus) pagoda tree bud

**Preparation and usage** To stop bleeding the charred herb is used (*huai hua tan* 槐花炭); to clear heat and cool the Liver, the unprocessed herb is used. The fruit of this plant, huái jiǎo 槐角 (Sophorae Fructus) is similar and can be used interchangeably.

**Contraindications** Caution in patients with bleeding from middle burner yang deficiency or yin deficiency with heat. Huái jiǎo 槐角 is contraindicated during pregnancy.

**Formulae** *Huai Hua San* (rectal bleeding, hemorrhoids from heat); *Hei Sheng San* (bleeding hemorrhoids)

### Cè Bǎi Yè (Platycladi Cacumen) Chinese arborvitae leaf

**Preparation and usage** In severe cases, up to 30 grams can be used. When used to stop bleeding in general, the charred herb is preferred (*ce bai tan* 侧柏炭); to stop bleeding from heat, alleviate cough and promote hair growth, the unprocessed herb is used. When applied topically to stimulate hair growth, the finely powdered herb is mixed with sesame oil and massaged firmly into the scalp. A layer can be secured with a night cap or scarf for retention while sleeping.

**Contraindications** Caution in patients with bleeding from blood stasis and those with middle burner yang deficiency.

**Formulae** *Si Sheng Wan* (bleeding from heat); *Bai Ye Tang* (bleeding from yang deficiency); *Wu Fa Wan* (alopecia following illness)

4 Appendix 6, p.108

| | Bai Ji 白及 | Xian He Cao 仙鹤草 | Zi Zhu 紫珠 | Zong Lu Pi 棕榈皮 | Xue Yu Tan 血余炭 | Ou Jie 藕节 | Tie Xian Cai 铁苋菜 | Ji Hua 檵花 | Ai Ye 艾叶 | Pao Jiang 炮姜 | Zao Xin Tu 灶心土 | | FUNCTIONS |
|---|---|---|---|---|---|---|---|---|---|---|---|---|---|
| △ Indication / ▲ Strong Indication / E External use / **E** Strong external indication / M Moxa | | | | | | | | | | | | | ○ Function / ● Strong Function |
| **abscess – breast, mastitis** | ○ | ● | △E○ | ● | | ○ | ○ | ○ | | | | | astringes bleeding |
| **abscess – Lung** | △ | | | | | | | | ○ | | | | calms a restless fetus |
| **abscesses & sores – skin** | E | | △E | | △ | | E | | ○ | ○ | ○ | | dispels cold |
| **anal fissure** | E | | | | ○ | | | | | | | | disperses blood stasis |
| **bleeding – epistaxis** | △ | △○ | △ | △E | ▲E | △ | △ | △ | △ | | △ | | kills parasites |
| **bleeding – gums & tongue** | ○ | △ | | △ | | | | | | | | | promotes healing |
| **bleeding – hematemesis** | ▲ | △ | ▲ | △ | △ | ▲ | △ | | ○ | △ | △ | | regulates menstruation |
| **bleeding – hematuria** | ● | △● | △○ | △● | ▲○ | △○ | ○ | ○ | ○ | ○ | ○ | | stops bleeding |
| **bleeding – hemoptysis** | ▲ | △○ | ▲ | △ | △ | ▲ | ○ | △○ | △ | | ○ | | stops diarrhea |
| **bleeding – hemorrhoids** | | △ | △ | △ | | | | | | △○ | | | stops pain |
| **bleeding – peptic ulcers** | ▲ | △ | △ | △ | △ | △ | | | | | ○ | | stops vomiting |
| **bleeding – postpartum** | | ▲ | | ▲ | △ | △ | | | | ▲○ | ○ | | warms the middle burner |
| **bleeding – pregnancy** | | | | | | | | | ▲○ | ○ | | | warms the uterus |
| **bleeding – rectal; damp heat** | | △ | | | | △ | | | | | | | |
| **bleeding – rectal; qi def.** | | ▲ | | △ | △ | △ | △ | | | | | | |
| **bleeding – rectal; yang def.** | | △ | | △ | | | | | | △ | ▲ | | |
| **bleeding – traumatic** | E | △ | E | | E | | E | E | | | | | |
| **bleeding – uterine; heat** | | △ | | △ | △ | △ | △ | | | | | | |
| **bleeding – uterine; yang qi def.** | | ▲ | | ▲ | △ | | | | ▲ | △ | | | |
| **burns & scalds** | E | | E | | | | | E | | | | | |
| **diarrhea – chronic, Spleen def.** | | △ | | | | | | △ | | △ | ▲ | | |
| **dysentery – amebic, acute** | | | | | | | △ | | | | | | |
| **dysenteric dis. – chronic; cold** | | ▲ | | △ | △ | △ | | △ | | | ▲ | | |
| **dysenteric dis. – chronic; heat** | | | | △ | △ | △ | ▲ | △ | | | | | **Domain** (✣) |
| **dysmenorrhea – deficient, cold** | ✣ | ✣ | ✣ | ✣ | | ✣ | ✣ | ✣ | △ M | | | | Lung |
| **dysuria – blood** | | △ | △ | △✣ | ▲ | △ | ✣ | | | | | | Large Intestine |
| **infertility – deficient, cold** | | | | | | | | | ▲M✣ | | | | Kidney |
| **leukorrhea – cold damp; Kid. def.** | ✣ | ✣ | ✣ | ✣ | ✣ | ✣ | ✣ | | △M✣ | ✣ | | | Liver |
| **malarial disorder** | | △ | | | | | ✣ | | | | | | Heart |
| **menses – irregular; yang def.** | | ✣ | | | | | | | △M✣ | ✣ | ✣ | | Spleen |
| **miscarriage – threatened; cold** | ✣ | | ✣ | | ✣ | ✣ | | ✣ | ▲ | | ✣ | | Stomach |
| **morning sickness – cold** | | | | | | | | | | | △ | | |
| **pain – abdominal; def., cold** | | | | | | | | | △ M | ▲ | | | |
| **pain – abdominal postpartum** | | | | | | | | | △ | ▲ | | | **Flavour, nature** (◆) |
| **pain – musculoskeletal** | | | | | | | | | M ◆ | | | | slightly toxic |
| **painful obst. – wind cold damp** | | | | | | | | | M ◆ | | ◆ | | acrid |
| **skin – eczema, dermatitis** | ◆ | ◆ | ◆ | ◆ | | ◆ | △E◆ | ◆ | E | ◆ | | | astringent |
| **skin – psoriasis** | ◆ | ◆ | ◆ | ◆ | ◆ | | △E | ◆ | ◆ | ◆ | | | bitter |
| **skin – itchy damp rash** | | | | | | | △E◆ | | △E | | | | slightly bitter |
| **trichomonas vaginitis** | ◆ | E | | | | ◆ | | | E | | | | sweet |
| **ulcers – gastric** | △◆ | | ◆ | | | | ◆ | | | | | | cool |
| **ulcers – skin, chronic** | E | ◆ | | ◆ | E◆ | ◆ | | ◆ | | | | | neutral |
| **vomiting, nausea – Spleen def.** | | | | | | | | | ◆ | ◆ | ▲◆ | | warm |
| **Standard dosage range (g)** | 3–9 | 9–15 | 9–15 | 3–9 | 6–9 | 9–15 | 15–30 | 6–9 | 3–9 | 3–6 | 15–30 | | |

### Bái Máo Gēn (Imperatae Rhizoma) woolly grass rhizome

**Preparation and usage** When the fresh herb is available, up to 60 grams can be used. Used unprocessed for optimum heat clearing action; the charred herb (*bai mao gen tan* 白茅根炭) is not as cool or moistening, but retains its ability to stop bleeding and is better tolerated by patients with deficiency.

**Contraindications** Bleeding from deficiency or cold. Caution in patients with middle burner yang qi deficiency.

**Formulae** *San Xian Yin* (cough and hemoptysis from Lung heat); *Mao Gen Yin Zi* (hematuria from yin deficiency with heat); *Mao Gen Tang* (vomiting from Stomach heat); *Shi Hui San* (bleeding from hot blood)

### Zhù Má Gēn (Boehmeriae Radix) ramie root

**Preparation and usage** When the fresh herb is available, 30–60 grams can be used. The juice squeezed from the fresh root can be applied to the skin for boils and infected lesions.

**Contraindications** Not suitable for bleeding or other conditions without heat in the blood or excess heat. Caution in patients with middle burner deficiency.

**Formulae** *Zhu Gen Tang* (threatened miscarriage from heat); *Zhu Gen San* (rectal or uterine bleeding from heat)

### Yáng Tí Gēn (Rumex japonicus Radix) Japan dock root

**Preparation and usage** When the fresh herb is available, 30–50 grams can be used. The fresh juice is best applied to parasitic skin infection.

**Contraindications** Middle burner yang qi deficiency and patterns with diarrhea.

**Formulae** *Yang Ti Gen San* (topically for damp itchy skin rashes); *Luo Li San* (tuberculous lymphadenitis)

### Bái Jí (Bletillae Rhizoma) bletilla rhizome

✿ This plant is listed in Appendix 2 of CITES[1] which permits limited trade with appropriate documentation.

**Preparation and usage** In severe cases up to 30 grams may be used in decoction, but is more effective when taken separately as powder for gastric and respiratory bleeding, at a dose of 1.5–3 grams in water, several times daily.

**Contraindications** Hemoptysis associated with acute external pathogenic invasion; early stage of Lung abscess; excess heat patterns of the Lungs and gastrointestinal tract with bleeding. Incompatible[2] with zhi fu zi (p.88), zhi chuan wu (p.94) and zhi cao wu (p.94).

**Formulae** *Bai Ji Pi Pa Wan* (hemoptysis from Lung yin deficiency); *Bai Ji San* (bleeding gastric ulcers); *Hua Rui Shi Bai Ji San* (hemoptysis with blood stasis); *Nei Xiao San†* (suppurative skin lesions); *Sheng Ji Gan Nong San†* (chronic superficial suppuration)

### Xiān Hè Cǎo (Agrimoniae Herba) agrimony

**Preparation and usage** In severe cases, up to 30–60 grams can be used in decoction. The fresh herb can be crushed and applied topically to bleeding wounds. For vaginal trichomonas, a strained decoction (120 grams of herb in one litre of water) cooled to body temperature, can be used as a douche or introduced via a soaked tampon or sponge, for 3–4 hours.

**Contraindications** This herb can cause nausea and vomiting in some patients, therefore should be used cautiously in those with middle burner weakness and phlegm damp patterns.

### Zǐ Zhū (Callicarpae formosanae Folium) callicarpa leaf

**Preparation and usage** When the fresh herb is available, 30–60 grams can be used in decoction. When taken directly as powder, the dose is 1.5–3 grams, several times daily.

**Contraindications** Caution in patients with bleeding from yang qi deficiency.

### Zōng Lǘ Pí (Trachycarpi Petiolus) trachycarpus palm fibre

**Preparation and usage** Always used in the charred form (*zong lu tan* 棕榈炭) to stop bleeding. When taken directly as powder the dose is 1–1.5 grams, several times daily.

**Contraindications** Bleeding associated with blood stasis, or in damp heat dysenteric disorder or leukorrhea.

**Formulae** *Shi Hui San* (bleeding from heat in the blood); *Gu Chong Tang* (uterine bleeding from Spleen qi deficiency); *Ru Sheng San* (uterine bleeding from yang deficiency); *Hei Sheng San* (bleeding hemorrhoids)

### Xuè Yú Tàn (Crinus carbonisatus) charred human hair

**Preparation and usage** When taken directly as powder the dose is 1–1.5 grams, several times daily. Can be powdered and blown into the nose or mouth for epistaxis and bleeding from the oral cavity.

**Contraindications** Caution in patients with weak middle burner qi. Often causes nausea.

**Formulae** *Hua Xue Dan* (various sites of bleeding with an element of blood stasis); *Bai Zhi San* (thin watery or bloody leukorrhea)

### Ǒu Jié (Nelumbinis Nodus rhizomatis) lotus rhizome node

**Preparation and usage** Up to 30 grams can be used in severe cases; when the fresh herb is available up to 60 grams can be used. The fresh juice squeezed from the root is also effective. When unprocessed or fresh, ou jie is used for bleeding from stasis and heat in the blood. Charred (*ou jie tan* 藕节炭) is slightly warm, more astringent and better for chronic bleeding associated from yang qi deficiency.

**Contraindications** None noted.

**Formulae** *Xiao Ji Yin Zi* (urinary bleeding from heat); *Bai Ji Pi Pa Wan* (hemoptysis from Lung yin deficiency); *Shu Xue Wan* (hemoptysis from Lung heat)

### Tiě Xiàn Cài (Acalyphae Herba) copperleaf herb

**Preparation and usage** When the fresh herb is available, 30–60 grams can be used in decoction. The liquid from a strong decoction, the juice pressed from the fresh plant or the bruised plant can be applied topically for skin diseases.

**Contraindications** Pregnancy. Caution in the elderly and debilitated.

### Jì Huā (Loropetalum chinensis Flos) Chinese fringe flower

**Preparation and usage** The flower, stem and roots are all used medically and have similar properties. The flower is used at a dose of 6–9 grams, the stem at 15–30 grams and the root at 30–60 grams. For burns and scalds, ji hua can be powdered, mixed with sesame oil or other suitable carriers and applied topically.

**Contraindications** Acute diarrhea and dysenteric disorder. Caution during pregnancy.

### Ài Yè (Artemisiae argyi Folium) mugwort leaf, moxa

This herb is placed in the internal warming group in some texts.

**Preparation and use** Unprocessed ai ye is used to warm the uterus, dispel cold and stop pain; when processed with vinegar (*cu chao ai ye* 醋炒艾叶) its ability to dispel cold, and stop pain and bleeding from cold is enhanced; when charred (*ai ye tan* 艾叶炭) its ability to stop bleeding is further enhanced. M refers to the use of moxa.

**Contraindications** Caution in patients with bleeding associated with yin deficiency. Ai ye is slightly toxic[3] and should not be used in too large a dose or for too long.

**Formulae** *Ai Fu Nuan Gong Wan* (infertility, dysmenorrhea and irregular menses from Kidney deficiency); *Jiao Ai Tang* (abnormal uterine bleeding from yang deficiency and instability of the *chōng mài* and *rèn mài*); *Si Sheng Wan* (bleeding from heat); *Bai Ye Tang* (bleeding from yang deficiency)

### Páo Jiāng (Zingiberis Rhizoma preparata) quick fried ginger

**Preparation and usage** Quick fried ginger is prepared by frying dried ginger at very high temperature until dark brown on the outside.

**Contraindications** Pregnancy, bleeding from yin deficiency or heat in the blood.

**Formulae** *Sheng Hua Tang* (postpartum blood stasis); *Ru Sheng San* (uterine bleeding from yang deficiency); *Xiao Yao San* (Liver qi constraint with blood deficiency); *Yang He Tang* (yin sores); *Hei Shen San* (postpartum blood stasis); *Da Yi Han Wan* (abdominal pain and diarrhea from Spleen yang deficiency)

---

| | Cang Zhu 苍术 | Hou Po 厚朴 | Huo Xiang 藿香 | Pei Lan 佩兰 | Sha Ren 砂仁 | Bai Dou Kou 白豆蔻 | Cao Dou Kou 草豆蔻 | Cao Guo 草果 |
|---|---|---|---|---|---|---|---|---|
| △ Indication / ▲ Strong Indication / E External Use / E Strong External Indication | | | | | | | | |
| **INDICATIONS** | | | | | | | | |
| abdominal distension | △ | ▲○ | △ | △ | ▲ | △ | △ | △ |
| alcohol – intoxication from | ○ | | | | | △ | | |
| appetite – loss of | △ | ▲ | △ | △ | △○ | ▲ | △ | |
| belching | | | | | △ | ▲ | | ○ |
| chest – stifling sensation in | △ | ▲● | △ | △ | △ | ▲ | △ | |
| common cold – summerdamp | | | ▲○ | ▲○ | | | | |
| common cold – summerheat | ● | | △ | ▲ | | △ | | |
| common cold – wind cold | △● | ○ | △ | | | | ○ | ○ |
| constipation – qi stag., phlegm | | △○ | | | ○ | ○ | | |
| cough – phlegm damp | ○ | ▲ | ○ | | | | | |
| damp blocking middle burner | ▲ | ▲ | ▲● | △ | △● | △○ | △ | △ |
| diarrhea – summerheat, damp | △○ | △ | ▲ | ▲ | △○ | ○ | △ | △ |
| diarrhea – Spleen qi def., damp | ▲ | | ○ | ○ | △○ | ○ | △ | |
| dysenteric dis. – chronic; def., cold | △ | △○ | | | △ | | △ | |
| eyes – green color blindness | △ | | | | ○ | ○ | ● | ● |
| eyes – night blindness | △ | | | | | | | |
| fatigue – damp obstruction | ▲ | △ | ▲ | △ | ▲ | ▲ | △ | △ |
| fever – damp, damp heat | | △ | △ | | △ | | | |
| fever & chills – alternating | | | | | | | | △ |
| fever & chills – simultaneous | △ | | △ | △ | | | | |
| food stagnation | | ▲ | | | △ | △ | | △ |
| headache – external; damp | △ | | △ | △ | | | | |
| hiccup | | | | | △ | △ | | |
| leukorrhea – damp, damp heat | ▲ | | | | | | | |
| malarial disorder – cold damp | | | | | | | △ | |
| miscarriage – threatened | | | | | △ | | | |
| morning sickness | | | △ | | ▲ | ▲ | | |
| muscle weakness & atrophy | ▲ | | | | | | | |
| nasosinusitis (*bi yuan*) | | | △ | | | | | |
| nausea – phlegm damp, cold | △ | △ | ▲ | △ | ▲ | △ | △ | △ |
| numbness – legs; damp heat | △ | | | | | | | |
| pain – abdominal, acute; damp | | ❖ | ▲❖ | ❖ | △ | △❖ | ▲ | △ |
| pain – abdominal., cold, food | | ▲❖ | | | △ | △ | ▲ | △ |
| pain – joint; wind damp; heat | ▲❖ | ❖ | ❖ | ❖ | ❖ | ❖ | | ❖ |
| pain – limbs; heavy & aching | ▲❖ | ❖ | ▲❖ | △❖ | ❖ | ▲❖ | ❖ | ❖ |
| pain – muscle aches; damp | ▲ | | ▲ | △ | | ▲ | | |
| painful obst. – wind damp; heat | ▲ | | | | | | | |
| plum pit qi (globus hystericus) | | ▲ | | | | | | |
| qi dynamic – blockage of | ▲◆ | ▲◆ | △◆ | △◆ | △◆ | △◆ | ▲◆ | △◆ |
| salivation – excessive, drooling | ◆ | ◆ | | △ | | | ▲ | |
| skin – tinea, ringworm | | | △E | ◆ | | | | |
| vomiting – phlegm damp, cold | △◆ | △◆ | ▲ | △ | ▲◆ | ▲◆ | △◆ | △◆ |
| wheezing – phlegm damp | | ▲ | ◆ | | | | | |
| **Standard dosage range (g)** | 6–12 | 3–9 | 6–12 | 6–9 | 3–6 | 3–6 | 3–6 | 3–6 |

○ Function ● Strong Function

**FUNCTIONS**
- alleviates food stagnation
- brightens the eyes
- calms a restless fetus
- checks malarial disorder
- directs qi downward
- dispels summerheat/damp
- dispels wind damp
- dries damp
- regulates qi
- releases the exterior
- stops vomiting
- strengthens the Spleen
- transforms damp
- transforms phlegm
- warms the middle burner

**Domain (❖)**
- Lung
- Large Intestine
- Spleen
- Stomach

**Flavour, nature (◆)**
- acrid
- bitter
- neutral
- warm
- slightly warm

**Zào Xīn Tǔ (Terra flava usta) baked earth from the center of an earthen wood fired stove**
Also known as fú lóng gān 伏龙肝.
**Preparation and usage** Cooked in a cloth bag for 30 minutes[1] prior to the other herbs.
**Contraindications** Bleeding from yin deficiency or vomiting from heat in the Stomach.
**Formulae** *Huang Tu Tang* (rectal bleeding from Spleen yang deficiency); *Bi He Yin* (vomiting from Stomach deficiency)

1 Appendix 6, p.108

**Substances from other groups**
Herbs from other groups with some hemostatic effect (main ones in bold) include hai piao xiao (p.2), chun pi (p.2), **ji guan hua** (p.2), wu bei zi (p.4), **chi shi zhi** (p.4), yu yu liang (p.4), jiang xiang (p.8), pu huang (p.8), shi wei (p.20), jing jie (p.28), **shan zhi zi** (p.32), ma bo (p.36), si ji qing (p.38), di jin cao (p.38), huang qin (p.42), he ye (p.46), dai zhe shi (p.48), guan zhong (p.52), **e jiao** (p.78), **mo han lian** (p.80), gui ban (p.80), huang yao zi (p.86), she mei (p.86), lu xian cao (p.94) and xue lian hua (p.94).

# 3.1 DAMPNESS – AROMATIC TRANSFORMING

**Cāng Zhú (Atractylodis Rhizoma) atractylodes rhizome**
Placed in the wind damp dispelling group in some texts.
**Preparation and usage** The unprocessed herb has the strongest damp drying and dispersing qualities. When stir fried (*chao cang zhu* 炒苍术), its ability to disperse acridity is moderated and the Spleen strengthening, middle burner harmonizing effect enhanced.
**Contraindications** Yin and blood deficiency patterns, constipated patients with dry stools, or in exterior pathogenic invasion and qi deficiency patterns with profuse sweating.
**Formulae** *Ping Wei San* (phlegm damp blocking the qi dynamic); *Cang Fu Dao Tan Tang* (amenorrhea from phlegm damp); *Yi Yi Ren Tang* (wind damp painful obstruction); *Bai Hu Jia Cang Zhu Tang* (acute damp heat painful obstruction); *Er Miao San* (weakness, numbness and atrophy of the legs from damp heat); *Dang Gui Nian Tong Tang* (damp heat leg pain and swelling); *Gu Chang Wan*† (chronic diarrhea from Spleen and Kidney yang deficiency); *Shen Zhu San* (wind cold damp common cold); *Yue Ju Wan* (abdominal bloating and reflux from the 'six stagnations')[1]; *Wan Dai Tang* (leukorrhea from Spleen deficiency with damp)

**Hòu Pò (Magnoliae officinalis Cortex) magnolia bark**
Other texts place this herb in the qi regulating group.
**Preparation and usage** Processing with ginger (*jiang hou po* 姜厚朴) enhances its ability to harmonize the middle burner and alleviate nausea and vomiting, and reduces its tendency to irritate the throat.
**Contraindications** Caution during pregnancy or in patients with Spleen qi deficiency.
**Formulae** *Ban Xia Hou Po Tang* (plum pit qi); *Hou Po Wen Zhong Tang* (cold damp in the middle burner); *Hou Po Cao Guo Tang* (damp malarial disorder); *Huo Po Xia Ling Tang* (lingering damp in the qi level); *Da Cheng Qi Tang* (*yáng míng* organ syndrome); *Ping Wei San* (phlegm damp blocking the qi dynamic); *Lian Po Yin* (vomiting and diarrhea from damp heat); *Su Zi Jiang Qi Tang* (chronic wheezing from Kidney deficiency with phlegm accumulation in the Lungs); *Shi Pi Yin* (edema and watery diarrhea from Spleen yang deficiency); *Zhi Shi Dao Zhi Wan* (food stagnation with constipation)

**Huò Xiāng (Pogostemonis/Agastaches Herba) patchouli**
**Preparation and usage** When the fresh herb is available, 15–30 grams can be used. It should only be cooked for a few minutes in a pot with a tight fitting lid to preserve the volatile oils. It can also be steeped in hot water and used as tea. The leaves (*huo xiang ye* 藿香叶) are best for releasing the exterior, whereas the stalks (*huo xiang geng* 藿香梗) are used for harmonizing the middle burner.
**Contraindications** Not suitable for conditions without damp.
**Formulae** *Huo Xiang Zheng Qi San* (summer damp common cold); *Huo Po Xia Ling Tang* (lingering damp in the qi level); *Gan Lu Xiao Du Dan* (damp heat febrile disease); *Huo Dan Wan* (chronic sinus congestion); *Xie Huang San* (mouth ulcers from hidden heat in the Spleen and Stomach)

**Pèi Lán (Eupatorii Herba) eupatorium**
**Preparation and usage** When the fresh herb is available, 15–30 grams can be used. It should only be cooked for a few minutes in a pot with a tight fitting lid to preserve the volatile oils.
**Contraindications** Not suitable for conditions without damp.

**Shā Rén (Amomi Fructus) amomum fruit**
Placed in the qi regulating group in some texts.
**Preparation and usage** Added at the end[2] of cooking. The seeds should be pounded in a mortar and pestle to break the hard outer shell before being added to the decoction, or ground to powder and added to the warm strained decoction. Can be steeped in hot water or a decoction of ginger and taken as tea.
**Contraindications** Caution in yin and blood deficiency patterns. Prolonged use alone can damage qi.
**Formulae** *Xiang Sha Liu Jun Zi Tang* (qi deficiency with phlegm damp); *Bi He Yin* (vomiting from Stomach deficiency); *Jian Pi Wan* (food stagnation and Spleen deficiency); *Dan Shen Yin* (chest and epigastric pain from blood stasis); *Yi Zhi San* (diarrhea from Spleen yang deficiency)

**Bái Dòu Kòu (Amomi Fructus rotundus) round cardamon**
Placed in the qi regulating group in some texts.
**Preparation and usage** Added at the end[3] of cooking. The seeds should be pounded in a mortar and pestle to break the hard outer shell before being added to the decoction, or ground to powder and added to the warm strained decoction.
**Contraindications** Yin and blood deficiency patterns. Prolonged use alone can damage qi.
**Formulae** *Bai Dou Kou Wan* (Spleen qi deficiency with damp blocking the qi dynamic); *Bai Dou Kou Tang* (vomiting from cold damp in the Stomach); *Ding Kou Li Zhong Wan* (acid reflux, abdominal pain and vomiting from yang deficiency); *San Ren Tang* (fever from damp heat in the qi level); *Huang Qin Hua Shi Tang* (damp heat in the qi level; heat greater than damp); *Huo Po Xia Ling Tang* (lingering damp in the qi level)

**Cǎo Dòu Kòu (Alpiniae katsumadai Semen) katsumada galangal seed**
Placed in the internal warming group in some texts.
**Preparation and usage** Added a minute or two before the end[4] of cooking. The seeds should be pounded in a mortar and pestle to break the hard outer shell before decoction.
**Contraindications** Yin and blood deficiency patterns.
**Formulae** *Hou Po Wen Zhong Tang* (cold damp in the middle burner); *Shi Pi Yin* (edema and watery diarrhea from Spleen yang deficiency)

**Cǎo Guǒ (Tsaoko Fructus) tsaoko fruit**
Placed in the internal warming group in some texts.
**Preparation and usage** Can sometimes aggravate vomiting; this can be alleviated by using the ginger-processed seeds (*jiang cao guo zi* 姜草果子). The fruit and seeds should be pounded in a mortar and pestle to break the hard outer shell before decoction.
**Contraindications** Yin and blood deficiency patterns. Caution in elderly and debilitated patients.
**Formulae** *Cao Guo Yin* (cold damp malarial disorder); *Jie Nüe Qi Bao Yin* (persistent cold damp malarial disorder); *Da Yuan Yin* (damp heat malarial disorder); *Qing Pi Yin* (phlegm heat malarial disorder); *Hou Po Cao Guo Tang* (damp malarial disorder); *Cao Guo Ping Wei San* (vomiting and abdominal pain from cold damp in the middle burner)

1 qi, blood, fire, food, damp, phlegm

2 Appendix 6, p.108
3 Ibid.
4 Ibid.

| △ Indication / ▲ Strong Indication / E External Use / E Strong External Indication — **INDICATIONS** | Fu Ling 茯苓 | Zhu Ling 猪苓 | Ze Xie 泽泻 | Che Qian Zi 车前子 | Yi Yi Ren 薏苡仁 | Han Fang Ji 汉防己 | Dong Gua Zi 冬瓜子 | Chi Xiao Dou 赤小豆 | Yu Mi Xu 玉米须 | Yin Chen Hao 茵陈蒿 | Jin Qian Cao 金钱草 | Hai Jin Sha 海金砂 | ○ Function / ● Strong Function — **FUNCTIONS** |
|---|---|---|---|---|---|---|---|---|---|---|---|---|---|
| abdominal distension | △ | | △ | | △ ● | △ | ○ | △ ○ | | | | | aids discharge of pus |
| abscesses & sores – skin | | | | | | | | △ E | ○ | E ● | △ E ○ | | aids Gallbladder function |
| abscess – Intestinal | | | | | ▲ | | ▲ | | ○ | | ○ | ○ | alleviates dysuria |
| abscess – Lung | | | | | ▲ | | ▲ | | | ● | | | alleviates jaundice |
| appetite – loss of | △ | | | ○ | △ | | | | | | | | brightens the eyes |
| ascites | ○ | | | | | △ | | | | | | | calms the shen |
| common cold – summerheat | | | | △ ○ | △ ○ | | ○ | △ | ○ | △ ○ | ○ | | clears damp heat |
| constipation – dryness | | | | | | | △ | ○ | | | ○ | | clears toxic heat |
| cough – heat, phlegm heat | | | | △ ○ | | | △ | | | | | | cools the Liver |
| diabetes (*xiao ke*) | | | | | ○ | ● | | | △ | | | | dispels wind damp |
| diarrhea – damp heat | | | △ | ▲ | △ | | | | | | ● | ○ | dissolves stones |
| diarrhea – Spleen qi def., damp | △ | △ | △ ○ | △ | ▲ | | | | | | | | drains Kidney fire |
| dizziness – phlegm damp | △ ○ | ● | ▲ ● | ○ | ○ | ○ | ○ | ○ | ○ | ○ | ○ | ○ | promotes urination |
| dysuria – damp heat | △ | △ | △ | ▲ ○ | △ ○ | | | △ | △ | | △ | ▲ | stops diarrhea |
| dysuria – during pregnancy | | △ | △ | | | | ○ | | | | | | stops pain |
| dysuria – stone, sand | ○ | | | △ | ○ | | | | △ | | ▲ | | strengthens the spleen |
| edema – eyes & fingers | ▲ | | | ○ | △ | | ○ | | | | | | transforms phlegm heat |
| edema – generalized | ▲ | ▲ | ▲ | ▲ | △ | △ | | △ | △ | | | △ | |
| edema – Kidney deficiency | △ | △ | ▲ | △ | | △ | | △ | △ | | | | |
| edema – knees, lower body | | | △ | △ | △ | ▲ | | △ | | | | | |
| edema – pregnancy | △ | △ | △ | | | | | | △ | | | | **Domain (❖)** |
| edema – Spleen deficiency | ▲ | | ❖ | | △ ❖ | △ | ❖ | | | | | △ | Lung |
| edema – wind, superficial | | | | | | ▲ | ❖ | | | | | | Large Intestine |
| eyes – red & sore; Liver heat | ❖ | ❖ | ❖ | △ ❖ | | ❖ | | | | | △ ❖ | | Kidney |
| eyes – weak, dry, blurry; def. | | ❖ | ❖ | △ | | ❖ | | | ❖ | | ❖ | ❖ | Bladder |
| fever – damp, damp heat | | | | △ ❖ | ▲ | | | | ❖ | △ ❖ | ❖ | | Liver |
| gallstones, cholecystitis | | | | | | | | | △ ❖ | △ ❖ | ▲ ❖ | △ | Gallbladder |
| hypertension | ❖ | | | △ | | | | ❖ | △ | | | | Heart |
| insomnia, much dreaming | △ | | | | | | ❖ | ❖ | | | | ❖ | Small Intestine |
| jaundice – damp heat | ❖ | △ | | | ❖ | ❖ | | △ | △ | ▲ ❖ | △ | △ | Spleen |
| jaundice – cold damp | | | | | ❖ | | ❖ | | △ | ▲ ❖ | | | Stomach |
| leukorrhea – Sp. qi def., damp | △ | △ | △ | △ | △ | | | ▲ | | | | | |
| memory – poor | △ | | | | | | | | | | | | |
| pain – & swelling, legs & knees | | | | | △ | ▲ | | | | | | | **Flavour, nature (◆)** |
| painful obst. – damp heat | | | | | △ | ▲ ◆ | | | | | | | acrid |
| painful obst. – wind damp | | | | | △ | ▲ ◆ | | | | | ◆ | | bitter |
| palpitations, anxiety | △ ◆ | ◆ | ◆ | | ◆ | | | | ◆ | | | ◆ | bland |
| skin – itchy damp/wind rash | | | | | | | | △ E | | E | ◆ | | salty |
| sperm – involuntary loss of | ◆ | ◆ | △ ◆ | ◆ | ◆ | | | ◆ | ◆ | | ◆ | ◆ | sweet |
| thin mucus disorders (*tan yin*) | △ | | △ | | | | | ◆ | | | | | sour |
| urination – difficult, scanty | △ ◆ | △ ◆ | ▲ | ▲ | △ | △ | | △ ◆ | △ | | | | neutral |
| urination – turbid | △ | △ | | | ◆ | | | | | ❖ | ◆ | △ | cool |
| warts – flat, plantar | | | ◆ | ◆ | △ | ◆ | ◆ | | | | | ◆ | cold |
| **Standard dosage range (g)** | 9–15 | 6–12 | 6–9 | 9–12 | 9–30 | 6–9 | 9–15 | 9–30 | 15–30 | 9–30 | 15–30 | 6–15 | |

Diuretic herbs eliminate damp by promoting urination and, by doing so, relieve edema, alleviate jaundice, ease dysuria and treat weeping skin lesions, all of which reflect damp pathologies. They can be broadly divided into four groups – those that specialize in edema, jaundice, dysuria or damp skin lesions. These are not precise divisions, however, as some herbs have multiple functions.

| edema | fu ling, zhu ling, ze xie, che qian zi, yi yi ren, han fang ji, dong gua zi, yu mi xu |
|---|---|
| jaundice | yin chen hao, jin qian cao, hai jin sha |
| dysuria | che qian zi, yu mi xu, hai jin sha, hua shi, mu tong, tong cao, qu mai, bian xu, di fu zi, shi wei, dong kui zi, deng xin cao, bi xie, dan zhu ye |
| weeping skin le-sions | chi xiao dou, jin qian cao, di fu zi, bi xie, ban bian lian |

## Fú Líng (Poria) hoelen, indian bread, tree root fungus

**Preparation and usage** For acute facial edema, up to 60 grams can be used. Specific activity varies depending on which part is used. The outer layer of the fungus (the "skin" – *fu ling pi* 茯苓皮) is better at promoting urination than tonifying and is used for edema. The light red variety (*chi fu ling* 赤茯苓) is better for clearing damp heat. The part closest to the penetrating pine root around which the fungus grows is known as the "spirit" of fu ling (*fu shen* 茯神) and is used for calming the *shén*.

**Contraindications** Excessive or frequent urination. Prolonged or excessive use may deplete fluids and damage yin.

**Formulae** *Wu Ling San* (general edema; edema in *tài yáng* pathology); *Zhen Wu Tang* (Spleen and Kidney yang deficiency edema); *Zhu Ling Tang* (Kidney yin deficiency with damp heat type dysuria); *Yin Chen Wu Ling San* (damp heat jaundice, damp greater than heat); *Ling Gui Zhu Gan Tang* (phlegm damp [thin mucus disorder] in the Intestines); *Si Jun Zi Tang* (Spleen qi deficiency); *Shen Ling Bai Zhu San* (Spleen qi deficiency edema and diarrhea); *Gui Zhi Fu Ling Wan* (blood stasis masses in the lower burner); *Gui Pi Tang* (*shén* disturbance and bleeding from Heart blood and Spleen qi deficiency); *An Shen Ding Zhi Wan* (qi deficiency shen disturbance); *Er Chen Tang* (phlegm); *Liu Wei Di Huang Wan* (Kidney yin deficiency)

## Zhū Líng (Polyporus) polyporus fungus

**Contraindications** Not suitable in the absence of damp or edema. Prolonged or excessive use (alone) can deplete fluids and damage yin.

**Formulae** *Zhu Ling Tang* (Kidney yin deficiency with damp heat type dysuria); *Wu Ling San* (general edema; edema in a *tài yáng* pathology); *Yin Chen Wu Ling San* (damp heat jaundice, damp greater than heat)

## Zé Xiè (Alismatis Rhizoma) alisma rhizome, water plantain

**Preparation and usage** Unprocessed for edema and urinary problems from heat; stir frying (*chao ze xie* 炒泽泻) warms it and renders it better for edema from Spleen deficiency; processing with salt (*yan ze xie* 盐泽泻) enhances its ability to influence the Kidneys and promote urination without damaging yin.

**Contraindications** Prolonged or excessive use (alone) may deplete fluids and damage yin.

**Formulae** *Ze Xie Tang* (dizziness from phlegm damp [thin mucus disorder]); *Wu Ling San* (general edema; edema in a *tài yáng* pathology); *Liu Wei Di Huang Wan* (Kidney yin deficiency); *Long Dan Xie Gan Tang* (damp heat in the Liver and Gallbladder); *Bi Xie Shen Shi Tang* (suppurative sores and discharge from damp heat in the lower burner; damp greater than heat); *Dang Gui Shao Yao San* (dysmenorrhea and premenstrual edema)

## Chē Qián Zǐ (Plantaginis Semen) plantago seed

**Preparation and usage** These tiny seeds contain a mucilaginous compound that is released during cooking, thus are best cooked in a cloth bag[1] to prevents the decoction from becoming too glutinous. Unprocessed seeds are best for edema, discharge and urinary problems from damp heat, and for transforming phlegm; stir frying (*chao che qian zi* 炒车前子) moderates their coldness and makes them easier on the Spleen – stir fried seeds are used for diarrhea and leukorrhea from Spleen deficiency.

**Contraindications** Pregnancy[2]. Prolonged or excessive use alone may deplete fluids and damage yin.

**Formulae** *Ba Zheng San* (damp heat dysuria); *Yi Huang Tang* (chronic leukorrhea from Spleen deficiency and damp heat); *Zhu Jing Tang* (weak vision from Liver and Kidney deficiency); *Ji Sheng Shen Qi Wan* (edema from Kidney yang deficiency); *Wan Dai Tang* (leukorrhea from Spleen deficiency with dampness); *Wu Zi Yan Zong Wan* (sperm disorders from Kidney deficiency)

## Yì Yǐ Rén (Coicis Semen) jobs' tears, coix seed

**Preparation and usage** Unprocessed yi yi ren is used for damp heat painful obstruction, abscesses, and other damp heat conditions. Stir frying (*chao yi ren* 炒苡仁) enhances its ability to strengthen the Spleen and stop diarrhea and leukorrhea from qi deficiency.

**Contraindications** Pregnancy[3].

**Formulae** *Yi Yi Fu Zi Bai Jiang Tang* (chronic Intestinal abscess); *Yi Yi Ren Tang* (wind damp joint pain); *Xuan Bi Tang* (wind damp heat painful obstruction); *Ma Xing Yi Gan Tang* (wind damp muscle pain); *Wei Jing Tang* (Lung abscess); *San Ren Tang* (lingering fever from damp heat in the qi level); *Si Miao Wan* (damp heat muscle weakness and atrophy); *Bi Xie Shen Shi Tang* (suppurative sores and discharge from damp heat in the lower burner; damp greater than heat); *Shen Ling Bai Zhu San* (Spleen qi deficiency edema and diarrhea)

## Hàn Fáng Jǐ (Stephaniae tetrandrae Radix) stephania root

Other texts place this herb in the wind damp dispelling group.

**Contraindications** Can easily damage Stomach qi, so should not be used for too long in qi deficiency patterns. Caution in patients with yin deficiency and in those without damp.

**Formulae** *Fang Ji Huang Qi Tang* (wind damp knee pain and edema); *Fang Ji Fu Ling Tang* (generalized edema); *Xuan Bi Tang* (wind damp heat painful obstruction); *Sang Zhi Tang* (shoulder pain and stiffness from wind damp); *Ji Jiao Li Huang Wan* (fluid accumulation in the Stomach and Intestines, ascites)

## Dōng Guā Zǐ (Benincasae Semen) wax gourd seed

Also known as dōng guā rén 冬瓜仁.

**Preparation and usage** Unprocessed seeds are used for internal abscesses; stir frying (*chao dong gua zi* 炒冬瓜子) enhances their ability to warm the Spleen and treat leukorrhea; stir frying with honey (*zhi dong gua zi* 炙冬瓜子) enhances their ability to transform phlegm and treat cough. The rind of this gourd (*dong gua pi* 冬瓜皮) is used as a diuretic for damp heat edema, in doses of 15–30 grams.

**Contraindications** Caution (unprocessed) in patients with middle burner deficiency and loose stools.

**Formulae** *Wei Jing Tang* (Lung abscess); *Da Huang Mu Dan Tang* (Intestinal abscess); *Kai Jin San* (anorectic dysenteric disorder)

## Chì Xiǎo Dòu (Phaseoli Semen) adzuki bean

**Preparation and usage** Can be boiled and strained, with the resulting liquid taken as a convenient treatment for acute damp heat dysuria.

**Contraindications** Caution during pregnancy[4].

**Formulae** *Chi Xiao Dou Tang* (edema of the lower body); *Ma Huang Lian Qiao Chi Xiao Dou Tang* (acute jaundice); *Xuan Du San* (topical formula for suppurative sores)

## Yù Mǐ Xū (Maydis Stigma) cornsilk

**Preparation and usage** When fresh Yu Mi Xu is available, the dose can be doubled. Can be used alone as tea for chronic nephritic edema in doses of 60 grams dry herb.

**Contraindications** None noted.

1 Appendix 6, p.109

2 Xu & Wang (2002) is the only source to assert a contraindication during pregnancy. See Appendix 1.1, p.98.
3 This contraindication is questionable. See Appendix 1.1, p.99.
4 This caution is questionable. See Appendix 1.2, p.99.

| INDICATIONS | Bian Xu 萹蓄 | Qu Mai 瞿麦 | Mu Tong 木通 | Tong Cao 通草 | Deng Xin Cao 灯心草 | Di Fu Zi 地肤子 | Dong Kui Zi 冬葵子 | Shi Wei 石苇 | Bi Xie 萆薢 | Hua Shi 滑石 | Ban Bian Lian 半边莲 | Dan Zhu Ye 淡竹叶 | FUNCTIONS |
|---|---|---|---|---|---|---|---|---|---|---|---|---|---|
| abscess – breast | ● | ● | ○ | | ○ | | △○ | ○ | | ● | | ○ | alleviates dysuria |
| abscesses & sores – skin | ○ | ○ | | | | ○ | | ○ | △ | ○ | △ E | | clears damp heat |
| amenorrhea – blood stasis | | △ | △○ | | ○ | | | | | | | ○ | clears Heart fire |
| ascites | | | △ | | | | | | | | △● | | clears toxic heat |
| bites & stings – insect & snake | | | | | | | | | | ○ | ▲ E | | dispels summerheat |
| bleeding – uterine | | | | | | | | △ | ○ | | | | dispels wind damp |
| bleeding – hematemesis | | ○ | | | | | | △ | | | | | invigorates blood |
| breast – distension & pain | ○ | | | | | | △ | | | | | | kills parasites |
| common cold – summerheat | | | | △ | | | ○ | | | ▲ | | | moistens the Intestines |
| constipation – dryness | | ● | ○ | | | | ▲○ | | | | | | promotes lactation |
| cough & wheeze – heat, phlegm | | ○ | | | | | | △ | | | | | promotes menstruation |
| diarrhea – damp heat | △○ | ○ | ○ | ○ | ○ | ○ | ○ | ○ | ○ | △○ | ○ | ○ | promotes urination |
| dysuria – damp heat | ▲ | ▲ | △ | △ | △ | △ | △ | △ | ● | ▲ | | △ | separates turbid & pure |
| dysuria – blood | △ | ▲ | △ | | | | △ | ▲○ | | | | | stops bleeding |
| dysuria – Heart fire | | ' | △ | △ | | | | ○ | | | | ▲ | stops cough |
| dysuria – stone, sand | △○ | △ | △ | | | ● | △ | | | △ | | | stops itch |
| dysuria – turbid | | | | | | | | | ▲ | | | | |
| ears – acute otitis | | | | | | | | | | E | | | |
| eczema, dermatitis, psoriasis | △ E | | | | | ▲ E | | | △ | E | △ E | | |
| edema – general | | | △ | △ | △ | | △ | △ | | | ▲ | | |
| edema – during pregnancy | | | | | | △ | △ | | | | | | |
| edema – acute nephritic | | | | | | | | | | | △ | | |
| fever – damp heat; lingering | | | | △ | | | | | | ▲ | | △ | |
| insomnia – Heart fire; Ht. → Kid. | | | △ | | △ | | | | | | | △ | |
| itch – generalized | △ | | | | | ▲ E | | | | | | | **Domain (✧)** |
| itch – vaginal, scrotal, anal | △ E | | ✧ | ✧ | | ▲ E | | ✧ | | | ✧ | | Lung |
| jaundice – damp heat | △ | | | | | | | ✧ | | | | | Large Intestine |
| lactation – insufficient | | | ▲ | △ | | ✧ | △ | | | | | | Kidney |
| leukorrhea – damp heat; def. | ✧ | ✧ | ✧ | | | ✧ | ✧ | ✧ | △ ✧ | ✧ | | | Bladder |
| night terrors in children – heat | | | | | △ | | | | ✧ | | | | Liver |
| painful obst. – damp heat | | ✧ | △ ✧ | | ✧ | | | | △ | | ✧ | ✧ | Heart |
| painful obst. – wind damp | | ✧ | △ ✧ | | ✧ | | | ✧ | △ | | ✧ | ✧ | Small Intestine |
| parasites – intestinal worms | △ | | | ✧ | | | | | ✧ | ✧ | | ✧ | Stomach |
| parasites – schistosomiasis | | | | | | | | | | | △ | | |
| skin – itchy damp rash | △ E | | | | | ▲ E | | | △ | E | △ E | | |
| skin – prickly heat | | | | | | | | | | E | | | **Flavour, nature (♦)** |
| skin – scabies | | | | | | E | | | | | ♦ | | acrid |
| skin – shingles | ♦ | ♦ | ♦ | | | ♦ | | ♦ | ♦ | | ▲ E | | bitter |
| skin – tinea, ringworm | E | | ♦ | ♦ | | | | | ♦ | E | ♦ | | bland |
| throat – sore, acute | | | | ♦ | △ E ♦ | ♦ | ♦ | ♦ | | ♦ | △ | △ | sweet |
| tumours – digestive tract, lymph | | | | | | | | | ♦ | | △ | | neutral |
| ulcers – mouth; Heart fire | ♦ | | △ ♦ | ♦ | ♦ | | | | | | | △ | cool |
| urination – turbid | | ♦ | | | | ♦ | ♦ | | ▲ | ♦ | ♦ | ♦ | cold |
| **Standard dosage range (g)** | 9–15 | 9–15 | 3–6 | 2–5 | 1–3 | 9–15 | 3–9 | 6–9 | 9–15 | 9–15 | 9–18 | 6–9 | |

Legend:
△ Indication
▲ Strong Indication
E External Use
**E** Strong External Indication
○ Function
● Strong Function

Yīn Chén Hāo (Artemisiae scopariae Herba) virgate wormwood, capillaris

**Contraindications** True jaundice should be distinguished from the yellowing of the skin or sallowness that can result from qi and blood deficiency, for which yin chen hao is contraindicated. Caution alone in yin type jaundice.

**Formulae** *Yin Chen Hao Tang* (damp heat jaundice); *Yin Chen Wu Ling San* (damp heat jaundice, damp greater than heat); *Yin Chen Si Ni Tang* (cold damp jaundice); *Gan Lu Xiao Du Dan* (damp heat febrile disease); *Dan Dao Pai Shi Tang* (gallstones from damp heat); *San Jin Tang* (urinary calculi)

Jīn Qián Cǎo (Lysimachiae/Desmodii Herba) lysimachia or desmodium

**Preparation and usage** If used as a tea on its own, up to 120 grams of the dried herb, or 250 grams of the fresh herb can be used per dose. To dissolve stones, it must be taken daily for at least one month.

**Contraindications** Caution in patients with Spleen deficiency.

**Formulae** *Dan Dao Pai Shi Tang* (gallstones from damp heat); *San Jin Tang* (urinary calculi); *San Jin Hu Tao Tang* (Kidney stones)

Hǎi Jīn Shā (Lygodii Spora) Japanese fern spores

**Preparation and usage** Should be decocted in a cloth bag[1] to prevent the spores from clouding the decoction and irritating the throat.

**Contraindications** Caution in Kidney yin deficiency.

**Formulae** *San Jin Tang* (urinary calculi); *San Jin Hu Tao Tang* (Kidney stones); *Hu Po San* (hematuria and urinary calculi)

Biǎn Xù (Polygoni avicularis Herba) knotweed

**Preparation and usage** If the fresh herb is available, up to 30 grams can be used.

**Contraindications** Caution in patient with urinary problems associated with Spleen qi deficiency, and in the absence of damp heat.

**Formulae** *Ba Zheng San* (damp heat dysuria)

Qú Mài (Dianthi Herba) Chinese pink, dianthus

**Contraindications** Pregnancy, and in patients with urinary problems associated with Spleen qi deficiency.

**Formulae** *Ba Zheng San* (damp heat dysuria); *Di Fu Zi Tang* (heat type dysuria); *San Jin Tang* (urinary calculi); *Shi Wei San*[2] (heat type dysuria)

Mù Tōng (Akebiae Caulis) akebia stem

**Contraindications** Caution during pregnancy, in the absence of damp heat, and in middle burner yang deficiency.

**Formulae** *Ba Zheng San* (damp heat dysuria); *Dao Chi San* (oral ulcers and dysuria from Heart fire); *Xiao Feng San* (itchy wind rash); *Xin Yi San* (wind cold headache and nasal congestion)

Tōng Cǎo (Tetrapanacis Medulla) rice paper plant pith

**Contraindications** Pregnancy. Caution in qi and yin deficiency and in the absence of damp heat.

**Formulae** *San Ren Tang* (fever from damp heat in the qi level); *Tong Ru Dan* (insufficient lactation); *Bai Ling Tiao Gan Tang* (infertility from blocked fallopian tubes or endometriosis); *Dang Gui Si Ni Tang* (numbness and pain in the extremities from cold in the channels)

Dēng Xīn Cǎo (Junci Medulla) juncus rush pith

**Contraindications** None noted.

**Formulae** *Ba Zheng San* (damp heat dysuria); *Xuan Qi San* (heat type dysuria); *Gu Jing Cao Tang* (visual disturbance and red sore eyes from Liver heat)

Dì Fū Zǐ (Kochiae Fructus) broom cyprus fruit

**Preparation and usage** Can be used alone as tea for dysuria during pregnancy.

**Contraindications** Scanty or concentrated urine from yin deficiency.

**Formulae** *Di Fu Zi Tang* (heat type dysuria)

Dōng Kuí Zǐ (Malvae Semen) mallow fruit

**Preparation and usage** Can be used alone as tea for dysuria and edema during pregnancy.

**Contraindications** Caution in pregnant women without edema or damp heat, and in patients with loose stools from Spleen deficiency.

**Formulae** *Kui Zi Fu Ling San* (generalized edema; edema during pregnancy); *Xuan Qi San* (heat type dysuria); *San Jin Tang* (urinary calculi)

Shí Weí (Pyrrosiae Folium) pyrossia leaf

**Preparation and usage** In severe cases up to 30 grams can be used.

**Contraindications** None noted.

**Formulae** *Shi Wei San*[3] (heat type dysuria); *Shi Wei San*[4] (stone dysuria)

Bì Xiè (Dioscoreae hypoglaucae Rhizoma) fish poison yam

**Contraindications** Caution in patients with Kidney yin deficiency.

**Formulae** *Bi Xie Fen Qing Yin* (turbid urine from Kidney deficiency); *Bi Xie Shen Shi Tang* (suppurative sores and discharge from damp heat in the lower burner; damp greater than heat); *Jin Gang Wan* (weakness and atrophy from Kidney deficiency); *Tu Fu Ling Gao* (syphilis and dysuria)

Huá Shí (Talcum) talcum; mineral composed primarily of magnesium silicate, $Mg_3(Si_4O_{10})(OH)_2$

**Preparation and usage** Should be cooked in a cloth bag and decocted for 30 minutes[5] prior to the other herbs. To treatment urinary calculi use 24–30 grams.

**Contraindications** Pregnancy[6], Spleen qi deficiency, when fluids are significantly damaged in a febrile disease, and in patients prone to involuntary seminal emission.

**Formulae** *Bai He Hua Shi San* (chronic fever and insomnia from lingering pathogenic heat in the qi level); *Huang Qin Hua Shi Tang* (damp heat febrile disease; heat greater than damp); *San Shi Tang* (acute heat in the qi level); *San Ren Tang* (lingering fever from damp heat in the qi level); *Hao Qin Qing Dan Tang* (damp heat in the *shào yáng* level); *Ba Zheng San* (damp heat dysuria); *Zhu Ling Tang* (Kidney yin deficiency with damp heat dysuria); *San Jin Hu Tao Tang* (Kidney stones); *Liu Yi San* (summerheat common cold); *Xuan Bi Tang* (wind damp heat painful obstruction)

Bàn Biān Lián (Lobeliae chinensis Herba) chinese lobelia

**Preparation and usage** When the fresh herb is available, 30–60 grams can be used.

**Contraindications** Edema from deficiency.

**Formulae** *Jing Wan Hong* (ointment for burns and non healing sores)

Dàn Zhú Yè (Lophatheri Herba) lophatherum leaves

Place in the heat clearing group in some texts.

**Contraindications** None noted.

**Formulae** *Xiao Ji Yin Zi* (blood dysuria)

Substances from other groups

Herbs from other groups with an effect on promoting urination to drain damp (the most important in bold) include yi mu cao (p.6), ze lan (p.6), pu huang (p.8), hu zhang (p.8), **lu lu tong** (p.8), luo de da (p.8), chuan niu xi (p.8), ma bian cao (p.10), **bai mao gen** (p.12), fu ping (p.26), **ma huang** (p.28), xiang ru (p.28), **zhu ye** (p.32), lu gen (p.32), pu gong ying (p.34), **tu fu ling** (p.34), **yu xing cao** (p.36), bai hua she she cao (p.36), quan shen (p.38), di jin cao (p.38), bai wei (p.44), **da fu pi** (p.64), **sang bai pi** (p.68), **ting li zi** (p.68), ai di cha (p.68), **huang qi** (p.74), bai zhu (p.74), ban zhi lian (p.86), wu jia pi (p.94) and di long (p.96).

---

1 Appendix 6, p.109
2 *Wai Tai Mi Yao* (Arcane Essentials from the Imperial Library)

3 *Wai Tai Mi Yao* (Arcane Essentials from the Imperial Library)
4 *Pu Ji Ben Shen Fang* (Formulas of Universal Benefit from My Practice)
5 Appendix 6, p.109
6 Xu & Wang (2002) is the only source to assert a contraindication during pregnancy. See Appendix 1.1, p.98

| △ Indication<br>▲ Strong Indication<br>E External Use<br>**E** Strong External Indication | Gua Di<br>瓜蒂 | Li Lu<br>藜芦 | Chang Shan<br>常山 | | | | | | | | | ○ Function<br>● Strong Function |
|---|---|---|---|---|---|---|---|---|---|---|---|---|
| **INDICATIONS** | | | | | | | | | | | | **FUNCTIONS** |
| chest – phlegm congestion | △ ○ | | △ | | | | | | | | | alleviates jaundice |
| consciousness – clouding of | | △ | ● | | | | | | | | | checks malarial disorder |
| food poisoning | △ ○ | △ | | | | | | | | | | clears damp heat |
| food stagnation – severe | △ ○ | ○ | △ ○ | | | | | | | | | induces vomiting |
| headache – external damp | E | ○ | ○ | | | | | | | | | kills parasites |
| jaundice – damp heat | E | | | | | | | | | | | |
| malaria – plasmodium | | | ▲ | | | | | | | | | |
| mania – phlegm fire | △ | | | | | | | | | | | |
| parasites – lice | | E | | | | | | | | | | |
| phlegm heat – constricting shen | ▲ | | | | | | | | | | | |
| poison – ingestion of | △ | △ | | | | | | | | | | |
| rhinitis – chronic | E | | | | | | | | | | | |
| seizures, epilepsy – phlegm heat | △ | △ | | | | | | | | | | |
| skin – scabies, tinea, ringworm | | E | | | | | | | | | | |
| throat – sore, acute | △ | △ | | | | | | | | | | |
| wheezing – phlegm heat | △ | | | | | | | | | | | |
| wind stroke – acute phase | | △ | | | | | | | | | | |
| | | | | | | | | | | | | |
| | | | | | | | | | | | | **Domain (❖)** |
| | | ❖ | ❖ | | | | | | | | | Lung |
| | | ❖ | ❖ | | | | | | | | | Liver |
| | | | ❖ | | | | | | | | | Heart |
| | ❖ | ❖ | | | | | | | | | | Stomach |
| | | | | | | | | | | | | |
| | | | | | | | | | | | | **Flavour, nature (♦)** |
| | | ♦ | ♦ | | | | | | | | | acrid |
| | ♦ | ♦ | ♦ | | | | | | | | | toxic |
| | ♦ | ♦ | ♦ | | | | | | | | | bitter |
| | ♦ | ♦ | ♦ | | | | | | | | | cold |
| **Standard dosage range (g)** | 2.5–5 | 0.3–0.9 | 6–9 | | | | | | | | | |

Emesis is induction of vomiting, a treatment reserved for poisoning, severe food stagnation and phlegm obstruction in the upper and middle burner. Quite popular in antiquity, this technique is rarely used anymore.

## Gūa Dì (Melo Pedicellus) melon stalk

Other texts place this herb in the phlegm transforming group.

**Preparation and usage** Taken directly in pill or powder, the dose is 0.3–1 gram. Can also be powdered and blown into the nose to stimulate secretion, and the external release of pathogens via the mucous membranes. This technique is used for severe damp type frontal and sinus headache and recalcitrant damp heat jaundice most visible in the face and eyes. A small amount of powder is applied to the nasal mucous membranes until a profuse yellow fluid is secreted. This herb is reasonably toxic and may cause side effects[1] within the standard dosage range.

**Contraindications** Pregnancy, postpartum, hemoptysis, hematemesis, in the debilitated and in those without excess in the upper burner.

**Formulae** *Gua Ding San* (powder blown in the nose for headache and jaundice); *Gua Di San* (severe food stagnation and phlegm accumulation in the chest; accidental poisoning)

## Lí Lú (Veratri nigri Radix et Rhizoma) veratrum root; black false hellebore

Other texts place this herb in the phlegm transforming group.

**Preparation and usage** Can be powdered and blown into the nose to restore from loss of consciousness. Can be mixed with a neutral carrier oil for topical application. This herb is very toxic and must be used with great caution. Side effects[2] may occur within the standard dosage range.

**Contraindications** Pregnancy, and debilitated or anemic patients. Incompatible[3] with dan shen (p.6), xi xin (p.28), xuan shen (p.40), chi shao (p.40), ku shen (p.42), ren shen (p.74), dang shen (p.74), bai shao (p.78), bei sha shen (p.80) and nan sha shen (p.80).

**Formulae** *Feng Tan Yin* (clouding of the consciousness from wind phlegm)

## Cháng Shān (Dichroeae Radix) dichroa root

Other texts place this herb in the anti–parasitic group.

**Preparation and usage** The unprocessed herb is used to induce vomiting; processing with wine (*jiu chang shan* 酒常山) reduced its emetic qualities, and is used to treat malaria. The unprocessed herb is quite toxic and may cause side effects[4] within the standard dosage range.

**Contraindications** Pregnancy. Caution in weak and debilitated patients.

**Formulae** *Jie Nüe Qi Bao Yin* (malarial disorder; true malaria)

---

1 Appendix 3.1, p.101

2 Ibid.
3 Appendix 2, p.100
4 Appendix 3.1, p.101

| △ Indication / ▲ Strong Indication / E External Use / **E** Strong External Indication — **INDICATIONS** | Liu Huang 硫磺 | Bai Fan 白矾 | She Chuang Zi 蛇床子 | Da Feng Zi 大风子 | Tu Jing Pi 土荆皮 | Mu Bie Zi 木鳖子 | Feng Fang 蜂房 | Lu Gan Shi 炉甘石 | Ban Mao 斑蝥 | Xue Jie 血竭 | Er Cha 儿茶 | ○ Function / ● Strong Function / ex. – Applied externally / int. – Used internally — **FUNCTIONS** |
|---|---|---|---|---|---|---|---|---|---|---|---|---|
| abscess – breast, mastitis | | ○ | | | | △E | E | | | ○ | ○ | astringes bleeding |
| abscesses & sores – skin | | | | | | △E | E | ○ | E | | | brightens the eyes |
| abscesses & sores – yin type | E | ○ | | | | E | | ○ | | | ○ | clears heat (ex.) |
| acne | E | ○ | ○ | E○ | ○ | E | | ○ | | | | dries damp (ex.) |
| alopecia | | | | | | | | | E○ | ○ | | invigorates blood |
| amenorrhea – blood stasis | ○ | ○ | ○ | ○ | ○ | ○ | ○ | | △ | △ | | kills parasites (ex.) |
| bleeding – various | ○ | E | | | | | | | | △ | E | opens the bowels (int.) |
| bleeding – traumatic | | E | | | | | | ○ | | E○ | E○ | promotes healing (ex.) |
| cancer | | ○ | | | | | △ | | △ | | | stops diarrhea |
| cervical lymphadenitis (luo li) | ○ | ○ | ● | ○ | ○ | △E | E | ○ | E | | | stops itch |
| constipation – yang deficient | ▲ | | | | | | | ○ | | ○ | | stops pain |
| diarrhea – chronic | | △○ | | | | | | | | | | transforms phlegm |
| dysmenorrhea – blood stasis | | | | | | ○ | ○ | | ○ | △ | | treats suppurative sores |
| eyes – pterygia, ulcers | ○ | | ○ | | | | | E | | | | warms Kidney yang (int.) |
| eyes – red & sore | | | | | | | | E○ | | | | wears away sores |
| fistula, anal | | E | | | | | | | | | | |
| hemorrhoids – bleeding, sore | | E | E | | | E | | | | E | | |
| impotence – Kidney yang def. | △ | | △ | | | | | | | | | **Domain (❖)** |
| infertility – Kidney yang def. | | ❖ | △ | | ❖ | | | | | ❖ | | Lung |
| itch – genital | E❖ | E❖ | E | | | | | | ❖ | | | Large Intestine |
| jaundice – damp heat | ❖ | △ | ❖ | ❖ | | | | | ❖ | | | Kidney |
| leprosy | | ❖ | | ▲❖ | | ❖ | ❖ | ❖ | ❖ | ❖ | | Liver |
| leukorrhea – cold damp | | | △ | | | | | | ❖ | | | Heart |
| nose – polyps; brandy nose | | E | | E | | | | | ❖ | | | Small Intestine |
| pain – & injury, trauma | | ❖ | | ❖ | ❖ | E❖ | | | | △E | △E | Spleen |
| pain – lower back, leg, knee | | | △ | | | ❖ | ❖ | ❖ | | | | Stomach |
| painful obst. – wind damp | | | △ | | | | △E | | | | | |
| parasites – round & tapeworms | | △ | | | | | △ | | | | | |
| seizures – wind phlegm | | △ | | | | | | | | | | **Flavour, nature (♦)** |
| skin – eczema | E♦ | **E** | E | ♦ | E♦ | ♦ | ♦ | **E** | ♦ | | E | toxic |
| skin – itchy damp rash | E | **E♦** | E | | E | | | **E** | | | E | slightly toxic |
| skin – itchy wind rash | E | | ♦ | | E♦ | | E | | ♦ | | E | acrid |
| skin – lichen simplex | E | E♦ | E | | E | | | | | | ♦ | astringent |
| skin – tinea | E | E | E♦ | E | E♦ | E♦ | E | | | | ♦ | bitter |
| skin – pompholyx eczema | E | E | E | | E | | | | | ♦ | | salty |
| skin – ringworm | E♦ | ♦ | E | | | | | | | | | sour |
| skin – rosacea | | | | E | | E | ♦ | ♦ | | ♦ | | sweet |
| skin – scabies | E | E | E | E | E | E♦ | E | | | | | slightly sweet |
| syphilitic sores; gumma | | | | E | | | ♦ | ♦ | | ♦ | E | neutral |
| toothache – severe | | | | | | ♦ | E | | | ♦ | | cool |
| trichomonal vaginitis | | ♦ | E | | | | | | ♦ | | | cold |
| ulcers – skin; chronic | | E | ♦ | | ♦ | | | E | E | **E** | E | warm |
| wheezing – Kidney deficient | △♦ | | | ♦ | | | | | | | | hot |
| **Internal dosage range (g)** | 1–3 | 0.6–1.5 | 3–9 | 0.3–1 | – | 0.5–1 | 2.5–4 | – | *see* p.25 | 1–1.5 | 1–3 | |

## Liú Huáng (Sulphur) sulphur

**Preparation and usage** For external use unprocessed sulphur is used, prepared as a paste or ointment. For internal use, processed sulphur is taken in pills or powders. To render it safe for internal use and less disagreeable, sulphur is processed with soy bean curd (*zhi liu huang* 制硫磺) which reduces its toxicity[1] and sulphurous odor.

**Contraindications** Pregnancy; yin deficiency with heat.

**Formulae** *Liu Huang Ruan Gao* (ointment for pruritus, scabies, rosacea etc.); *Chou Ling Dan*† (topical formula for stubborn itchy ringworm); *Ban Liu Wan* (constipation from yang deficiency); *Xing Pi Wan* (chronic childhood convulsions from Spleen deficiency)

## Bái Fán (Alumen) alum, a mineral composed of aluminium and potassium, with the chemical composition $KAl(SO_4)_2$

**Preparation and usage** Used internally in pills or powders only.

**Contraindications** For internal use in weak patients or in those without damp heat or phlegm heat.

**Formulae** *Er Yan San* (topical powder for ear infection); *Hua Chong Wan*† (intestinal parasites); *Bai Jin Wan* (seizures or manic behavior from wind phlegm); *She Chuang Zi San* (a wash for itching from numerous causes)

## Shé Chuáng Zǐ (Cnidii Fructus) cnidium seeds

**Preparation and usage** For external washes, 15–30 grams is used.

**Contraindications** For internal use in patients with yin deficiency and heat, or damp heat in the lower burner.

**Formulae** *She Chuang Zi San* (a wash for itching from numerous causes); *Zan Yu Dan* (impotence and infertility from Kidney yang deficiency)

## Dà Fēng Zǐ (Hydnocarpi Semen) chaulmoogra seeds

**Preparation and usage** This herb is very toxic[2] and rarely, if ever, used internally any more. In previous times it was the main treatment available for leprosy, but has been superseded for this. When prepared for external use, it can be roasted, crushed and mixed with a suitable carrier such as lard or sorbolene.

**Contraindications** Pregnancy; yin deficiency; heat in the blood.

## Tǔ Jīng Pí (Pseudolaricis Cortex) golden larch bark

Also known as tǔ jīn pí 土槿皮.

**Preparation and usage** Only used externally in alcohol or vinegar tinctures, or ointments.

**Contraindications** Not suitable for internal use.

**Formulae** *Tu Jin Pi Ding* (tincture for tinea)

## Mù Biē Zǐ (Momordicae Semen) momordica seeds

**Preparation and usage** Used internally in pills or powders only, in which the defatted product (*mu bie zi shuang* 木鳖子霜) is used. Side effects[3] may occur within the standard dosage range and caution is required when used internally. For external use the ground seeds are mixed with vinegar or a suitable carrier, such as lard or sorbolene.

**Contraindications** Pregnancy; qi and blood deficiency; middle burner deficiency.

**Formulae** *Wu Long Gao* (ointment for toxic sores)

## Fēng Fáng (Vespae Nidus) wasp nest

**Preparation and usage** Used internally for cancer (lymphatic, nasopharyngeal, breast) or severe pain it can be decocted, but is thought better in pill or powders with a dose of 1–2 grams, twice daily. This substance is toxic[4] and must be used with caution internally.

**Contraindications** Qi and blood deficiency; sores that have already ruptured; patients with impaired renal function.

**Formulae** *Feng Fang Gao*† (ointment for cervical lymphadenitis and scrophula); *Xuan Du San* (topical formula for suppurative sores)

## Lú Gān Shí (Calamina) calamine, a zinc carbonate mineral with the chemical composition $ZnCO_3$

**Preparation and usage** Only used externally or as a fine powder suspended in sterile saline.

**Contraindications** Not suitable for internal use.

**Formulae** *Lu Gan Shi San* (inflammation and ulceration of the eyes)

## Bān Máo (Mylabris) cantharides beetle, blister beetle

**Preparation and usage** For external use the ground beetle is steeped in alcohol or vinegar and prepared as a tincture. Rarely used internally due to its toxicity[5], but when ingested to treat cancer (liver, digestive tract) it was traditionally stir fried with rice (*mi ban mao* 米斑蝥) and used in pills or powder with a dosage range of 0.03–0.06 grams.

**Contraindications** Pregnancy and in weak or debilitated patients.

**Formulae** *Ban Mao Ding* (tincture for alopecia); *Chou Ling Dan*† (topical formula for stubborn itchy ringworm)

## Xuè Jié (Daemonoropis Resina) resinous secretion of Daemonorops palm

**Preparation and usage** Only used in pills or powder.

**Contraindications** Internally during pregnancy or menstruation, and in patients without blood stasis.

**Formulae** *Xue Jie San* (chronic non healing ulcers and sores); *Sheng Ji Yu Hong Gao*† (ointment for suppurative and inflamed skin lesions); *Qi Li San*† (traumatic injury)

## Ér Chá (Catechu) a paste made from a concentrated decoction of the bark and twigs of the tree Acacia catechu

**Preparation and usage** Mostly used in pill or powder form, although it can be decocted, in which case it should be cooked in a cloth bag[6].

**Contraindications** None noted.

**Formulae** *Sheng Ji San*† (chronic non healing ulcers and sores); *Qi Li San*† (traumatic injury)

## Substances from other groups

Substances from other groups that are used externally to heal wounds and treat skin conditions include hai piao xiao (p.2), chi shi zhi (p.4), ru xiang (p.6), mo yao (p.6), di bie chong (p.10), di yu (p.12), bai ji (p.14), shi gao (p.32), han shui shi (p.32), si ji qing (p.38), chan su (p.50), da suan (p.52), mao zhua cao (p.54) and long gu (p.72).

## Endnotes

† These formulae traditionally contain items from endangered animal species and/or obsolete toxic substances, and are unavailable in their original form.

---

1 Appendix 3.1, p.101
2 Ibid.
3 Ibid.

4 Ibid.
5 Ibid.
6 Appendix 6, p.109

| INDICATIONS | Bo He 薄荷 | Niu Bang Zi 牛蒡子 | Chan Tui 蝉蜕 | Sang Ye 桑叶 | Ju Hua 菊花 | Man Jing Zi 蔓荆子 | Mu Zei 木贼 | Dan Dou Chi 淡豆豉 | Fu Ping 浮萍 | Ge Gen 葛根 | Chai Hu 柴胡 | Sheng Ma 升麻 | FUNCTIONS |
|---|---|---|---|---|---|---|---|---|---|---|---|---|---|
| abscesses & sores – skin | | ▲ | ○ | ○ | △ ● | ○ | ○ | | | | | | brightens the eyes |
| bleeding – vomiting, uterine; heat | | | | △○ | ○ | | | | | | | | calms the Liver |
| common cold – wind cold | | ○ | | | | | | △ | | △ | | ○ | clears toxic heat |
| constipation – wind heat | | △ | | ● | ○ | | | | | | | | cools the Liver |
| convulsions – febrile in children | ○ | | ▲ | ● | | | | | | | | | cools the Lungs |
| cough – wind heat, Lung heat | △ | △ | | ▲ | | | ○ | | | | | | dispels wind damp |
| diabetes (xiao ke) | ● | ● | ● | ○ | ○ | ○ | ○ | | | ▲ | | | dispels wind heat |
| diarrhea – qi deficiency | ○ | | | | | | | | | ▲ | △ ● | △ | dredges the Liver |
| diarrhea – acute; damp heat | △○ | ● | ○ | | | | | | | △ | | | eases the throat |
| dizziness, vertigo – yang ↑ | | | | △ | △ | △ | | | | ○ | | | generates fluids |
| edema – wind heat; acute | | | | | | | | | ▲ | | ● | | harmonizes shào yáng |
| eyes – corneal opacity, cataract | | | △ | | | | △ | | ○ | | | | promotes sweating |
| eyes – excessive lacrimation | | | | | △ | △ | △ | | ○ | | | | promotes urination |
| eyes – red, sore, itchy | △ | | △ | △ | ▲ | ▲ | ▲ | | | ○ | ○ | ○ | raises yang & sinking qi |
| fever & chills – alternating | | | | | | | | | | ○ | ▲ | | releases the muscle layer |
| fever – low grade, lingering | △ | △ | | | △ | | | ▲ | | △○ | ▲ | △ | stops diarrhea |
| fever – acute, wind heat | ▲ | △ | ● | △ | △ | | | △ | △○ | △ | ▲ | △ | stops itch |
| headache – ascendant yang | | | ○ | △ | △ | △ | | | | | | | stops spasm |
| headache – temporal, migraine | ○ | ○ | | | ○ | ▲ | | ● | | ○ | △ ● | ○ | vents lingering pathogens |
| headache – qi constraint, tension | △○ | ○ | ● | | | | | | ○ | ○ | ▲ | ● | vents rashes |
| headache – Stomach heat | | | | | | | | | | | | △ | |
| headache – wind heat | △ | | | △ | △ | ▲ | | △ | | △ | △ | △ | |
| insomnia, irritability – post fever | | | | | | | | △ | | | | | |
| lingering path. – qi, nutritive | △ | △ | | | △ | | | ▲ | | △ | | △ | |
| lingering path. – shao yang | | | | | | | | | | | ▲ | | **Domain (✣)** |
| malarial disorder | ✣ | ✣ | ✣ | ✣ | ✣ | | | ✣ | ✣ | | ▲ | ✣ | Lung |
| measles – inadequate rash in | △ | △ | ▲ | | | | | △ | | ▲ | | ▲✣ | Large Intestine |
| menstruation – irregular | | | | | | ✣ | | | ✣ | | ▲ | | Bladder |
| mumps – wind heat, toxic heat | ✣ | △ | ✣ | ✣ | ✣ | ✣ | ✣ | | | | ✣ | | Liver |
| night terrors in children – heat | | | △ | | | | ✣ | | | | ✣ | | Gallbladder |
| prolapse – rectal, uterine, ptosis | | | | | | | | | | ✣ | ▲ | ▲✣ | Spleen |
| pain – abdomen; heat; qi const. | △ | ✣ | | | | ✣ | | ✣ | | ✣ | △ | ✣ | Stomach |
| pain – chest; qi stag., constraint | △ | | | | | | | | | | ▲ | | |
| pain – hypochondriac; qi const. | △ | | | | | | | | | | ▲ | | |
| pain – neck, & stiffness | | | | | | | | | | ▲ | | | **Flavour, nature (♦)** |
| painful obst. – wind damp | ♦ | ♦ | | | ♦ | △♦ | | ♦ | ♦ | ♦ | ♦ | ♦ | acrid |
| skin – itchy wind rash; urticaria | △♦ | △ | ▲♦ | ♦ | ♦ | ♦ | | | | △ | ♦ | △ | bitter |
| spasm & cramp – skeletal mm. | | | △ | | | | | | ♦ | | | | slightly bitter |
| throat – sore, acute | △ | ▲ | △♦ | △♦ | ♦ | | ♦ | ♦ | | ♦ | | △♦ | sweet |
| toothache – Stomach fire | | | ♦ | | | △ | | | | | | ▲ | salty |
| ulcers – mouth; heat | | △ | | | | | ♦ | | | | | △ | neutral |
| voice – hoarse, loss of | ♦ | | ▲ | | ♦ | | | ♦ | | ♦ | ♦ | ♦ | cool |
| vomiting – acute; damp heat | △ | ♦ | ♦ | ♦ | | | | | ♦ | | | | cold |
| **Standard dosage range (g)** | 3-9 | 3-9 | 3-9 | 6-9 | 6-15 | 6-12 | 3-9 | 6-12 | 3-9 | 9-18 | 3-12 | 3-9 | |

△ Indication
▲ Strong Indication
E External Use
**E** Strong External Indication
○ Function
● Strong Function

### Bò Hé (Mentha haplocalycis Herba) mint

**Preparation and usage** To dispel wind heat, doses at the top of the range are used; to regulate qi, smaller doses, 3-4 grams, are used. Should be added to the hot decoction at the end[1] of cooking. Mint leaves are best for clearing the exterior; the stalk (*bo he geng* 薄荷梗) is best for regulating Liver qi. When the fresh herb is used the dose is 15–30 grams.

**Contraindications** Ascendant Liver yang, or sweating from qi deficiency.

**Formulae** *Sang Ju Yin* (wind heat cough); *Yin Qiao San* (wind heat common cold); *Zhu Ye Liu Bang Tang* (early stage wind rash and measles); *Cang Er Zi San* (nasal congestion; chronic sinus congestion); *Xiao Yao San* (Liver qi constraint with blood deficiency); *Gan Lu Xiao Du Dan* (damp heat febrile disease)

### Niú Bàng Zǐ (Arctii Fructus) burdock seed

**Preparation and usage** Should be broken up in a mortar and pestle before decoction. Stir frying (*chao niu bang zi* 炒牛蒡子) reduces its bitter coldness and makes it acceptable for patients with Spleen deficiency.

**Contraindications** Middle burner deficiency with diarrhea.

**Formulae** *Zhu Ye Liu Bang Tang* (early stage wind rash and measles); *Gua Lou Niu Bang Tang* (acute mastitis and breast abscess); *Niu Bang Jie Ji Tang* (early stage boils and sores); *Niu Bang Tang* (toxic heat sore throat and erysipelas); *Yin Qiao San* (wind heat common cold); *Pu Ji Xiao Du Yin* (toxic heat in the throat and head)

### Chán Tuì (Cicadae Periostracum) cicada shell

**Preparation and usage** To alleviate muscular spasms or convulsions, 15–30 grams can be used.

**Contraindications** Caution during pregnancy.

**Formulae** *Zhu Ye Liu Bang Tang* (early stage of wind rash and measles); *Chan Ju San* (wind heat eye disorders); *Xiao Feng San* (itchy wind rash); *Tian Zhu Huang San* (infantile convulsions from phlegm heat)

### Sāng Yè (Mori Folium) mulberry leaf

**Preparation and usage** Mostly used unprocessed, but for dry or heat type cough, with the honey-processed leaf (*zhi sang ye* 炙桑叶) can be used. When used alone externally as an eyewash, 30–120 grams can be used. When used for bleeding from heat in the blood, 15–30 grams must be used.

**Contraindications** None noted.

**Formulae** *Sang Ju Yin* (wind heat cough); *Sang Xing Tang* (dry wind heat common cold); *Qing Zao Jiu Fei Tang* (Lung dryness cough)

### Jú Huā (Chrysanthemi Flos) chrysanthemum flower

**Preparation and usage** For wind heat common cold, the yellow flower is used (*huang ju hua* 黄菊花). For visual problems and to calm the Liver, the white flower (*bai ju hua* 白菊花) is preferred.

**Contraindications** Headache from yang deficiency or when the patient has aversion to cold. Caution in patients with poor appetite and diarrhea from Spleen qi deficiency.

**Formulae** *Sang Ju Yin* (wind heat cough); *Qi Ju Di Huang Wan* (Liver and Kidney yin deficiency); *Ji Li Ju Hua Tang* (dizziness and headache from ascendant Liver yang)

### Màn Jīng Zǐ (Viticis Fructus) vitex fruit

**Preparation and usage** Stir frying (*chao man jing zi* 炒蔓菁子) reduces its acrid dispersal, while enhancing its ability to alleviate headache and sore eyes.

**Contraindications** Headache and dizziness from blood deficiency. Caution in patients with Stomach deficiency.

**Formulae** *Yi Qi Cong Ming Tang* (qi deficiency type visual disorders); *Qiang Huo Sheng Shi Tang* (wind damp headache)

### Mù Zéi (Equiseti hiemalis Herba) equisetum

**Contraindications** Caution during pregnancy or in patients with qi and blood deficiency visual problems.

### Dàn Dòu Chǐ (Sojae Semen preparata) prepared soybean

**Preparation and usage** These beans are prepared by steaming and fermenting with other herbs. Depending on the herbs used, the temperature of the final product can be cold or warm. Most commonly qing hao (p.44) and sang ye (this page) are used, resulting in the cool product noted here, also known as *xiāng dòu chǐ* 香豆豉 or *qīng dòu chǐ* 清豆豉. In some parts of China, ma huang is used resulting in a warm product (also known as *wēn dòu chǐ* 温豆豉), used for wind cold common cold, as in *Cong Chi Tang*, below.

**Contraindications** None noted.

**Formulae** *Yin Qiao San* (wind heat common cold); *Cong Chi Tang* (early stage of wind cold common cold); *Zhi Zi Chi Tang* (lingering heat in the chest); *Lian Po Yin* (vomiting and diarrhea from damp heat); *Huo Po Xia Ling Tang* (lingering damp in the qi level)

### Fú Píng (Spirodelae Herba) duckweed

**Contraindications** Sweating from qi deficiency.

### Gé Gēn (Puerariae Radix) kudzu root

**Preparation and usage** Roasting ge gen (*wēi ge gen* 煨葛根) enhances its ability to raise Spleen yang and is used for treating chronic diarrhea.

**Contraindications** Sweating from qi deficiency or fully expressed rashes. Caution (unprocessed) in patients with cold in the middle burner.

**Formulae** *Chai Ge Jie Ji Tang* (external wind in the muscle layer with internal heat); *Ge Gen Tang* (wind cold neck pain); *Sheng Ma Ge Gen Tang* (weak expression of rash); *Ge Gen Qin Lian Tang* (damp heat diarrhea); *Yu Quan Wan* (diabetes); *Qi Wei Bai Zhu San* (chronic diarrhea from Spleen qi deficiency)

### Chái Hú (Bupleuri Radix) bupleurum root

**Preparation and usage** For a mild to moderate wind heat fever, 9–12 grams is sufficient. To allay a persistent high fever, 15–30 grams[2] of the unprocessed herb can be used for a few days; it should be cooked for 30–45 minutes, or until the original liquid volume of the decoction is reduced by 75%. To dredge the Liver, 6–9 grams of the suitably processed herb is used; to raise sinking qi and to guide the action of other herbs to the ears and eyes, 3-6 grams is used. Processing with vinegar (*cu chai hu* 醋柴胡) reduces its dispersing and yang raising action and enhances its ability to regulate Liver qi and stop pain; processing with wine (*jiu chai hu* 酒柴胡) enhances its ability to raise yang qi.

**Contraindications** Caution in patients with yin deficiency and ascendant Liver yang. Can aggravate headaches and cause nausea and vomiting in some patients with latent ascendant yang, although processing with vinegar and the cooking method for fever noted above, can help counteract this.

**Formulae** *Chai Ge Jie Ji Tang* (external wind in the muscle layer with internal heat); *Jing Fang Bai Du San* (wind cold common cold); *Qing Pi Yin* (phlegm heat malarial disorder); *Si Ni San* (Liver qi constraint); *Chai Hu Shu Gan San* (Liver qi constraint); *Xiao Chai Hu Tang* (*shào yáng* syndrome); *Da Chai Hu Tang* (*shào yáng* and *yáng míng* syndrome); *Chai Hu Jia Long Gu Mu Li Tang* (simultaneous *tài yáng, shào yáng* and *yáng míng* syndrome); *Long Dan Xie Gan Tang* (damp heat in the Liver and Gallbladder); *Xue Fu Zhu Yu Tang* (qi and blood stasis); *Bu Zhong Yi Qi Tang* (Spleen qi deficiency fever and prolapse); & 18+ more in Appendix 7.

### Shēng Má (Cimicifugae Rhizoma) cimicifuga

**Preparation and usage** To expel external pathogens the unprocessed herb is used; when used in small doses, 3-6 grams, and processed with honey (*zhi sheng ma* 炙升麻) its ability to raise yang qi is enhanced.

**Contraindications** Yin deficiency with heat and ascendant yang, headache from ascendant yang, wheezing from obstructed Lung qi, and following the full expression of rashes.

**Formulae** *Sheng Ma Ge Gen Tang* (weak expression of rash); *Qing Wei San* (headache and oral ulcers from Stomach heat); *Pu Ji Xiao Du Yin* (toxic heat in the throat and head); *Lian Qiao Bai Du San* (mumps and suppurative sores from toxic heat); *Bu Zhong Yi Qi Tang* (Spleen qi deficiency fever and prolapse)

### Substances from other groups

Substances from other groups that can dispel wind heat include gu jing cao (p.32), jin yin hua (p.34), lian qiao (p.34) and qian hu (p.56).

---

1 Appendix 6, p.108

2 *Shi Yong Zhong Yao Xue* (1985)

Legend:
- △ Indication
- ▲ Strong Indication
- E External Use
- E Strong External Indication
- ○ Function
- ● Strong Function

| INDICATIONS | Ma Huang 麻黄 | Gui Zhi 桂枝 | Zi Su Ye 紫苏叶 | Jing Jie 荆芥 | Fang Feng 防风 | Bai Zhi 白芷 | Gao Ben 藁本 | Xi Xin 细辛 | Sheng Jiang 生姜 | Cong Bai 葱白 | Xiang Ru 香薷 | Xin Yi Hua 辛夷花 | FUNCTIONS |
|---|---|---|---|---|---|---|---|---|---|---|---|---|---|
| abdominal distension | | | ▲ | | | ○ | | | | | △ | | aids discharge of pus |
| abscesses & sores – skin, early | | | ○ | △ | △ | ▲ | | | ○ | E | | | alleviates toxicity |
| abscesses & sores – yin type | ▲● | | | | | | | | | | | | alleviates wheezing |
| amenorrhea – cold & bld. stasis | | △ | ○ | | | | | | | | | | calms a restless fetus |
| bleeding – Intestinal wind | | | | △ | | ● | | ○ | | | | ● | clears the nose & sinuses |
| bleeding – general, mild | | | | △ | | | | | | ○ | | | dispels summerdamp |
| common cold – summerdamp | | ○ | | ○ | ○ | | | | | | ▲ | | dispels wind |
| common cold – WC, no sweat | ▲○ | △ | △○ | △ | △ | △ | △○ | △○ | △○ | △○ | △ | △○ | dispels wind cold |
| common cold – WC, sweating | | ▲ | | △ | △○ | ○ | ○ | | | | | | dispels wind damp |
| common cold – wind heat | | | | △ | △ | △● | | | | | | △ | dries damp |
| cough – phlegm damp | △● | ○ | △ | | | | | ▲ | ▲ | ○ | ○ | | promotes sweating |
| cough – wind cold | ▲○ | | △ | | | | | △ | △ | | ○ | | promotes urination |
| diabetes (xiao ke) | | ▲ | ○ | | | | | | | | | | regulates qi |
| diarrhea – acute, with abd. pain | | ● | △ | | △ | | | | | △ | △ | | releases the muscle layer |
| dysmenorrhea – cold & bld. stasis | | ▲ | | ○ | | | | | | | | | stops itch |
| edema – acute onset; nephritis | ▲ | △ | | | ○ | ○ | ○ | ● | | | △ | | stops pain |
| fever & chills – simultaneous | △ | △ | △ | △ | △○ | △ | | △ | △ | △ | △ | | stops spasm |
| food & herb poisoning | | ▲ | | | | | | | △● | | | | stops vomiting |
| headache – frontal; sinus | | ○ | | | △ | ▲ | △ | △○ | ○ | | △ | △ | transforms phlegm damp |
| headache – occipital | △ | ● | | | △ | △ | | △ | | ○ | | | unblocks yang |
| headache – vertex | | | | ○ | △ | △ | ▲ | | | | | | vents rashes |
| leukorrhea – damp; damp heat | | ○ | | | | ▲ | | | | | | | warms the channels |
| masses – lower abdomen | | △ | | | | | | | ○ | ○ | | | warms the Lungs |
| measles – inadequate rash in | | ○ | | △ | | | | | | ○ | | | warms the middle burner |
| miscarriage – threatened | | | △ | | | | | | | | | | |
| morning sickness | | | ▲ | | | | | | △ | | | | |
| nasosinusitis (bi yuan) | △ | | | | | ▲ | | △ | △ | △ | | ▲ | **Domain (❖)** |
| nausea, vomiting | ❖ | ❖ | △❖ | ❖ | | ❖ | | ❖ | ▲❖ | ❖ | △❖ | ❖ | Lung |
| pain – abdominal, cold | | ▲ | | | | | | △❖ | | △ | | | Kidney |
| pain – abdominal, Liv. → Sp. | ❖ | ❖ | | | ▲❖ | ❖ | | | | | | | Bladder |
| pain – chest; cold, phlegm | | △ | | ❖ | ❖ | | | | | | | | Liver |
| pain – facial (neuralgia) | | ❖ | | | | △ | | ▲❖ | | | | | Heart |
| pain – muscle; generalized | △ | ▲ | ❖ | | △❖ | ❖ | △ | △ | ❖ | | △ | | Spleen |
| pain – shoulder & arm | | ▲ | | | | ❖ | | | ❖ | ❖ | ❖ | ❖ | Stomach |
| painful obst. – wind cold damp | △ | ▲ | | | ▲ | △ | △ | △ | | | | | |
| palpitations – phlegm; yang def. | | △ | | | | | | | | | | | |
| skin – itchy wind rash; urticaria | | | | ▲ | ▲ | △ | | | | | | | **Flavour, nature (♦)** |
| sweating – spontaneous; qi def. | ♦ | △ | | | | ♦ | | | ♦ | | | | slightly toxic |
| spasm, cramp, tremor | ♦ | ♦ | ♦ | ♦ | △♦ | ♦ | ♦ | ♦ | ♦ | ♦ | ♦ | ♦ | acrid |
| thin mucus disorders (tan yin) | ♦ | △♦ | | | | | | △ | △ | | | | slightly bitter |
| toothache, jaw pain – cold | | ♦ | | | ♦ | △ | △ | ▲ | | | | | sweet |
| wheeze – wind, cold, heat excess | ▲♦ | ♦ | ♦ | | | ♦ | ♦ | ♦ | | ♦ | | ♦ | warm |
| wheeze – phlegm damp | ▲ | | | ♦ | ♦ | | | | △ | ♦ | | ♦ | slightly warm |
| **Standard dosage range (g)** | 2-9 | 3-9 | 6-9 | 3-9 | 6-9 | 3-9 | 3-9 | 1-3 | 3-9 | 3-9 | 3-9 | 3-9 | |

## Má Huáng (Ephedrae Herba) ephedra stem

**Preparation and usage** Unprocessed ma huang is a strong diaphoretic, reserved for excess conditions and robust patients without sweating (when diaphoresis is desired), edema, wheezing from excess and inhibited urination. Boiling first and skimming the scum off the decoction before adding the other herbs reduces the likelihood of side effects. Stir frying with honey (*zhi ma huang* 炙麻黄) moderates its dispersing action and promotes its action of directing Lung qi downwards and moistening the Lungs. This form is used for wheezing and cough from deficiency, heat or dryness, and for surface conditions in weak or debilitated patients.

**Contraindications** Night sweats from yin deficiency and wheezing from Kidneys failing to grasp qi. Not suitable unprocessed when used for patients with Lung deficiency and defensive qi deficiency with sweating, wheezing or edema. Caution in hypertensive patients. Avoid concurrent use in patients taking cardiac glycoside medication such as digoxin/digitalis. Side effects[1] are likely to occur with inappropriate or recreational application and in high doses. Not suitable for prolonged use.

**Formulae** *Ma Huang Tang* (wind cold); *Ma Huang Fu Zi Xi Xin Tang* (wind cold in a patient with yang deficiency); *Ma Xing Shi Gan Tang* (cough and wheeze from Lung heat); *Ma Xing Yi Gan Tang* (wind damp painful obstruction); *Xiao Qing Long Tang* (wind cold with thin phlegm congestion); *Ding Chuan Tang* (wheezing from phlegm heat); *Yue Bi Jia Zhu Tang* (acute wind edema); *Yang He Tang* (yin sores)

## Guì Zhī (Cinnamomi Ramulus) cinnamon twigs

**Preparation and usage** Mostly used unprocessed, however stir frying with honey (*zhi gui zhi* 炙桂枝) enhances its ability to treat middle burner yang deficiency. For painful conditions such as wind cold damp painful obstruction, up to 30 grams can be used with care for short periods of time (a few weeks).

**Contraindications** Pregnancy, heat patterns, heat type painful obstruction (alone), yin deficiency, ascendant yang, or for patients with bleeding disorders from heat. Caution in women with menorrhagia.

**Formulae** *Gui Zhi Tang* (nutritive defensive qi disharmony; exterior deficiency common cold); *Gui Zhi Fu Zi Tang* (cold damp painful obstruction); *Gui Zhi Fu Ling Wan* (blood stasis masses in the lower burner); *Gui Zhi Shao Yao Zhi Mu Tang* (painful obstruction; heat concentrated in a joint); *Gui Zhi Jia Long Gu Mu Li Tang* (sweating and *shén* disturbance from disruption to the Heart Kidney axis); *Ling Gui Zhu Gan Tang* (phlegm damp [thin mucus] in the Stomach and Intestines); *Zhi Shi Xie Bai Gui Zhi Tang* (chest painful obstruction; angina); *Wu Ling San* (edema in *tài yáng* syndrome); *Wen Jing Tang* (infertility and dysmenorrhea from *chōng mài / rèn mài* deficiency)

## Zǐ Sū Yè (Perillae Folium) perilla leaf

**Preparation and usage** Cook no longer than 5–8 minutes[2]. For food poisoning from seafood, 30–60 grams can be used. For external use, a strong decoction, or the crushed fresh leaf, can be applied topically.

**Contraindications** Exterior heat patterns, qi deficiency with sweating from wei qi deficiency, or fetal restlessness from heat in the blood or qi deficiency.

**Formulae** *Xing Su San* (wind dryness cough); *Xiang Su San* (wind cold with constrained qi); *Shen Su Yin* (wind cold with qi deficiency); *Ban Xia Hou Po Tang* (plum pit qi)

## Jīng Jiè (Schizonepetae Herba) schizonepeta stem or bud

**Preparation and usage** Cook no longer than 5–8 minutes[3]. To clear wind from the exterior use unprocessed jing jie; to stop bleeding use charred jing jie (*jing jie tan* 荆芥炭).

**Contraindications** Contraindicated (unprocessed) in the absence of external wind pathogens or in sweating from exterior deficiency.

**Formulae** *Jing Fang Bai Du San* (wind cold common cold); *Yin Qiao San* (wind heat common cold); *Niu Bang Jie Ji Tang* (early stage boils and sores); *Huai Hua San* (bleeding hemorrhoids; Intestinal wind); *Jiao Ai Tang* (chronic uterine bleeding); *Xiao Feng San* (itchy wind rash)

## Fáng Fēng (Saposhnikovae Radix) siler root

**Preparation and usage** Stir frying (*chao fang feng* 炒防风) enhances its ability to raise Spleen yang, harmonize the Liver and Spleen, and treat mouth ulcers, diarrhea and abdominal pain; for rectal bleeding from Intestinal wind, charred fang feng (*fang feng tan* 防风炭) is used.

**Contraindications** Spasms and tremors associated with yin and blood deficiency or heat, and in the absence of pathogenic wind, cold or dampness.

**Formulae** *Fang Feng Tang* (wind damp painful obstruction; wind predominant); *Jing Fang Bai Du San* (wind cold common cold); *Fang Feng Tong Sheng San* (combined internal and external excess patterns); *Tong Xie Yao Fang* (abdominal pain and diarrhea from Liver Spleen disharmony); *Yu Zhen San* (tetanic spasm); *Xie Huang San* (mouth ulcers from hidden heat in the Spleen); *Yu Ping Feng San* (poor immunity and sweating from wei qi deficiency); *Xiao Feng San* (itchy wind rash)

## Bái Zhǐ (Angelicae dahuricae Radix) angelica root

**Preparation and usage** The finely powdered herb may be blown into the nose to alleviate congestion.

**Contraindications** Blood and yin deficiency patterns, and heat in the blood. Not suitable following rupture of acute abscesses and boils. This herb is very drying, and side effects[4] may occur at doses of 30 grams.

**Formulae** *Bai Zhi San* (thin watery or bloody leukorrhea); *Chuan Xiong Cha Tiao San* (wind cold headache); *Cang Er Zi San* (nasal congestion; chronic sinus congestion); *Xian Fang Huo Ming Yin*† (toxic heat boils and sores); *Jin Huang San* (topical treatment for boils and burns)

## Gǎo Běn (Ligustici Rhizoma) Chinese lovage root

**Contraindications** Headache from heat, ascendant yang, blood or yin deficiency.

**Formulae** *Qiang Huo Sheng Shi Tang* (wind damp headache); *Xin Yin San* (wind cold headache and nasal congestion)

## Xì Xīn (Asari Herba) Chinese wild ginger

**Preparation and usage** When used in pills or powders the daily dose is 1–1.5 grams per day; in decoction 1.5–3 grams.

**Contraindications** Sweating from qi deficiency, headache from yin and blood deficiency with ascendant yang, and cough from Lung heat or yin deficiency. Toxic effects[5] may occur at doses of 15 grams. Incompatible[6] with li lu (p.22).

**Formulae** *Ma Huang Fu Zi Xi Xin Tang* (wind cold in a patient with yang deficiency); *Xiao Qing Long Tang* (wind cold with thin phlegm congestion); *Chuan Xiong Cha Tiao San* (wind cold headache); *Du Huo Ji Sheng Tang* (wind damp painful obstruction with Liver and Kidney deficiency); *Dang Gui Si Ni Tang* (numbness and pain in the extremities from cold in the channels); *Bi Yun San* (inhaled powder for nasal congestion)

## Shēng Jiāng (Zingiberis Rhizoma recens) ginger root

**Preparation and usage** Roasting fresh ginger root in hot ashes (*wei jiang* 煨姜) reduces its dispersing nature while enhancing its ability to warm the middle burner and stop nausea. The peel of ginger root (*sheng jiang pi* 生姜皮) is used to promote urination and reduce edema.

**Contraindications** Sweating from qi and yin deficiency, and yin deficiency with heat patterns.

**Formulae** *Sheng Jiang Xie Xin Tang* (heat and pathological fluids blocking the qi dynamic); *Xiao Ban Xia Tang* (nausea & vomiting); *Ju Pi Zhu Ru Tang* (vomiting from heat in the Stomach); *Bai Dou Kou Tang* (vomiting from cold damp in the Stomach); *Er Chen Tang* (phlegm); *Gui Zhi Tang* (ying wei disharmony; exterior deficiency common cold); *Wu Pi San* (superficial upper body edema)

## Cōng Bái (Allii fistulosi Bulbus) scallion/spring onion

**Contraindications** Sweating from qi deficiency.

**Formulae** *Cong Chi Tang* (early stage of common cold); *Bai Tong Tang* (abdominal pain from cold blocking the middle burner); *Jia Jian Wei Rui Tang* (wind heat in a patient with underlying yin deficiency)

---

1 Appendix 3.2, p.104
2 Appendix 6, p.108
3 Ibid.

4 Appendix 3.2, p.103
5 Appendix 3.2, p.104
6 Appendix 2, p.100

| INDICATIONS | Shan Zha 山楂 | Shen Qu 神曲 | Mai Ya 麦芽 | Gu Ya 谷芽 | Lai Fu Zi 莱菔子 | Ji Nei Jin 鸡内金 | E Wei 阿魏 | FUNCTIONS |
|---|---|---|---|---|---|---|---|---|
| abdominal distension | △ | ▲ | △ | △ | ▲○ | △ | △ | directs qi downward |
| accumulation disorder (gan ji) | △○ | | | | | △ | | disperses blood stasis |
| acid reflux, heartburn | | ▲ | △ | △ | △ | △ | ▲○ | dissipates masses |
| appetite – loss of | △ | △ | ▲ | ▲ | △ | △○ | △ | dissolves stones |
| belching | △ | ▲ | △○ | △ | ▲ | △ | △ | moves qi |
| breast – distension & pain | | | △● | | | | | reduces lactation |
| cardiovascular disease | △ | | | | | ○ | | restrains urine |
| cough – phlegm damp | | ○ | ○ | ○ | ▲ | | | strengthens digestion |
| diarrhea | △ | △ | △ | △ | △○ | △ | | transforms phlegm |
| dysenteric disorder | ▲ | | | | | | △ | |
| dysmenorrhea – blood stasis | △ | | | | | | | |
| dysuria – stone, sand | | | | | | ▲ | | |
| flatulence | △ | △ | △ | △ | △ | △ | ▲ | |
| food stagnation (carbohydrate) | | △ | ▲ | ▲ | | | | |
| food stagnation (general) | △ | ▲ | △ | △ | ▲ | △ | △ | |
| food stagnation (protein, fats) | ▲ | | | | △ | △ | | |
| gallstones | | | | | | ▲ | | |
| hypercholesterolemia | △ | | | | | | | |
| hypertension | △ | | | △ | | | | |
| indigestion | △ | ▲ | △ | △ | ▲ | △ | △ | |
| lactation – excessive | | | ▲ | | | | | |
| lactation – to reduce; weaning | | | ▲ | | | | | |
| Liver & Stomach disharmony | | | △ | | | | | |
| malarial disorder | | | | | | | △ | |
| masses – abdominal | △ | | | | | | ▲ E | |
| pain – abdominal | △ | △ | △ | △ | ▲ | △ | ▲ | |
| pain – abdominal; Liv → Sp. | | | △ | | | △ | | **Domain (❖)** |
| pain – chest, angina; bld. stasis | △ | | | ❖ | | | | Lung |
| pain – hypochondriac | | | △ | | | ❖ | | Bladder |
| pain – postpartum abdominal | ▲❖ | | ❖ | | | ❖ | | Liver |
| pain – testicular | △ | | | | | ❖ | | Small Intestine |
| placenta, lochia – retention of | △❖ | ❖ | ❖ | ❖ | ❖ | ❖ | ❖ | Spleen |
| reflux in infants | △❖ | ❖ | △❖ | ❖ | ❖ | ❖ | ❖ | Stomach |
| sperm – involuntary loss of | | | | | | △ | | |
| ulcers – mouth | | | | | | △ | | |
| urination – enuresis | | | | | | ▲ | | **Flavour, nature (◆)** |
| urination – incontinence of | | ◆ | | | ◆ | ▲ | ◆ | acrid |
| urination – nocturia | | | | | | ▲ | ◆ | bitter |
| vomiting of milk in infants | ◆ | ◆ | △◆ | ◆ | ◆ | ◆ | | sweet |
| wheezing – phlegm damp | ◆ | | | | ▲ | | | sour |
| | | ◆ | | ◆ | ◆ | ◆ | | neutral |
| | | ◆ | | | | | ◆ | warm |
| | ◆ | | | | | | | slightly warm |
| **Standard dosage range (g)** | 9–15 | 6–15 | 9–15 | 9–15 | 6–9 | 3–9 | 1–1.5 | |

Legend:
△ Indication
▲ Strong Indication
E External Use
**E** Strong External Indication
○ Function
● Strong Function

**Xiāng Rú (Moslae Herba) aromatic madder**

**Preparation and usage** To promote sweating and treat summerdamp patterns, cook for 5–10 minutes and take cool; when used for edema it cook for 15–20 minutes.

**Contraindications** Sweating from qi deficiency, and summerheat patterns with high fever and sweating.

**Formulae** *Xiang Ru San* (summerdamp common cold)

**Xīn Yí Huā (Magnoliae Flos) magnolia flower**

**Preparation and usage** Should be decocted in a cloth bag[1] as the small hairs can irritate the throat. Can be powdered and blown into the nose.

1 Appendix 6, p.109

**Contraindications** Yin deficiency with heat. Caution during pregnancy[2].

**Formulae** *Xin Yi San* (wind cold headache and nasal congestion); *Cang Er Zi San* (nasal congestion; chronic sinus congestion)

## Substances from other groups

Substances from other groups that can dispel wind cold include huo xiang (p.16), dan dou chi (p.26), qiang huo (p.90) and du huo (p.90).

2 Bensky et al (2004) 3rd ed.

# 7. FOOD STAGNATION RELIEVING – DIGESTIVES

**Shān Zhā (Crataegi Fructus) hawthorn fruit**

**Preparation and usage** In severe cases up to 30 grams can be used. Unprocessed for hypertension; mostly stir fried (*chao shan zha* 炒山楂) for food stagnation; cooking until black on the outside (*jiao shan zha* 焦山楂) or charring (*shan zha tan* 山楂炭) enhances its ability to stop diarrhea and dispel blood stasis.

**Contraindications** Pregnancy[1]. Caution in patients with middle burner yang deficiency and in those with an excess of gastric acid.

**Formulae** *Bao He Wan* (food stagnation); *E Wei Wan* (food stagnation with copious flatulence); *Fei Er Wan* (accumulation disorder with fever and heat in infants); *Du Sheng San* (dysmenorrhea and postpartum abdominal pain from blood stasis)

**Shén Qū (Massa medicata fermentata) medicated leaven[2]**

**Preparation and usage** When used to assist the absorption of minerals (as in *Ci Zhu Wan*), the unprocessed material is preferred; when used for food stagnation it is usually stir fried or charred. Stir frying (*chao shen qu* 炒神曲) enhances its ability to strengthen the Spleen and harmonize the middle burner in addition to reducing food stagnation[3]; when charred (*jiao shen qu* 焦神曲) its ability to stop diarrhea is enhanced.

**Contraindications** Stomach fire and Spleen yin deficiency. Caution during pregnancy.

**Formulae** *Zhi Shi Dao Zhi Wan* (food stagnation with constipation); *Jian Pi Wan* (food stagnation and Spleen deficiency); *Yue Ju Wan* (abdominal bloating and reflux from the 'six stagnations')[4]; *Ci Zhu Wan†* (insomnia and palpitations from disruption to the Heart Kidney axis)

**Mài Yá (Hordei Fructus germinantus) sprouted barley**

**Preparation and usage** When used to restrain lactation, 30–60 grams should be used. To strengthen the Spleen and Stomach and regulate Liver qi the unprocessed herb is used; to alleviate food stagnation and restrain lactation the stir fried form (*chao mai ya* 炒麦芽) is used.

**Contraindications** High doses in women who wish to continue lactating (low doses, below 9 grams, will not affect lactation).

**Formulae** *Jian Pi Wan* (food stagnation and Spleen deficiency); *Zhi Shi Xiao Pi Wan* (epigastric blockage with Spleen deficiency); *Fei Er Wan* (accumulation disorder with fever and heat in infants); *Zhen Gan Xi Feng Tang* (ascendant Liver yang)

**Gǔ Yá (Setariae [Oryzae] Fructus germinatus) sprouted rice/millet**

**Preparation and usage** In severe cases up to 30 grams may be used. Unprocessed gu ya is best for harmonizing the middle burner; the stir fried form (*chao gu ya* 炒谷芽) is traditionally considered better for alleviating food stagnation[5].

**Contraindications** None noted.

1 Bensky et al (2004) 3rd ed. is the only source to assert a contraindication during pregnancy. See Appendix 1, p.99.

2 A fermented product composed of a mixture of wheat flour, bran and various herbs, including xing ren p.68, qing hao p.44, chi xiao dou p.18, and others depending on production region.

3 The traditional claim is questioned in Bensky 2004 (p.499) who states that current research shows that the unprocessed form is best for aiding digestion of starches.

4 qi, blood, fire, food, damp, phlegm

5 See footnote 3.

**Lái Fú Zǐ (Raphani Semen) radish seeds**

**Preparation and usage** The seeds should be pounded in a mortar and pestle to break the hard outer shell before use. Unprocessed lai fu zi raises yang qi and can cause vomiting. This property was utilized historically to quickly expel wind phlegm, but is rarely used anymore. Stir frying (*chao lai fu zi* 炒莱菔子) until the seeds pop, enhances their ability to direct qi downward and transform phlegm. Stir fried lai fu zi is less likely to cause vomiting. This is the form used internally in modern practice.

**Contraindications** The absence of excess in the form of food stagnation or phlegm; wheezing and cough from Lung and Kidney deficiency. Caution in patients with food stagnation as well as qi and blood deficiency. Long term use depletes qi. Antagonistic[6] to ren shen (p.74). Some texts[7] extend this list to include shu di huang (p.78) and zhi he shou wu (p.78). The strong pungency of lai fu zi is thought to negate the tonic effects of the other herbs.

**Formulae** *Bao He Wan* (food stagnation); *San Zi Yang Qin Tang* (wheezing and cough from phlegm accumulation in the Lungs); *Gu Zhi Zeng Sheng Wan* (bony proliferation, osteophytes)

**Jī Nèi Jīn (Gigeriae galli Endothelium corneum) epithelial lining of a chickens gizzard**

**Preparation and usage** Generally considered most effective when taken as a power, in which case the dose is 1.5–3 grams. When treating stones, the unprocessed material is used; stir frying (*chao ji nei jin* 炒鸡内金) enhances its ability to alleviate food stagnation; charring (*nei jin tan* 内金炭) enhances its ability to secure the Kidneys and reduce enuresis.

**Contraindications** Caution in patients with Spleen deficiency in the absence of food stagnation.

**Formulae** *Yi Pi Bing* (loss of appetite and diarrhea from Spleen deficiency); *Tu Su Zi San* (enuresis from Kidney deficiency); *San Jin Hu Tao Tang* (Kidney stones); *Yu Ye Tang* (diabetes)

**Ē Wèi (Ferulae Resina) Chinese asafoetida**

**Preparation and usage** Not suitable for decoction; used in powder or pill form only. Can be applied topically, ground and adhered to a sticky plaster, for abdominal masses.

**Contraindications** Pregnancy; middle burner qi deficiency.

**Formulae** *E Wei Wan* (food stagnation with copious flatulence); *E Wei Hua Pi Gao†* (topical plaster for masses)

## Substances from other groups

Herbs from other groups that have a effect on food stagnation include e zhu (p.10), san leng (p.10), shui hong hua zi (p.10), hou po (p.16), jin qiao mai (p.38), zhi shi (p.64) and qing pi (p.64).

## Endnotes

† These formulae traditionally contain items from endangered animal species and/or obsolete toxic substances, and are unavailable in their original form.

6 Appendix 2, p.100
7 Bensky et al (2004) 3rd ed.; *Shi Yong Zhong Yao Xue* (1985)

**Legend**

- △ Indication
- ▲ Strong Indication
- E External Use
- **E** Strong External Indication
- ○ Function
- ● Strong Function
- Domain (✧)
- Flavour, nature (♦)

| Indication | Shi Gao 石膏 | Han Shui Shi 寒水石 | Zhi Mu 知母 | Shan Zhi Zi 山栀子 | Zhu Ye 竹叶 | Xia Ku Cao 夏枯草 | Tian Hua Fen 天花粉 | Lu Gen 芦根 | Lian Zi Xin 莲子心 | Qing Xiang Zi 青葙子 | Gu Jing Cao 谷精草 | Mi Meng Hua 密蒙花 | Function / Domain / Flavour |
|---|---|---|---|---|---|---|---|---|---|---|---|---|---|
| abscess – breast, mastitis | | | | | | △ | ▲E○ | | | | | | aids discharge of pus |
| abscess – Lung | | | | | | | | ▲ | | ○ | ○ | ○ | brightens the eyes |
| abscesses & sores – skin | | | | △● | | | △E○ | | | | | | clears damp & toxic heat |
| bleeding – hemoptysis | | | ● | △ | | | △ | △ | | | | | clears deficient heat |
| bleeding – heat in the blood | | | | △○ | ● | | | | △○ | | | | clears Heart fire |
| breast – cysts & lumps | ● | ○ | ○ | ○ | | ▲ | △○ | ○ | | | | | clears Stomach heat/fire |
| burns & scalds | E | E | | E○ | | | | | | | | | cools the blood |
| cervical lymphadenitis (luo li) | | | | | | ▲○ | | | | ○ | | ○ | cools the Liver |
| cough – Lung heat, fire | ▲● | | △○ | ○ | | | △○ | ▲● | | | | | cools the Lungs |
| cough – wind heat | | | | | | | | ▲ | | | ○ | | dispels wind heat |
| cough – yin deficiency, dry | | | △ | | | | ● | △ | | | | | dissipates masses |
| diabetes (xiao ke) | | | △○ | | | | ▲● | ○ | | | | | generates fluids |
| dizziness, vertigo – yang↑ | | | ○ | | | △ | | | | | | | nourishes yin |
| dysuria – damp heat; bld. | ○ | ○ | | ▲ | △ | | | △ | | | | | promotes healing |
| dysuria – Heart fire | | | | | △○ | | | ○ | | | | | promotes urination |
| eyes – corneal opacity, cataract | | | | | | | | | | ▲○ | ▲○ | ▲○ | reduces visual opacity |
| eyes – photophobia, lacrimation | | | | ○ | | | | | | ▲ | ▲ | ▲ | stops bleeding |
| eyes – red & sore; wind heat, fire | | E | | △ | | △ | | ○ | | ▲ | ▲ | ▲ | stops vomiting |
| fever – qi level | ▲○ | △ | ▲ | △ | ○ | | △ | △ | | | | | vents from the qi level |
| fever – high | ▲ | △ | △ | | | | △ | △ | | | | | |
| fever – bone steaming; yin def. | | | △ | | | | | | | | | | |
| fever – lingering, low grade | △ | | ▲ | ▲ | ▲ | | | | | | | | |
| headache – Liver fire, yang↑ | | | | | | △ | | | | | | | **Domain (✧)** |
| headache – Stomach heat | △✧ | | ✧ | ✧ | | | ✧ | ✧ | | | | | Lung |
| headache – wind heat | | ✧ | ✧ | | | | | | | △ | △ | | Kidney |
| hemorrhoids – heat, damp heat | | | | E | | ✧ | △ | | | ✧ | ✧ | ✧ | Liver |
| hypertension – Liver heat | | | | | | ▲✧ | | | △ | △ | | | Gallbladder |
| insomnia – Heart fire | | ✧ | | △✧ | ▲✧ | | | | △✧ | | | | Heart |
| irritability – Heart fire | | | | ▲ | ▲✧ | | | | △ | | | | Small Intestine |
| jaundice – damp heat | | | | ▲✧ | | | | | | | | | Triple Burner |
| measles – inadequate rash in | ✧ | ✧ | ✧ | ✧ | ✧ | | ✧ | △✧ | | | ✧ | | Stomach |
| nodules, masses – phlegm fire | | | | | | ▲ | | | | | | | |
| skin – eczema; chronic ulcers | E | E | | | | | | | | | | | |
| skin – rash, purpura, in fever | △ | | | | | | | | | | | | **Flavour, nature (♦)** |
| sweating – night sweats | ♦ | ♦ | △ | | | ♦ | | | | | | | acrid |
| thirst – severe, from heat | ▲ | △ | △♦ | ♦ | △ | ♦ | ▲♦ | △ | ♦ | ♦ | | | bitter |
| throat – sore; acute | | E | | | ♦ | | | | | | △ | | bland |
| throat – sore; chronic, dry | | ♦ | △ | | | | | | | | | | salty |
| thyroid – nodules, goitre | ♦ | | ♦ | | ♦ | ▲ | △♦ | ♦ | | | ♦ | ♦ | sweet |
| toothache – Stomach fire | △ | | | | | | | △ | | | △♦ | | neutral |
| ulcers – mouth | △ | | △ | △ | △ | | | | △ | ♦ | | ♦ | cool |
| vomiting, nausea – St. heat | △ | | ♦ | △♦ | ♦ | ♦ | ♦ | ▲♦ | ♦ | ♦ | | | cold |
| wheezing – Lung heat | △♦ | ♦ | | | | | | | | | | | very cold |
| **Standard dosage range (g)** | 15–60 | 9–15 | 6–12 | 6–9 | 6–15 | 9–15 | 9–15 | 15–30 | 1.5–3 | 6–15 | 6–9 | 6–9 | |

### Shí Gāo (Gypsum Fibrosum) gypsum, CaSO₄

**Preparation and usage** When decocted, shi gao should be broken into pieces and cooked for 30–60 minutes[1] before the other herbs are added. For external use, it is calcined (*duan shi gao* 煅石膏) and pulverized to powder.

**Contraindications** Middle burner yang deficiency, heat and fever from yin deficiency.

**Formulae** *Bai Hu Tang* (acute qi level fever); *Bai Hu Jia Ren Shen Tang* (qi level heat with fluid damage); *Zhu Ye Shi Gao Tang* (lingering heat in the qi level); *Qing Dai Shi Gao Tang* (febrile rash); *Qing Wen Bai Du Yin* (high fever and delirium from heat in the qi and blood levels); *Da Qing Long Tang* (wind cold with internal heat); *Ma Xing Shi Gan Tang* (cough and wheeze from Lung heat); *Yu Nü Jian* (oral pathology from Stomach fire); *Xiao Feng San* (itchy skin disorders from heat in the blood)

### Hán Shuǐ Shí (Glauberitum) calcitum, CaCO₃

**Preparation and usage** When decocted, han shui shi should be broken into pieces and cooked for 30–60 minutes[2] before the other herbs are added. For external and topical use, it is pulverized to powder.

**Contraindications** Middle burner yang deficiency.

**Formulae** *San Shi Tang* (acute heat in the qi level); *Zi Xue Dan*† (febrile convulsions); *Feng Yin Tang* (seizures and tremors from phlegm heat affecting the Heart); *Chan Su Gao* (topical paste for toxic sores and tumours)

### Zhī Mǔ (Anemarrhenae Rhizoma) anemarrhena rhizome

**Preparation and usage** To clear acute and excess heat, the unprocessed herb is used; to clear heat from deficiency and direct the action of the herb towards the Kidneys and lower burner, salt processed zhi mu (*yan zhi mu* 盐知母) is used.

**Contraindications** Middle burner yang deficiency patterns, especially with diarrhea and poor appetite.

**Formulae** *Bai Hu Tang* (acute qi level fever); *Bai Hu Jia Ren Shen Tang* (qi level heat with fluid damage); *Gui Zhi Shao Yao Zhi Mu Tang* (painful obstruction; heat concentrated in a joint); *Zhi Bai Di Huang Wan* (Kidney yin deficiency with heat); *Da Bu Yin Wan* (bone steaming fever from Kidney yin deficiency); *Yu Ye Tang* (diabetes); *Sheng Xian Tang* (sinking da qi); *Suan Zao Ren Tang* (insomnia from Liver yin blood deficiency); *Xiao Ru Tang*† (early stage breast abscess and mastitis); *Er Xian Tang* (hypertension and menopausal symptoms from Kidney yin and yang deficiency)

### Shān Zhī Zǐ (Gardeniae Fructus) cape jasmine fruit

**Preparation and usage** Unprocessed shan zhi zi is used to clear heat; for nausea and vomiting it can be processed with ginger (*jiang zhi zi* 姜栀子); stir frying until charred on the outside (*zhi zi tan* 栀子炭) is best for bleeding. The seeds inside the shell are thought better for cooling the Heart and alleviating irritability; the shell of the fruit is thought better for clearing qi level heat.

**Contraindications** Middle burner yang deficiency patterns, especially with diarrhea and poor appetite.

**Formulae** *Zhi Zi Chi Tang* (lingering heat in the chest); *Dan Zhi Xiao Yao San* (Liver qi constraint with heat); *Zhi Zi Bai Pi Tang* (damp heat jaundice); *Yin Chen Hao Tang* (damp heat jaundice); *Lian Po Yin* (vomiting and diarrhea from damp heat); *Yue Ju Wan* (abdominal bloating and reflux from the 'six stagnations')[3]; *Qing Wen Bai Du Yin* (high fever and delirium from heat in the qi and blood levels); *Huang Lian Jie Du Tang* (local and systemic toxic heat patterns); *Ba Zheng San* (damp heat dysuria); *Xiao Ji Yin Zi* (blood dysuria); *Shi Hui San* (bleeding from heat in the blood); *Xuan Bi Tang* (wind damp heat painful obstruction)

### Zhú Yè (Phyllostachys nigrae Folium) bamboo leaves

Often confused with dàn zhú yè 淡竹叶 (Lophatheri Herba), p.20, a plant that closely resembles bamboo. They are similar in action and can be used interchangeably, but zhú yè is better at clearing and venting heat from the Heart and upper burner, while dàn zhú yè is better able to promote urination and ease dysuria.

**Preparation and usage** If the fresh herb is available 15-30 grams may be used. Do not cook for longer than 10–15 minutes[4].

**Contraindications** Fever and bone steaming associated with heat from yin deficiency.

**Formulae** *Zhu Ye Shi Gao Tang* (lingering heat in the qi level); *Zhu Ye Liu Bang Tang* (early stage of wind rash and measles); *San Ren Tang* (lingering damp heat in the qi level); *Qing Ying Tang*† (heat in the nutritive level); *Yin Qiao San* (wind heat common cold); *Dao Chi San* (oral ulcers and dysuria from Heart fire)

### Xià Kū Cǎo (Prunellae Spica) selfheal spike

**Preparation and usage** This herb is commercially prepared as a syrup with various additional herbs depending on the manufacturer, for long term use in lymphadenopathy, nodular swellings, hypertension and thyroid disorders.

**Contraindications** Caution in patients with middle burner yang qi deficiency.

**Formulae** *Xia Ku Cao Gao* (nodular phlegm type swellings); *Xia Ku Cao San* (visual disturbances from Liver yin deficiency); *Nei Xiao Luo Li Wan* (neck lumps and scrofula from phlegm); *Lian Qiao Jin Bei Jian* (breast abscess); *Gou Teng Di Long Tang* (chronic migraine type headache from Liver heat)

### Tiān Huā Fěn (Trichosanthes Radix) trichosanthes root

Also known as guā lóu gēn 栝楼根.

**Contraindications** Caution in patients with middle burner yang qi deficiency.

**Formulae** *Sha Shen Mai Dong Tang* (Lung and Stomach dryness); *Bei Mu Gua Lou San* (cough with sticky phlegm); *Gua Lou Niu Bang Tang* (acute mastitis and breast abscess); *Yu Ye Tang* (diabetes); *Xian Fang Huo Ming Yin*† (toxic heat boils and sores); *Fu Yuan Huo Xue Tang*† (traumatic blood stasis); *Jin Huang San* (topical treatment for boils and burns)

### Lú Gēn (Phragmitis Rhizoma) reed rhizome

Also known as wěi gēn 苇根.

**Preparation and usage** Dried lu gen should be soaked in cold water for at least an hour to rehydrate before cooking. When the fresh herb (*xian lu gen* 鲜芦根) is available double or triple the standard dose can be used. The fresh herb is better at clearing heat and generating fluids than the dried herb.

**Contraindications** Caution in patients with middle burner yang qi deficiency.

**Formulae** *Wei Jing Tang* (Lung abscess); *Sang Ju Yin* (wind heat cough); *Yin Qiao San* (wind heat common cold); *Lian Po Yin* (vomiting and diarrhea from damp heat)

### Lián Zǐ Xīn (Nelumbinis Plumula) lotus plumule

**Contraindications** None noted.

**Formulae** *Niu Huang Shang Qing Wan*† (ulceration and pain of the oral cavity, eyes and throat from fire)

### Qīng Xiāng Zǐ (Celosia Semen) celosia seeds

**Contraindications** Patients with elevated eye pressure and glaucoma. Caution in visual disorders from Liver and Kidney deficiency.

**Formulae** *Bai Ji Li San* (wind heat eye disorders); *Zhen Zhu San* (painful eyes and visual disturbances from Liver deficiency with heat)

### Gǔ Jīng Cǎo (Eriocauli Flos) pipewort

**Contraindications** Visual disorders from yin and blood deficiency.

**Formulae** *Gu Jing Cao Tang* (visual disturbance and red sore eyes from Liver heat)

### Mì Méng Huā (Buddlejae Flos) buddleia flower bud

**Contraindications** None noted.

**Formulae** *Mi Meng Hua San* (visual disturbance and red sore eyes from Liver heat)

### Endnotes

† These formulae traditionally contain items from endangered animal species and/or obsolete toxic substances, and are unavailable in their original form.

---

1 Appendix 6, p.108
2 Ibid.
3 qi, blood, fire, food, damp, phlegm

---

4 Appendix 6, p.108

Legend:
△ Indication
▲ Strong Indication
E External Use
E Strong External Indication
○ Function
● Strong Function
Domain (✥)
Flavour, nature (♦)

| INDICATIONS | Jin Yin Hua 金银花 | Lian Qiao 连翘 | Zi Hua Di Ding 紫花地丁 | Pu Gong Ying 蒲公英 | Da Qing Ye 大青叶 | Ban Lan Gen 板蓝根 | Bai Jiang Cao 败酱草 | Hong Teng 红藤 | Bai Tou Weng 白头翁 | Ma Chi Xian 马齿苋 | Chuan Xin Lian 穿心莲 | Tu Fu Ling 土茯苓 | FUNCTIONS |
|---|---|---|---|---|---|---|---|---|---|---|---|---|---|
| abscesses & sores – skin | ▲ | ▲ | ▲ E | ▲ | | | △ E ○ | △ | | △ E | △ E | △ | aids discharge of pus |
| abscesses – recurrent, chronic | | | | ○ | | | | | | | ○ | ▲ | alleviates dysuria |
| abscess – breast; mastitis | △ E ○ | ▲ | △ | ▲ E ○ | △ | △ | | △ | ○ | ○ | ○ | ○ | clears damp heat |
| abscess – Intestinal | △ ● | △ ● | △ ○ | ▲ ○ | ● | ● | ▲ ○ | ▲ ○ | ○ | ○ | ● | ○ | clears toxic heat |
| abscess – Liver | △ | △ | △ | △ | △ ○ | △ | ▲ | △ | | ○ | | | cools the blood |
| abscess – Lung | △ | △ | | △ ○ | | | △ | | | | △ | | cools the Liver |
| abscess – pelvic | △ ○ | △ ○ | | ▲ | △ | △ | ▲ | ▲ | | | | | dispels wind heat |
| amenorrhea – blood stasis | | ○ | | | | | | ○ | △ ○ | | | | dissipates masses |
| bites & stings – insect & snake | | | E | | | | | ○ | ○ | E | E | | invigorates blood |
| bleeding – hematemesis, nose | | | | ○ | △ | | | | | | | ○ | promotes urination |
| bleeding – purpura; heat in bld. | △ | △ | | | | ▲ | | | ● | ○ | ○ | | stops dysentery |
| bleeding – uterine, hematuria | | | | | | | ○ | ○ | | △ | | | stops pain |
| cholecystitis | | | | ▲ | △ ○ | △ | | | | | | | transforms maculae |
| common cold – wind heat | ▲ | ▲ | | | △ | △ | | | | | △ | | |
| cough & wheeze – Lung heat | | | | | | △ | | | | | ▲ | | |
| dysentery – amoebic | | | | | | | | | ▲ | | | | |
| dysentery – bacterial | △ | △ | | | △ | | | | ▲ | ▲ | △ | | |
| dysmenorrhea – blood stasis | | | | | | | △ | △ | | | | | |
| dysuria – damp heat | ▲ | △ | | △ | | | | | | ▲ | △ | △ | |
| dysuria – turbid | | | | | | | | | | | | ▲ | |
| encephalitis, infectious | | | | | ▲ | ▲ | | | | | | | |
| erysipelas | △ | △ | ▲ E | △ | ▲ | ▲ | | | | △ | | | |
| eyes – red & sore | △ | △ | △ | △ | | | △ | | | | | | |
| fever – epidemic febrile disease | △ | △ | | | ▲ | ▲ | | | | | | | **Domain (✥)** |
| fever – high, in warm disease | △ ✥ | △ ✥ | | | ▲ ✥ | ▲ ✥ | | | | | ✥ | | Lung |
| hepatitis – acute | △ ✥ | | | ▲ | ▲ | ▲ | ✥ | ✥ | ✥ | ✥ | ✥ | △ | Large Intestine |
| itch – vulvitis, genital, anal | | | ✥ | ✥ | | | ✥ | ✥ | E | ✥ | | ✥ | Liver |
| jaundice – damp heat | | ✥ | △ | ▲ | △ | △ | | | | | | △ | Gallbladder |
| leukorrhea – damp heat | | ✥ | ✥ | | ✥ | ✥ | | | △ | △ | | | Heart |
| mumps | △ | △ | △ | | ▲ | ▲ | | | | | ✥ | | Small Intestine |
| nodules, masses – phlegm heat | ✥ | ▲ | | △ ✥ | ✥ | ✥ | ✥ | | | | ✥ | ✥ | Stomach |
| nodules, masses – blood stasis | | | | | | | △ | △ | | | | | |
| pain – chest & abdominal | | | | | | | △ | △ | | | | | |
| pain – postpartum abdominal | | | | | | | △ | △ | | | | | **Flavour, nature (♦)** |
| painful obst. – wind damp heat | | | ♦ | | | | ♦ | △ | | | | △ | acrid |
| parasites – round & pinworms | | ♦ | ♦ | ♦ | ♦ | ♦ | ♦ | △ ♦ | ♦ | | ♦ | | bitter |
| Pericardium – heat entering | | △ | | | △ | △ | | | | | | ♦ | bland |
| skin – eczema, psoriasis | △ | △ | | ▲ | | | | | | △ ♦ | E | ▲ | sour |
| skin – maculopapular rash, heat | ♦ | △ | | ♦ | ▲ | | | | | | ♦ | | sweet |
| skin – rash, purpura, in fever | △ | △ | | | ▲ | | | ♦ | | | ♦ | | neutral |
| syphilis | | ♦ | | | | | ♦ | | | | | ▲ | cool |
| throat – sore; acute, with pus | △ ♦ | △ | △ ♦ | △ ♦ | △ | ▲ ♦ | | | ♦ | ♦ | △ ♦ | | cold |
| warm diseases – early stage of | ▲ | ▲ | | △ | ▲ ♦ | ▲ | | | | | △ | | very cold |
| **Standard dosage range (g)** | 6–21 | 6–15 | 15–30 | 9–30 | 9–15 | 9–15 | 6–15 | 9–15 | 6–15 | 9–15 | 6–15 | 15–60 | |

### Jīn Yín Huā (Lonicerae Flos) honeysuckle flower

**Preparation and usage** Smaller doses, at the lower end of the dosage range, are used to release the exterior and dispel wind heat; large doses, at the top of the dosage range are necessary to clear toxic heat. For severe suppuration, up to 60 grams can be used. The herb is used unprocessed for most applications, however, it can be charred (*yin hua tan* 银花炭) for bloody dysenteric disorder. Following rupture and drainage of suppurating lesions, the dose should be reduced, or the herb ceased altogether to prevent its coldness from congealing qi and blood.

**Contraindications** Caution in patients with middle burner yang deficiency.

**Formulae** *Yin Qiao San* (wind heat common cold); *Qing Luo Yin* (summerheat common cold); *Qing Ying Tang*† (heat in the nutritive level); *Xian Fang Huo Ming Yin*† (toxic heat abscesses and sores); *Lian Qiao Bai Du San* (mumps and suppurative sores from toxic heat); *Wu Wei Xiao Du Yin* (toxic heat abscesses and sores); *Qing Chang Yin* (Intestinal abscess); *Si Miao Yong An Tang* (peripheral ulceration and necrosis from heat and blood stasis); *Tu Fu Ling Gao* (syphilis and dysuria); *Xiao Ru Tang*† (early stage breast abscess and mastitis)

### Lián Qiào (Forsythiae Fructus) forsythia fruit

**Preparation and usage** Following rupture and drainage of suppurating lesions, the dose should be reduced or the herb ceased to prevent congealing qi and blood due to bitterness.

**Contraindications** Lesions that have already ruptured. Caution in middle burner yang deficiency.

**Formulae** *Lian Qiao Jin Bei Jian* (breast abscess); *Lian Qiao Bai Du San* (mumps and suppurative sores from toxic heat); *Ma Huang Lian Qiao Chi Xiao Dou Tang* (early stage damp heat jaundice); *Yin Qiao San* (wind heat common cold); *Qing Ying Tang*† (heat in the nutritive level); *Bao He Wan* (food stagnation); *Pu Ji Xiao Du Yin* (toxic heat in the throat and head); *Hai Zao Yu Hu Tang* (goitre; firm masses in the neck)

### Zǐ Huā Dì Dīng (Violae Herba) viola

**Preparation and usage** In severe cases up to 60 grams of dried herb can be used for a week or so. For external use the fresh herb or fresh juice extracted from the herb is best.

**Contraindications** Yin sores.

**Formulae** *Wu Wei Xiao Du Yin* (toxic heat abscesses and sores); *Hong Teng Jian* (Intestinal abscess)

### Pú Gōng Yīng (Taraxaci Herba) dandelion

**Preparation and usage** When the fresh herb is available, double or triple the standard dose can be used in decoction. For mastitis and breast abscess, a poultice can be prepared from the fresh herb or the dregs left following decoction and applied warm topically.

**Contraindications** Patients without excess heat pathology. Caution in patients with middle burner yang deficiency. While generally well tolerated, large doses can cause diarrhea.

**Formulae** *Lian Qiao Jin Bei Jian* (breast abscess); *Wu Wei Xiao Du Yin* (toxic heat abscesses and sores); *Lan Wei Jie Du Tang* (Intestinal abscess; appendicitis); *Chuan Xin Lian Kang Yan Pian* (prepared medicine for sore throat, boils and sores and cough from Lung heat)

### Dà Qīng Yè (Isatidis Folium) dyers woad leaf

**Contraindications** Patients without excess heat pathology; middle burner yang deficiency.

**Formulae** *Shui Niu Jiao Da Qing Tang*† (rash and purpura from heat in the blood)

### Bǎn Lán Gēn (Isatidis/Baphicacanthis Radix) dyers woad root, baphicacanthus root

**Preparation and usage** In severe cases up to 30 grams can be used.

**Contraindications** Patients without excess heat pathology; middle burner yang deficiency.

**Formulae** *Fu Fang Nan Ban Lan Gen Pian* (toxic heat patterns); *Pu Ji Xiao Du Yin* (toxic heat in the throat and head)

### Bài Jiàng Cǎo (Patriniae Herba) patrinia

**Contraindications** Caution during pregnancy, in the absence of heat and blood stasis, and middle burner yang deficiency.

**Formulae** *Yi Yi Fu Zi Bai Jiang San* (suppurating or encapsulated Intestinal abscess with few heat signs); *Chang Yong Tang* (acute Intestinal abscess)

### Hóng Téng (Sargentodoxae Caulis) sargentodoxa vine

**Preparation and usage** In severe cases, up to 30 grams can be used. This herb is commonly prepared as an alcohol extract for blood stasis and painful conditions.

**Contraindications** Caution during pregnancy.

**Formulae** *Hong Teng Jian* (Intestinal abscess); *Lian Qiao Jin Bei Jian* (breast abscess); *Fei Zi Guan Zhong Tang* (hookworms)

### Bái Tóu Wēng (Pulsatillae Radix) pulsatilla root

**Preparation and usage** In severe cases of amebic dysentery, up to 30 grams of the dried herb can be used. Can also be used as retention enema. Effective against other amebic infections, including Trichomonas. Only the dried herb is suitable for ingestion, as the fresh herb contains components (broken down during drying and storage) that can cause toxic reactions. The aerial parts of the plant are similarly toxic.

**Contraindications** Chronic cold or deficiency type dysenteric disorder and diarrhea patterns.

**Formulae** *Bai Tou Weng Tang* (damp heat dysenteric disorder with bleeding); *Bai Tou Weng Jia Gan Cao E Jiao Tang* (postpartum blood deficient type dysenteric disorder)

### Mǎ Chǐ Xiàn (Portulacae Herba) purslane

**Preparation and usage** When the fresh herb is available, 30–60 grams can be used.

**Contraindications** Pregnancy[1], and chronic cold or deficiency type dysenteric disorder and diarrhea patterns.

### Chuān Xīn Lián (Andrographitis Herba) andrographis

**Preparation and usage** This herb is extremely bitter and unpalatable, and best delivered in pills or capsules. Not suitable for prolonged use (more than a few weeks) as its bitterness easily damages Stomach qi.

**Contraindications** Absence of excess heat pathology or in patients with middle burner yang deficiency.

**Formulae** *Chuan Xin Lian Kang Yan Pian* (prepared medicine for sore throat, boils and sores and cough from Lung heat)

### Tǔ Fú Líng (Smilacis glabrae Rhizoma) smooth greenbrier rhizome

**Contraindications** Liver and Kidney yin deficiency patterns. Traditionally, the drinking of tea while taking this herb was avoided, as it was thought to aggravate hair loss.

**Formulae** *Tu Fu Ling Gao* (syphilis and dysuria); *Jian Pi Chu Shi Wan* (weeping skin lesions from Spleen deficiency with damp in the muscles)

### Endnotes

† These formulae traditionally contain items from endangered animal species and/or obsolete toxic substances, and are unavailable in their original form.

1 Bensky et al (2004) 3rd ed., is the only source to assert a contraindication during pregnancy. See Appendix 1.1, p.98.

△ Indication
▲ Strong Indication
E External Use
**E** Strong External Indication

○ Function
● Strong Function

| INDICATIONS | Yu Xing Cao 鱼腥草 | Ma Bo 马勃 | Shan Dou Gen 山豆根 | She Gan 射干 | Bai Hua She She Cao 白花蛇舌草 | Ji Gu Cao 鸡骨草 | Gui Zhen Cao 鬼针草 | Hu Er Cao 虎耳草 | Chui Pen Cao 垂盆草 | Ya Dan Zi 鸦胆子 | Qing Dai 青黛 | Chong Lou 重楼 | FUNCTIONS |
|---|---|---|---|---|---|---|---|---|---|---|---|---|---|
| abscesses & sores – skin | △EO | | △E | | ▲O | | | △ | △E | | △E | ▲E | aids discharge of pus |
| abscess – breast, mastitis | O | | | | | △E | | | | | | △ | alleviates dysuria |
| abscess – Intestinal | | | | ▲ | | O | △ | | O | | | | alleviates jaundice |
| abscess – Lung | ▲O | O | O | O | ● | O | O | △O | O | O | ● | O | clears toxic heat |
| bites & stings – insect | | | | | | △E | O | | | O | | | cools the blood |
| bleeding – oral, traumatic | | E | | | | O | | | | | O | E | cools the Liver |
| bleeding – heat in the blood | ● | O | | | | | | △ | | | △O | | cools the Lungs |
| burns & scalds | | | | | | O | | E | △E | | | | dredges the Liver |
| cervix – inflammation of | | ● | △E● | ● | | | | | | | | | eases the throat |
| convulsions – febrile in children | | | | O | | | | | | | △ | △ | expels phlegm |
| cough – with hemoptysis | △ | | | | | | | | | | ▲O | O | extinguishes wind |
| cough – Lung heat | ▲ | △ | △ | △ | O | | O | | | | △ | | invigorates blood |
| cough – Liver invading Lungs | | | | | | | | | O | | ▲ | | kills parasites |
| cough – phlegm damp | O | | | △ | O | | | | | | | | promotes urination |
| cough – phlegm heat | ▲ | O | | △ | | | | | | | △ | | stops bleeding |
| diarrhea – damp heat | △ | | | | | | △ | | O | | | | stops dysentery |
| dysenteric dis. – damp heat | △ | | | | | | △ | | | △ | O | | transforms maculae |
| dysentery – amebic, recurrent | | | | | | | | | | ▲ | | | |
| dysuria – damp heat | ▲ | | | | ▲ | | △ | | | | | | |
| ears – acute otitis | | | | | | | | ▲E | | | | | |
| edema – acute nephritic | △ | | | △ | | | | | | | | | |
| gingivitis – Lung & Stomach fire | | | △ | | | | | | | | | | **Domain (❖)** |
| hemorrhoids – painful | E❖ | ❖ | ❖ | ❖ | | | E❖ | E❖ | | | ❖ | | Lung |
| hepatitis – acute & chronic | | | | | ❖ | ▲ | △❖ | | ▲ | ❖ | | | Large Intestine |
| jaundice – damp heat | ❖ | | △ | △ | | ▲ | | | ▲ | | | | Bladder |
| malarial disorder – chronic | | | | | | ❖ | ❖ | | ❖ | △❖ | ❖ | ❖ | Liver |
| mumps | | | | | △ | ❖ | | ❖ | ❖ | | △E | | Gallbladder |
| oral cavity – inflammation of | | | △E | | ❖ | | | | ❖ | | | | Small Intestine |
| pain – & injury, trauma | | | ❖ | | ❖ | | | | | | ❖ | △ | Stomach |
| pain – hypochondriac | | | | | | △ | △ | | △ | | | | |
| pain – joint, with stiffness | | | | | | △ | △ | | | | | | |
| painful obst. – wind damp | | | | | | △ | △ | | | | | | **Flavour, nature (♦)** |
| seizures & tremors | | | | | | | | | | ♦ | | △ | toxic |
| skin – eczema | | | ♦ | | | | | △E♦ | | | ♦ | ♦ | slightly toxic |
| skin – itchy wind rash; urticaria | ♦ | ♦ | | | | | E | △E♦ | | | | | acrid |
| skin – maculopapular rash, heat | | | ♦ | ♦ | ♦ | ♦ | ♦ | ♦ | | | ▲ | ♦ | bitter |
| skin – rash, purpura in fever | | | | | | | | | ♦ | | ▲ | | bland |
| snakebite | △E | | | △ | | | △E | △E | △E | | ♦ | ▲ | salty |
| throat – sore; acute, with pus | | ▲ | ▲ | ▲ | △ | | △ | | △♦ | | △E | △ | sour |
| tumours – lung, digestive tract | | | △E | | ▲♦ | ♦ | △ | | ♦ | △ | | | sweet |
| ulcers – skin, chronic | | ♦ | | | | | | E | | | | | neutral |
| ulcers – mouth | ♦ | | △E | | | ♦ | | | ♦ | | △E | ♦ | cool |
| warts & corns | | | ♦ | ♦ | ♦ | | | ♦ | | E♦ | ♦ | | cold |
| **Standard dosage range (g)** | 15–30 | 1.5–6 | 3–9 | 3–9 | 15–60 | 15–30 | 15–30 | 9–15 | 15–30 | 0.5–2 | 1.5–3 | 3–9 | |

## Yú Xīng Cǎo (Houttuyniae Herba) houttuynia

**Preparation and usage** Should be cooked for no longer than 5 minutes[1]. If the fresh herb is available, up to 60 grams can be used. When applied topically, the bruised fresh herb or briefly decocted dried herb can be used.

**Contraindications** Middle burner yang deficiency and yin sores.

**Formulae** *Fu Fang Yu Xing Cao Pian* (sore throat from wind heat)

## Mǎ Bó (Lasiosphaerae/Calvatiae) puffball fruiting body

**Preparation and usage** This herb is cooked in a cloth bag[2] to prevent the tiny spores from irritating the throat, or used in pills and powder. It can be blown onto bleeding areas with a straw.

**Contraindications** None noted.

**Formulae** *Pu Ji Xiao Du Yin* (toxic heat in the throat and head); *She Gan Tang* (sore throat from Lung heat)

## Shān Dòu Gēn (Sophorae tonkinensis Radix) sophora root

**Contraindications** Middle burner yang deficiency patterns, especially with diarrhea and poor appetite. Do not exceed the recommended dosage range or toxic effects[3] may occur.

**Formulae** *Qing Liang San* (sore throat from fire or toxic heat); *Zi Cao Xiao Du Yin* (measles and sore throat from toxic heat)

## Shè Gān (Belamacandae Rhizoma) belamcanda rhizome

**Preparation and usage** Can be stir fried (*chao she gan* 炒射干) to moderate its bitter coldness and make it less likely to aggravate diarrhea in weak or older patients.

**Contraindications** Pregnancy or middle burner yang deficiency.

**Formulae** *She Gan Ma Huang Tang* (wheezing and cough from phlegm clogging the Lungs); *She Gan Xiao Du Yin* (phlegm heat blocking the throat); *She Gan Tang* (sore throat from Lung heat)

## Bái Huā Shé Shé Cǎo (Hedyotis diffusae Herba) 白花蛇舌草; hedyotis, oldenlandia

**Preparation and usage** If the fresh herb is available, up to 120 grams can be used for general toxic heat conditions. For treating cancers, 60–120 grams of the dried herb and up to 240 grams of fresh herb, can be used[4].

**Contraindications** Pregnancy[5], middle burner yang deficiency or yin sores.

## Jī Gǔ Cǎo (Abri Herba) Canton love pea vine

**Contraindications** None noted.

## Guǐ Zhēn Cǎo (Bidens bipinnata Herba) bidens

**Preparation and usage** When the fresh herb is available, up to 60 grams can be used.

**Contraindications** None noted.

## Hǔ Ěr Cǎo (Saxifraga stolonifera Herba) saxifrage

**Preparation and usage** When the fresh herb is available, up to 60 grams can be used. This herb is classified as slightly toxic, but no supporting evidence could be found to support this claim. See Appendix 3.2, 102.

**Contraindications** None noted

## Chuí Pén Cǎo (Sedi Herba) hanging stonecrop, sedum

**Preparation and usage** When the fresh herb is available, 50–100 grams per dose may be used.

**Contraindications** Yin sores or yin jaundice.

## Yā Dǎn Zǐ (Bruceae Fructus) java brucea fruit

**Preparation and usage** Traditionally, the dose was expressed in fruit. For malaria, 10–15 fruits constituted one dose; for chronic relapsing dysenteric disorder, 10–30 fruits[6]. Suitable for short term use only (several days at a time), during the symptomatic or febrile phase. Not suitable for decoction; only used in capsules, or traditionally, wrapped in a longan fruit or date to mitigate the intense bitterness.

**Contraindications** Pregnancy, small children, patients with middle burner yang deficiency, gastrointestinal bleeding, chronic renal failure or impaired hepatic function.

## Qīng Dài (Indigo Naturalis) indigo

**Preparation and usage** Not suitable for decoction; used in pills or powders only and taken separately to any other decocted herbs. Do not exceed the recommended dosage range or toxic effects[7] may occur.

**Contraindications** The absence of excess heat pathology, and middle burner yang deficiency.

**Formulae** *Qing Dai Hai Shi Wan* (phlegm heat in the Lungs); *Qing Dai Shi Gao Tang* (febrile rash); *Liang Jing Wan*† (childhood febrile convulsions); *Dang Gui Long Hui Wan* (Liver fire with constipation); *Dai Ge San* (cough and hemoptysis from Lung heat and Liver fire invading the Lungs); *Qing Yin Wan*† (hoarse voice, loss of voice and sore throat from Lung fire); *Bi Yun San* (inhaled powder for nasal congestion)

## Chóng Lóu (Paridis Rhizoma) paris rhizome

Also known as zǎo xiū 蚤休 and qī yè yī zhī huā 七叶一枝花.

**Contraindications** Pregnancy, in patients with an absence of excess heat, or yin sores. Caution in deficient patients.

**Formulae** *Niu Huang Jie Du Wan* (toxic heat sores, ulcers and throat pain)

### Endnotes

† These formulae traditionally contain items from endangered animal species and/or obsolete toxic substances, and are unavailable in their original form.

---

1 Appendix 6, p.108
2 Appendix 6, p.109
3 Appendix 3.2, p.104
4 *Shi Yong Zhong Yao Xue* (1985)
5 Xu & Wang (2002) is the only source to assert a contraindication during pregnancy. See Appendix 1.1, p.98

---

6 *Zhong Yao Xue* (2000)
7 Appendix 3.2, p.104

**Legend:**
△ Indication
▲ Strong Indication
E External Use
**E** Strong External Indication
○ Function
● Strong Function

| INDICATIONS | Quan Shen 拳参 | Bai Lian 白蔹 | Lou Lu 漏芦 | Si Ji Qing 四季青 | Jin Qiao Mai 金荞麦 | Di Jin Cao 地锦草 | Qian Li Guang 千里光 | Di Er Cao 地耳草 | Qing Ye Dan 青叶胆 | Feng Wei Cao 凤尾草 | Liu Yue Xue 六月雪 | Ye Ju Hua 野菊花 | FUNCTIONS |
|---|---|---|---|---|---|---|---|---|---|---|---|---|---|
| abdominal distension | | | | | △○ | | | | | | | | alleviates food stagnation |
| abscess – breast, mastitis | | | △ | | | ○ | | △○ | ○ | | | | alleviates jaundice |
| abscess – Intestinal | | | | | | | △○ | | | | | ○ | brightens the eyes |
| abscess – Lung | | | | ○ | △ | ○ | | △ | | ○ | | | cools the blood |
| abscesses & sores – skin | △ | △E | △ | △ | △ | △E | △○ | △E | | | △ | △ | cools the Liver |
| bleeding – blood stasis | | | | | | △ | | | | | ○ | | dispels wind damp |
| bleeding – hematuria | | | | | | △○ | | ○ | | △ | | | invigorates blood |
| bleeding – heat in the blood | △ | ○ | | ○ | | | | | | | | | promotes healing |
| bleeding – gastrointestinal | △ | | ○ | | | △ | | | | △ | | | promotes lactation |
| bleeding – traumatic | E○ | | | △E | | △○ | | | | | | | promotes urination |
| bleeding – uterine | | | | ○ | | △○ | | | | | | | stops bleeding |
| burns & scalds | | E | | E | ○ | | | | | | | | strengthens the Spleen |
| cervical lymphadenitis (luo li) | | E | | | △ | | | | | | | | |
| cough – Lung heat | | | | △ | △ | | | | | | | | |
| dysenteric dis. – damp heat | △ | | | △ | △ | △ | △ | | | △ | △ | | |
| dysuria – damp heat | | | | △ | | △ | | | | △ | △ | | |
| edema – damp heat | △ | | | | | | | | | | △ | | |
| eyes – red & sore | | | | | | | △ | | | | △ | ▲ | |
| hepatitis – acute | | | | | | △ | | △ | △ | △ | | | |
| indigestion, food stagnation | | | | | △ | | | | | | | | |
| jaundice – damp heat | | | | | | △ | | △ | △ | △ | | | |
| lactation – insufficient | | | △ | | | | | | | | | | |
| leukorrhea – damp heat | | | | | | | | | | △ | △ | | |
| pain – & injury from trauma | | | | | | | | △E | | | | | |
| pain – hypochondriac | | | | | | △ | | △ | △ | △ | | | |
| pain – lower back & legs | | | | | | | | | | | △ | | **Domain (❖)** |
| painful obst. – wind damp | | | | ❖ | ❖ | | ❖ | | | | △❖ | | Lung |
| skin – eczema | ❖ | | | △E | | ❖ | △❖ | △E | | ❖ | ❖ | △E | Large Intestine |
| snakebite | | | | | △E | △E | | △E | | ❖ | | | Bladder |
| throat – sore; acute, with pus | ❖ | ❖ | | | ▲ | ❖ | ❖ | ❖ | ❖ | ❖ | △❖ | △❖ | Liver |
| tumours – various | | | | | | | | ❖ | ❖ | △ | | | Gallbladder |
| ulcers – skin, chronic | | △E❖ | | △E❖ | | | | | | | | ❖ | Heart |
| ulcers – mouth | △E | | | | | ❖ | | | | | | | Spleen |
| | ❖ | ❖ | ❖ | | | ❖ | ❖ | | | | | | Stomach |
| | | | | | | | | | | | | | |
| | | | | | | | | | | | | | |
| | | | | | | | | | | | | | |
| | | | | | | | | | | | | | **Flavour, nature (♦)** |
| | | ♦ | | | | ♦ | | | | | ♦ | ♦ | acrid |
| | | | | ♦ | | | | | | | | | astringent |
| | ♦ | ♦ | ♦ | ♦ | ♦ | | ♦ | ♦ | ♦ | ♦ | ♦ | ♦ | bitter |
| | | | | | ♦ | ♦ | | ♦ | | | | | neutral |
| | ♦ | ♦ | | | | | | | | | ♦ | ♦ | cool |
| | | | ♦ | ♦ | | | ♦ | | | ♦ | | | cold |
| **Standard dosage range (g)** | 3–9 | 3–9 | 6–12 | 9–30 | 15–30 | 15–30 | 9–15 | 15–30 | 9–15 | 9–21 | 9–15 | 9–15 | |

Quán Shēn (Bistortae Rhizoma) bistort rhizome

**Contraindications** The absence of excess heat pathology, middle burner yang deficiency or yin sores.

Bái Liàn (Ampelopsis Radix) ampelopsis root

**Preparation and usage** Can be decocted, with the resulting liquid boiled down and thickened with honey for topical application, or powdered and mixed with sesame oil.

**Contraindications** Middle burner yang deficiency. Incompatible[1] with zhi fu zi (p.88) and zhi chuan wu (p.94).

**Formulae** *Bai Lian San* (topical powder for chronic ulcers)

Lòu Lú (Rhapontici Radix) rhaphonticum root

**Contraindications** Pregnancy or insufficient lactation from qi and blood deficiency.

**Formulae** *Zhong Ru Tang* (insufficient lactation from Stomach heat or yin deficiency)

Sì Jì Qīng (Ilicis chinensis Folium) Chinese holly leaf

**Contraindications** Middle burner yang deficiency.

Jīn Qiáo Mài (Fagopyrum dibotrys Radix) perennial buckwheat root

**Contraindications** None noted.

Dì Jǐn Cǎo (Euphorbia humifusa Herba) creeping euphorbia

❂ Euphorbia species are listed in Appendix 2 of CITES[2] which permits limited trade with appropriate documentation.

**Preparation and usage** When the fresh herb is available, 30–60 grams can be used. The crushed fresh plant is best applied topically.

**Contraindications** None noted.

Qiān Lǐ Guāng (Senecio scandens Herba) climbing groundsel

**Preparation and usage** When the fresh herb is available, up to 30 grams can be used.

**Contraindications** Middle burner yang deficiency.

Dì Ěr Cǎo (Hypericum japonicum Herba) matted St John's wort

**Preparation and usage** When the fresh herb is available, up to 60 grams can be used.

**Contraindications** None noted.

Qīng Yè Dǎn (Swertia mileensis Herba) swertia

**Contraindications** None noted.

Fèng Wěi Cǎo (Pteris multifida Herba) spider brake fern

**Contraindications** None noted.

Liù Yuè Xuě (Serissa japonica Herba) snowrose; Japanese boxthorn

**Contraindications** None noted.

Yě Jú Huā (Chrysanthemi indici Flos) wild chrysanthemum flower

**Contraindications** None noted.

**Formulae** *Wu Wei Xiao Du Yin* (toxic heat abscesses and sores); *Bi Min Gan Wan* (prepared medicine for hayfever and rhinitis)

## Substances from other groups

There are a large number of herbs (the most important in bold) with varying degrees of toxic heat clearing action, including yi mu cao (p.6), **hu zhang** (p.8), luo de da (p.8), ma bian cao (p.10), **da ji** (p.12), xiao ji (p.12), zhu ma gen (p.12), yang ti gen (p.12), zi zhu (p.14), tie xian cai (p.14), ji hua (p.14), jin qian cao (p.18), chi xiao dou (p.18), ban bian lian (p.20), sheng ma (p.26), niu bang zi (p.26), **xuan shen** (p.40), zi cao (p.40), **shui niu jiao** (p.40), huang qin (p.42), **huang lian** (p.42), huang bai (p.42), san ke zhen (p.42), ma wei lian (p.42), bai wei (p.44), lu dou, guan zhong (p.52), **da huang** (p.60), mang xiao (p.60), sheng he shou wu (p.78), ren dong teng (p.92), xi xian cao (p.92), luo shi teng (p.92), lao guan cao (p.92), ling yang jiao (p.96), **niu huang** (p.96), quan xie (p.96), wu gong (p.96), bai jiang cao (p.96), and all the anticancer herbs on p.86.

---

1 Appendix 2, p.100
2 Appendix 4, p.105

| INDICATIONS | Shui Niu Jiao 水牛角 | Sheng Di Huang 生地黃 | Xuan Shen 玄参 | Mu Dan Pi 牡丹皮 | Chi Shao 赤芍 | Zi Cao 紫草 | FUNCTIONS |
|---|---|---|---|---|---|---|---|
| abscesses & sores – skin | △● | | △● | △ | ▲ | △ E ○ | clears toxic heat |
| abscess – Intestinal | ● | ● | ○ | ▲○ | △○ | ○ | cools the blood |
| amenorrhea – blood stasis | | | △○ | △○ | | | cools the Liver |
| bleeding – heat in the blood | ▲ | ▲ | △● | ▲ | △ | △ | dissipates masses |
| Buerger's disease – toxic heat | | | ▲○ | | △ | | eases the throat |
| burns & scalds | | ○ | | | | E | generates fluids |
| constipation – dry | | ▲ | ▲ | ○ | ○ | △ | invigorates blood |
| convulsions – febrile | ▲ | ● | ○ | | | | nourishes yin |
| delirium – in high fever | ▲ | △ | △ | | ○ | | stops pain |
| diabetes (*xiao ke*) | | ▲ | | | | ○ | vents rashes |
| dysmenorrhea – blood stasis | | | | ▲ | ▲ | | |
| dysuria – heat; blood | | | | | △ | | |
| dysuria – Heart fire | | △ | | | | | |
| eczema, dermatitis – hot blood | | △ | | | ▲ | △ E | |
| eyes – red & sore; Liver fire | | | | ▲ | ▲ | | |
| fever – shen disturbance in high | ▲ | △ | △ | | | | |
| fever – lingering, low grade | | ▲ | △ | △ | | | |
| fever – menstrual, menopausal | | | | ▲ | | | |
| fever – high | ▲ | △ | △ | | | | |
| fever – yin def., bone steaming | | △ | △ | ▲ | | | |
| headache – blood stasis | | | | | △ | | |
| heat in the blood level | ▲ | ▲ | △ | △ | △ | △ | |
| heat in the nutritive level | ▲ | ▲ | △ | △ | △ | △ | |
| hemiplegia | | | | ▲ | | | |
| itch – vaginal | | | | | | E | |
| masses – abdominal; bld. stasis | | | | △ | ▲ | | |
| measles – inadequate rash in | | | | | | ▲ | |
| menstruation – irregular, short | | △ | | ▲ | △ | | |
| nodules & masses – phlegm | | | ▲ | | | | **Domain (✣)** |
| pain – & injury from trauma | | | ✣ | △ | ▲ | | Lung |
| pain – chest & hypochondriac | | ✣ | ✣ | △ ✣ | ▲ | | Kidney |
| pain – postpartum abdominal | ✣ | ✣ | | △ ✣ | △ ✣ | ✣ | Liver |
| Pericardium – heat entering | ▲ ✣ | △ ✣ | △ | ✣ | | ✣ | Heart |
| post concussion syndrome | ✣ | | ✣ | | △ | | Stomach |
| restlessness, insomnia | | △ | △ | | | | |
| skin – itchy skin rash; urticaria | | ▲ | | | ▲ | △ | |
| skin – lesions, hot blood | ▲ | ▲ | △ | | ▲ | △ E | |
| skin – rash, purpura; febrile | ▲ | ▲ | △ | △ ♦ | △ | ▲ | **Flavour, nature (♦)** |
| sweating – night; post febrile | | ▲ ♦ | ♦ | ♦ | ♦ | | acrid |
| thirst, irritability – post febrile | ♦ | △ | △ ♦ | | | | bitter |
| throat – sore, acute | △ | ♦ | ▲ ♦ | | | △ ♦ | salty |
| throat – sore; chronic, dry | | △ | ▲ | ♦ | ♦ | | sweet |
| thyroid – benign nodules | | ♦ | ▲ ♦ | | | ♦ | cool |
| | | | | | | | cold |
| **Standard dosage range (g)** | *see* p.41 | 12–30 | 9–18 | 6–12 | 6–15 | 3–9 | |

△ Indication
▲ Strong Indication
E External Use
**E** Strong External Indication

○ Function
● Strong Function

### Shuǐ Niú Jiǎo (Bubali Cornu) water buffalo horn

**Preparation and usage** Water buffalo horn replaces rhinoceros horn. Most commonly used as powder or in pills in doses of 6–15 grams per day. Can also be decocted in doses of 15-30 grams, in which case the horn should be shaved into fine strips or grated, and cooked for several hours[1, 2].

**Contraindications** Middle burner yang deficiency.

**Formulae** *Shui Niu Jiao Di Huang Tang*† (heat in the blood); *Shui Niu Jiao Da Qing Tang*† (rash and purpura from heat in the blood); *An Gong Niu Huang Wan*† (delirium, loss of consciousness and high fever from heat affecting the Pericardium); *Qing Ying Tang*† (heat in the nutritive level); *Hua Ban Tang*† (purpura from heat in the blood); *Zhi Bao Dan*† (febrile convulsions); *Qian Gen Wan*† (rectal bleeding from damp heat); *Shi Hu Ye Guang Wan*† (visual weakness from Liver and Kidney yin deficiency)

### Shēng Dì Huáng (Rehmanniae Radix) raw rehmannia root

**Preparation and usage** The unprocessed root is used to clear heat and generate fluids; processing with wine (*jiu sheng di* 酒生地) moderates its richness and renders it less likely to cause bloating and indigestion; to stop bleeding the charred herb is used (*sheng di tan* 生地炭).

**Contraindications** Middle burner deficiency with damp. Easily causes bloating, loose stools and loss of appetite. Digestive side effects can be offset somewhat by combining with sha ren (p.16) or processing with wine (above).

**Formulae** *Shui Niu Jiao Di Huang Tang*† (heat in the blood); *Qing Ying Tang*† (heat in the nutritive level); *Qing Hao Bie Jia Tang* (yin deficiency fever); *Bai He Di Huang Tang* (post febrile irritability and insomnia); *Ku Shen Di Huang Tang* (damp heat rectal bleeding and hemorrhoids); *Long Dan Xie Gan Tang* (Liver fire; Liver Gallbladder damp heat); *Si Sheng Wan* (bleeding from heat in the blood); *Dang Gui Liu Huang Tang* (night sweats from yin deficiency); *Xiao Feng San* (itchy skin disorders from heat in the blood); *Ai Fu Nuan Gong Wan* (infertility, dysmenorrhea and irregular menses from Kidney deficiency); *Yi Wei Tang* (Stomach yin deficiency); *Zeng Ye Tang* (constipation and dryness from fluid damage due to heat); *San Jia Fu Mai Tang* (tremor and spasm from post febrile yin deficiency); *Dao Chi San* (oral ulcers and dysuria from Heart fire); *Wu Jing Jian Wan* (memory problems and profound debility from essence deficiency); *Zhi Gan Cao Tang* (arrhythmia from Heart qi deficiency); *Tian Wang Bu Xin Dan* (insomnia and shen disturbance from Heart and Kidney yin deficiency); & 40+ more in Appendix 7.

### Xuán Shēn (Scrophulariae Radix) ningpo figwort

**Contraindications** Cold damp blocking the middle burner. Incompatible[3] with li lu (p.22).

**Formulae** *Xuan Shen Gan Jie Tang* (chronic sore throat from yin deficiency); *Pu Ji Xiao Du Yin* (toxic heat in the throat and head); *Qing Ying Tang*† (heat in the nutritive level); *Qing Wen Bai Du Yin* (high fever and delirium from heat in the qi and blood levels); *Hua Ban Tang*† (purpura from heat in the blood); *Bai He Gu Jin Tang* (chronic cough from Lung yin deficiency); *Si Miao Yong An Tang* (peripheral ulceration and necrosis from heat and blood stasis); *Xiao Luo Wan* (phlegm masses); *Feng Fang Gao*† (ointment for cervical lymphadenitis and scrophula); *Zeng Ye Tang* (constipation and dryness from fluid damage due to heat)

### Mǔ Dān Pí (Moutan Cortex) tree peony root bark

**Preparation and usage** The unprocessed herb is used to clear heat and cool the blood; processing with wine (*jiu dan pi* 酒丹皮) enhances its ability to invigorate blood and disperse blood stasis; charred mu dan pi (*dan pi tan* 丹皮炭) is used to stop bleeding.

**Contraindications** Pregnancy, patients with blood deficiency and cold, and in those with menorrhagia not associated with blood stasis or heat in the blood.

**Formulae** *Dan Zhi Xiao Yao San* (Liver qi constraint with heat); *Da Huang Mu Dan Tang* (Intestinal abscess); *Shui Niu Jiao Di Huang Tang*† (heat in the blood); *Qing Hao Bie Jia Tang* (yin deficiency fever); *Gui Zhi Fu Ling Wan* (blood stasis masses in the lower burner); *Shi Hui San* (bleeding from hot blood); *Xuan Yu Tong Jing Tang* (premenstrual fever, short cycle and dysmenorrhea from qi constraint with heat in the blood); *Liu Wei Di Huang Wan* (Kidney yin deficiency); *Wen Jing Tang* (infertility and dysmenorrhea from *chōng mài* / *rèn mài* deficiency)

### Chì Sháo (Paeoniae Radix rubra) red peony root

Other texts place this herb in the blood invigorating group.

**Preparation and usage** Used unprocessed to cool the blood; processing with wine (*jiu chi shao* 酒赤芍) enhances its ability to invigorate blood; processing with vinegar (*cu chi shao* 醋赤芍) enhances its ability to stop pain.

**Contraindications** Yang deficiency. Incompatible[4] with li lu (p.22).

**Formulae** *Shui Niu Jiao Di Huang Tang*† (heat in the blood); *Zi Xue Tang* (blood stasis type amenorrhea and dysmenorrhea); *Gui Zhi Fu Ling Wan* (blood stasis masses in the lower burner); *Xue Fu Zhu Yu Tang* (qi and blood stasis); *Ge Xia Zhu Yu Tang* (abdominal masses from blood stasis); *Bu Yang Huan Wu Tang* (hemiplegia from qi deficiency with blood stasis); *Jie Gu Dan* (slow healing broken bones); *Bai Ling Tiao Gan Tang* (infertility from blocked fallopian tubes or endometriosis); *Xian Fang Huo Ming Yin*† (early stage superficial toxic heat type abscesses and sores); *Juan Bi Tang* (wind damp painful obstruction); *Qin Jiao Ji Sheng Tang* (postpartum joint pain from blood deficiency with wind); *Si Wu Xiao Feng Yin* (itchy wind rash); *Wu Long Gao* (ointment for toxic sores)

### Zǐ Cǎo (Arnebiae/Lithospermi Radix) arnebia or lithospermum root

**Preparation and usage** When applied externally to treat conditions such as eczema, dermatitis, suppurative skin infections, vaginal pruritus and burns, finely powdered zi cao is steeped in a suitable oil base, typically sesame oil (1:2) for a few days. The solids are drained from the oil and discarded, and the oil is applied to the affected area.

**Contraindications** Middle burner yang deficiency with loss of appetite and diarrhea.

**Formulae** *Sheng Ji Yu Hong Gao*† (topical ointment for suppurative and inflamed skin lesions); *Zi Cao You* (topical ointment for burns); *Zi Cao Xiao Du Yin* (measles and sore throat from toxic heat)

### Substances from other groups

Herbs from other groups that can cool the blood (most important in bold) include **dan shen** (p.6), qian cao gen (p.12), xiao ji (p.12), da ji (p.12), di yu (p.12), huai hua mi (p.12), ce bai ye (p.12), **bai mao gen** (p.12), zhu ma gen (p.12), yang ti gen (p.12), shan zhi zi (p.32), da qing ye (p.34), hu er cao (p.36), **qing dai** (p.36), di gu pi (p.44), yin chai hu (p.44), bai wei (p.44), **qing hao** (p.44), dai zhi shi (p.48), jue ming zi (p.48), da huang (p.60), **mo han lian** (p.80) and huang yao zi (p.86).

### Endnotes

† These formulae traditionally contain items from endangered animal species and/or obsolete toxic substances, and are unavailable in their original form.

1 *Zhong Yao Xue* (2000)
2 Appendix 6, p.108
3 Appendix 2, p.100
4 Appendix 2, p.100

**Legend (Indications):** △ Indication · ▲ Strong Indication · E External Use · **E** Strong External Indication

**Legend (Functions):** ○ Function · ● Strong Function

| INDICATIONS | Huang Qin 黄芩 | Huang Bai 黄柏 | Huang Lian 黄连 | Long Dan Cao 龙胆草 | Ku Shen 苦参 | Bai Xian Pi 白鲜皮 | Qin Pi 秦皮 | San Ke Zhen 三棵针 | Ma Wei Lian 马尾连 | FUNCTIONS |
|---|---|---|---|---|---|---|---|---|---|---|
| abscesses & sores – skin | △E○ | △E | ▲E | △ | | △ | | △ | △ | calms a restless fetus |
| acid reflux, heartburn – St. heat | △ | ○ | ▲ | △ | | | | | | clears deficient heat |
| bleeding – epistaxis | ▲ | | △○ | | | | | | | clears Heart fire |
| bleeding – hematemesis | ▲ | | △○ | | | | | | | clears Stomach heat/fire |
| bleeding – hematuria | △○ | △○ | ▲● | | | | | ○ | ○ | clears toxic heat |
| bleeding – hemoptysis | ▲ | | △ | ● | | | ○ | | | cools the Liver |
| bleeding – rectal | ▲ | △ | △ | | △○ | ○ | | | | dispels wind |
| bleeding – uterine | △ | ▲ | | | ○ | | | | | kills parasites |
| burns & scalds | E○ | E | E | | | | | | | stops bleeding |
| cough – Lung heat | ▲ | | | | ● | ● | △ | | △ | stops itch |
| delirium – in high fever | | | △ | | | | | | | |
| diarrhea – damp heat | △ | ▲ | ▲ | | △ | | ▲ | | | |
| dysenteric dis. – damp heat | △ | ▲ | ▲ | | △ | | ▲ | △ | △ | |
| dysuria – damp heat | △ | ▲ | | △ | △ | | | | | |
| eczema – damp heat | △ | △E | E | △ | ▲E | ▲E | | △E | | |
| ears – acute otitis | | | | ▲ | | | | | | |
| ears – tinnitus, ↓hearing; Liver fire | | | | ▲ | | | | | | |
| eyes – red & sore | △ | △ | △ | ▲ | | | ▲ | △ | △ | |
| fever – bone steaming, yin def. | | △ | | | | | | | | |
| fever – damp heat | △ | | △ | | | | | | | |
| fever – high | △ | | ▲ | | | | | | | |
| headache – Liver fire; yang↑ | △ | | | ▲ | | | | | | |
| hypertension – Liver fire; yang↑ | ▲ | | | △ | | | | | | |
| insomnia – Heart fire | | | ▲ | | | | | | | |
| irritability – Heart fire | △ | | ▲ | | | | | | | |
| itch – genitals, skin; damp heat | | ▲E | | △ | ▲E | ▲E | | | | |
| jaundice – damp heat | ▲ | △ | | ▲ | △ | △ | | △ | △ | |
| leukorrhea – damp heat | | ▲ | | ▲ | △ | △ | △ | | | |
| Liver heat becoming wind | | | | ▲ | | | | | | **Domain (❖)** |
| miscarriage – threatened | ▲❖ | | | | | | | ❖ | | Lung |
| muscle weakness & atrophy | ❖ | ▲❖ | ❖ | | ❖ | | ❖ | ❖ | ❖ | Large Intestine |
| numbness – legs, with swelling | | △❖ | | | | | | | | Kidney |
| pain – ear | | ❖ | | ▲ | ❖ | | | | | Bladder |
| pain – testicular | | | ❖ | △❖ | ❖ | | ❖ | ❖ | | Liver |
| painful obst. – damp heat | ❖ | | | ❖ | | △ | △❖ | | | Gallbladder |
| skin – scabies, tinea, ringworm | | | ❖ | | E❖ | E | | ❖ | | Heart |
| skin – itchy wind rash; urticaria | | | | | ▲ | ▲❖ | | | | Spleen |
| skin – itchy damp rash | △❖ | △E | E❖ | △❖ | ▲E❖ | ▲E❖ | | △E❖ | | Stomach |
| sweating – night, from yin def. | | △ | | | | | | | | |
| throat – sore, acute | △ | △ | ▲ | △ | | | | △ | | |
| toothache – Stomach heat | | | ▲ | | | | | | | **Flavour, nature (♦)** |
| ulcers – mouth | △♦ | △♦ | ▲♦ | ♦ | ♦ | ♦ | | ♦ | ♦ | bitter |
| vomiting, nausea – St. heat | △♦ | ♦ | ▲♦ | △♦ | ♦ | ♦ | ♦ | ♦ | ♦ | cold |
| **Standard dosage range (g)** | 3–12 | 3–12 | 3–9 | 3–9 | 3–9 | 6–15 | 6–12 | 9–15 | 6–12 | |

## Huáng Qín (Scutellariae Radix) baical skullcap root

**Preparation and usage** Unprocessed huang qin is used to clear damp heat and toxic heat; stir frying (*chao huang qin* 炒黄芩) enhances its ability to calm a restless fetus; processing with wine (*jiu huang qin* 酒黄芩) enhances its ability to clear heat from the Lungs; to stop bleeding the charred root is used (*huang qin tan* 黄芩炭).

**Contraindications** Middle burner yang deficiency.

**Formulae** *Huang Qin Hua Shi Tang* (damp heat in the qi level); *Huang Lian Jie Du Tang* (local and systemic toxic heat); *Pu Ji Xiao Du Yin* (toxic heat in throat and the head); *Ge Gen Qin Lian Tang* (damp heat diarrhea); *Xiao Chai Hu Tang* (*shào yáng* syndrome); *Hao Qin Qing Dan Tang* (damp heat in the *shào yáng* level); *Qing Qi Hua Tan Wan* (phlegm heat in the Lungs); *Dang Gui San* (threatened miscarriage from heat); *Dang Gui Liu Huang Tang* (night sweats from yin deficiency); *Gu Jing Wan* (uterine bleeding from yin deficiency with heat); *Bai Ji San* (bleeding gastric ulcers); *Meng Shi Gun Tang Wan* (phlegm fire type mental disorders, mania, severe palpitations or seizures); *Qing Xin Lian Zi Yin* (persistent or recurrent dysuria from Heart fire with qi and yin deficiency); *Ban Xia Xie Xin Tang* (mixed heat and cold blocking the qi dynamic)

## Huáng Bǎi (Phellodendri Cortex) phellodendron bark

**Preparation and usage** Unprocessed huang bai is used to clear damp heat and toxic heat; processing with salt (*yan huang bai* 盐黄柏) enhances its ability to clear heat from deficiency and focus its action in the Kidneys; processing with wine (*jiu huang bai* 酒黄柏) focuses its action in the upper burner and face; the herb is charred (*huang bai tan* 黄柏炭) to stop bleeding.

**Contraindications** Middle burner yang deficiency patterns.

**Formulae** *Zhi Zi Bai Pi Tang* (damp heat jaundice); *Bai Tou Weng Tang* (damp heat dysenteric disorder with bleeding); *Yi Huang Tang* (damp heat leukorrhea); *Er Miao San* (weakness, swelling, numbness and atrophy of the legs from damp heat); *Huang Lian Jie Du Tang* (local and systemic toxic heat patterns); *Zhi Bai Di Huang Wan* (Kidney yin deficiency with heat); *Da Bu Yin Wan* (Kidney yin deficiency type bone steaming); *Dang Gui Liu Huang Tang* (night sweats from yin deficiency); *Er Xian Tang* (hypertension and menopausal symptoms from Kidney yin and yang deficiency); *Hu Qian Wan*† (weakness and atrophy of the legs from Liver and Kidney deficiency); *Jin Huang San* (topical treatment for boils and burns)

## Huáng Lián (Coptidis Rhizoma) coptis rhizome

**Preparation and usage** Unprocessed huang lian clears heat from the Heart and Large Intestine; processing with wine (*jiu huang lian* 酒黄连) leads the herb's action to the upper burner and head moderating its intense bitter coldness; processing with ginger (*jiang huang lian* 姜黄连) focuses its action on the middle burner to cool Stomach heat and alleviate nausea and vomiting; processing with wu zhu yu p.88 (*yu huang lian* 萸黄连) enhances its ability to direct qi downwards and is used to treat heartburn, reflux and heat from Liver qi constraint; processing with pig bile (*zhu dan chao huang lian* 猪胆炒黄连) increases its ability to purge Liver and Gallbladder fire via the bowel.

**Contraindications** Middle burner yang deficiency and cold patterns. Caution in patients with yin deficiency.

**Formulae** *Huang Lian Jie Du Tang* (local and systemic toxic heat patterns); *Huang Lian E Jiao Tang* (post febrile yin damage with insomnia); *Lian Po Yin* (vomiting and diarrhea from damp heat); *Xiang Lian Wan* (tenesmus in dysenteric disorder); *Bai Tou Weng Tang* (damp heat dysenteric disorder with bleeding); *Shao Yao Tang* (damp heat dysenteric disorder with abdominal pain); *Ge Gen Qin Lian Tang* (damp heat diarrhea); *Ban Xia Xie Xin Tang* (mixed heat and cold blocking the qi dynamic); *Zuo Jin Wan* (acid reflux from Liver invading the Stomach); *Xiao Xian Xiong Tang* (focal chest wall and pleuritic pain from phlegm heat); *Qing Wei San* (oral pathology from Stomach fire)

## Lóng Dǎn Cǎo (Gentianae Radix) Chinese gentian root

**Preparation and usage** Processed with wine (*jiu long dan cao* 酒龙胆草) to moderate its intense coldness and tendency to freeze and constrict qi and blood movement. This form also guides the action of the herb to the upper body and head, and enhances its ability to stop pain.

**Contraindications** Middle burner yang deficiency and in patients with yin deficiency.

**Formulae** *Long Dan Xie Gan Tang* (Liver fire; Liver Gallbladder damp heat); *Dang Gui Long Hui Wan* (Liver fire with constipation); *Liang Jing Wan*† (childhood febrile convulsions); *Ling Yang Jiao San*[1]† (eye pain and visual disorders from Liver fire); *Gu Jing Cao Tang* (visual disturbance and red sore eyes from Liver heat); *Zhen Ni Tang* (vomiting from Liver fire invading the Stomach)

## Kǔ Shēn (Sophorae flavescentis Radix) sophora root

**Preparation and usage** Used externally as a wash for itchy skin diseases, 30–50 grams is used. Can be stir fried (*chao ku shen* 炒苦参) to moderate its bitter coldness, and make it a bit easier on the Spleen and Stomach when ingested.

**Contraindications** Middle burner yang deficiency patterns. Caution in patients with yin deficiency and damaged fluids. Incompatible[2] with li lu (p.22).

**Formulae** *Xiang Shen Wan* (damp heat dysenteric disorder); *Xiao Feng San* (itching, redness and weeping lesions from damp heat in the skin); *Ku Shen Di Huang Tang* (damp heat rectal bleeding and hemorrhoids); *Dang Gui Nian Tong Tang* (damp heat leg pain and swelling); *She Chuang Zi San* (a wash for itching from numerous causes)

## Bái Xiān Pí (Dictamni Cortex) Chinese dittany root bark

**Preparation and usage** When used externally as a wash for itchy skin diseases, 30–50 grams is used. Can also be powdered and mixed with a suitable carrier such as lanoline or sorbolene.

**Contraindications** Caution used internally in patients with middle burner yang deficiency.

**Formulae** *Si Wu Xiao Feng Yin* (itchy wind rash); *Bai Bu Gao* (ointment for itchy psoriasis)

## Qín Pí (Fraxini Cortex) Korean ash bark

**Preparation and usage** Usually used unprocessed, but can be charred (*qin pi tan* 秦皮炭) to enhance its astringency and ability to stop bleeding in dysenteric disorder.

**Contraindications** Middle burner yang deficiency patterns.

**Formulae** *Bai Tou Weng Tang* (damp heat dysenteric disorder with bleeding); *Bai Tou Weng Jia Gan Cao E Jiao Tang* (postpartum blood deficient type dysenteric disorder); *Chang Yong Tang* (acute Intestinal abscess)

## Sān Kē Zhēn (Berberidis Radix) barberry root

**Contraindications** Middle burner yang deficiency and cold patterns. Caution in patients with yin deficiency.

## Mǎ Wěi Lián (Thalictri Radix et Rhizoma) thalictri root

**Contraindications** None noted.

## Substances from other groups

Herbs from other groups that can clear damp heat (the most important in bold) include chun pi (p.2), yu jin (p.8), hu zhang (p.8), **di yu** (p.12), huai hua mi (p.12), che qian zi (p.18), yi yi ren (p.18), dong gua zi (p.18), yu mi xu (p.18), **yin chen hao** (p.18), jin qian cao (p.18), di fu zi (p.20), **hua shi** (p.20), gua di (p.22), jin yin hua (p.34), **pu gong ying** (p.34), **bai tou weng** (p.34), ma chi xian (p.34), chuan xin lian (p.34), **tu fu ling** (p.34), hu huang lian (p.44), shi da gong lao (p.44) and da huang (p.60).

## Endnotes

† These formulae traditionally contain items from endangered animal species and/or obsolete toxic substances, and are unavailable in their original form.

1 *He Ji Ju Fang* (Imperial Grace Formulary of the Tai Ping Era)
2 Appendix 2, p.100

| INDICATIONS | Di Gu Pi 地骨皮 | Yin Chai Hu 银柴胡 | Bai Wei 白薇 | Qing Hao 青蒿 | Hu Huang Lian 胡黄连 | Shi Da Gong Lao 十大功劳 | | | | | | | FUNCTIONS |
|---|---|---|---|---|---|---|---|---|---|---|---|---|---|
| abscesses & sores – skin | | | △E○ | | △ | △ | | | | | | | alleviates dysuria |
| accumulation disorder | △ | ▲ | | ● | ▲ | | | | | | | | checks malarial disorder |
| bleeding – epistaxis | △ | | | △ | ○ | ○ | | | | | | | clears damp heat |
| bleeding – hematemesis | △● | ○ | ○ | ● | ○ | ○ | | | | | | | clears deficient heat |
| bleeding – hematuria | △ | | ○ | | | | | | | | | | clears toxic heat |
| bleeding – hemoptysis | △○ | | | | | ▲ | | | | | | | cools the Lungs |
| bleeding – skin, purpura | ● | ○ | ○ | △● | | | | | | | | | cools the blood |
| common cold – summerheat | | | | ▲○ | | | | | | | | | dispels summerheat |
| cough – Lung heat | ▲ | | △○ | | | | | | | | | | promotes urination |
| cough – Lung yin deficiency | | | | ● | | ▲ | | | | | | | vents lingering pathogens |
| diabetes | △ | | | | | | | | | | | | |
| dysenteric dis. – damp heat | | | | | △ | △ | | | | | | | |
| dysuria – damp heat, bld. | | | △ | | | | | | | | | | |
| dysuria – in pregnancy | | | △ | | | | | | | | | | |
| eyes – red & sore | | | | △ | | △ | | | | | | | |
| fever & chills – alternating | | | | ▲ | | | | | | | | | |
| fever – bone steaming; yin def. | ▲ | △ | △ | ▲ | △ | △ | | | | | | | |
| fever – infantile gan syndrome | △ | ▲ | | | △ | | | | | | | | |
| fever – lingering, low grade | ▲ | △ | △ | ▲ | | | | | | | | | |
| fever – postpartum | | | ▲ | | | | | | | | | | |
| fever – summerheat | | | | △ | | | | | | | | | |
| fever – yin deficiency | ▲ | △ | ▲ | △ | △ | △ | | | | | | | |
| hemorrhoids – painful | | | | | △ E | | | | | | | | |
| hypertension | | △ | | | | | | | | | | | |
| lingering pathogen – *shao yang* | | | | ▲ | | | | | | | | | |
| lingering pathogen – nutritive | | | | ▲ | | | | | | | | | |
| malarial disorder | | △ | | ▲ | | | | | | | | | **Domain (❖)** |
| malaria – plasmodium | ❖ | | | ▲ | | ❖ | | | | | | | Lung |
| snakebite | | | △ E | | ❖ | | | | | | | | Large Intestine |
| skin – itchy wind rash; urticaria | ❖ | | | E | | ❖ | | | | | | | Kidney |
| sweating – night sweats | ▲ | △ ❖ | ❖ | ▲ ❖ | △ ❖ | | | | | | | | Liver |
| throat – sore; chronic, dry | | | △ | ❖ | | | | | | | | | Gallbladder |
| tuberculosis | | | | | ❖ | ▲ | | | | | | | Heart |
| | | ❖ | ❖ | ❖ | ❖ | | | | | | | | Stomach |
| | | | | | | | | | | | | | |
| | | | | | | | | | | | | | |
| | | | | | | | | | | | | | **Flavour, nature (◆)** |
| | | | | ◆ | | | | | | | | | acrid |
| | | ◆ | | ◆ | ◆ | ◆ | | | | | | | bitter |
| | | | ◆ | | | | | | | | | | salty |
| | ◆ | ◆ | | | | | | | | | | | sweet |
| | | ◆ | | | | ◆ | | | | | | | cool |
| | ◆ | | ◆ | ◆ | ◆ | | | | | | | | cold |
| **Standard dosage range (g)** | 6–15 | 3–9 | 6–15 | 6–15 | 3–9 | 9–15 | | | | | | | |

Legend:
△ Indication
▲ Strong Indication
E External Use
E Strong External Indication

○ Function
● Strong Function

### Dì Gǔ Pí (Lycii Cortex) wolfberry root bark

**Contraindications** Fever associated with wind cold invasion, Spleen qi deficiency patterns.

**Formulae** *Qing Gu San* (yin deficiency fever and bone steaming); *Di Gu Pi San* (night sweats and bone steaming from yin deficiency); *Xie Bai San* (Lung heat cough); *Bai Bu Tang* (chronic cough from Lung qi and yin deficiency)

### Yín Chái Hú (Stellariae Radix) stellaria root

**Contraindications** Fever associated with wind cold invasion, blood deficiency patterns without heat.

**Formulae** *Qing Gu San* (yin deficiency fever and bone steaming); *Di Gu Pi San* (night sweats and bone steaming from yin deficiency)

### Bái Wěi (Cynanchi atrati Radix) swallowwort root

**Preparation and usage** Usually used unprocessed, but can be stir fried (*chao bai wei* 炒白薇) to moderate its coldness and make it easier on the Spleen and Stomach.

**Contraindications** Caution in middle burner deficiency.

**Formulae** *Bai Wei Tang* (persistent low grade fever from yin deficiency); *Jia Jian Wei Rui Tang* (wind heat common cold in a patient with underlying yin deficiency)

### Qīng Hāo (Artemisiae annuae Herba) sweet wormwood

**Preparation and usage** Do not cook for longer than 5–10 minutes[1].

**Contraindications** Generally very well tolerated, but be careful when using high doses in patients with Spleen qi deficiency and loose stools.

**Formulae** *Qing Hao Bie Jia Tang* (post febrile yin deficient low grade fever); *Qing Gu San* (yin deficiency fever and bone steaming); *Hao Qin Qing Dan Tang* (damp heat in the *shào yáng*)

### Hú Huáng Lián (Picrorhizae Rhizoma) picrorhiza rhizome

**Contraindications** Caution in middle burner deficiency.

**Formulae** *Qing Gu San* (yin deficiency fever and bone steaming); *Fei Er Wan* (accumulation disorder with fever and heat in infants)

### Shí Dà Gōng Láo (Mahonia Folium) mahonia leaf

**Preparation and usage** This herb needs to be taken long term to be effective in chronic Lung deficiency patterns, but its bitter coolness can weaken the Spleen and Stomach. To offset this it can be prepared as a syrup with dates (da zao p.74) and honey, and taken in addition to a suitable constitutional prescription.

**Contraindications** Middle burner yang deficiency.

### Substances from other groups

Herbs from other groups that can clear heat from deficiency include fu xiao mai (p.2), nuo dao gen xu (p.2), zhi mu (p.32), huang bai (p.42), tian dong (p.80), shi hu (p.80), nu zhen zi (p.80), gui ban (p.80) and bie jia (p.80).

---

1 Appendix 6, p.108

| | He Ye 荷叶 | Lü Dou 绿豆 | Xi Gua 西瓜 | Bian Dou 扁豆 | | | | | | | | | FUNCTIONS |
|---|---|---|---|---|---|---|---|---|---|---|---|---|---|
| △ Indication / ▲ Strong Indication / E External Use / E Strong External Indication — ○ Function / ● Strong Function | | | | | | | | | | | | | |
| **INDICATIONS** | | | | | | | | | | | | | |
| abdominal distension | △ | ○ | | △ ○ | | | | | | | | | alleviates toxicity |
| abscesses & sores – skin | | △ E ○ | | | | | | | | | | | clears toxic heat |
| antidote to toxic herbs | ○ | ▲ | | | | | | | | | | | stops bleeding |
| appetite – loss of | | | | △ ○ | | | | | | | | | stops diarrhea |
| bleeding – epistaxis | △ | ○ | ○ | | | | | | | | | | stops thirst |
| bleeding – heat in the blood | △ | | | ○ | | | | | | | | | strengthens the Spleen |
| bleeding – hematemesis | △ | | | ○ | | | | | | | | | transforms damp |
| bleeding – rectal | △ | | | | | | | | | | | | |
| bleeding – uterine | △ | | | | | | | | | | | | |
| common cold – summerheat | △ | △ | △ | ▲ | | | | | | | | | |
| diarrhea – summerheat | △ | | | ▲ | | | | | | | | | |
| diarrhea – Spleen qi def. | △ | | | ▲ | | | | | | | | | |
| dysenteric dis. – damp heat | △ | | | | | | | | | | | | |
| edema – wind; acute | △ | | | | | | | | | | | | |
| erysipelas, cellulitis | | △ | | | | | | | | | | | |
| fever – summerheat | △ | | | | | | | | | | | | |
| head distension – acute | △ | | | | | | | | | | | | |
| headache – summerheat, acute | △ | | | | | | | | | | | | |
| irritability – summerheat | △ | △ | △ | | | | | | | | | | |
| leukorrhea – Sp. qi def; damp | | | | ▲ | | | | | | | | | |
| measles – prevention of | | △ | | | | | | | | | | | |
| pain – abdominal | | | | △ | | | | | | | | | |
| poisoning – food | | | | ▲ | | | | | | | | | |
| poisoning – aconite, croton seed | | ▲ | | | | | | | | | | | |
| poisoning – alcohol | | △ | | △ | | | | | | | | | |
| thirst in summerheat attack | | △ | ▲ | | | | | | | | | | |
| vomiting, nausea | | | | △ | | | | | | | | | |
| | | | | | | | | | | | | | |
| | | | | | | | | | | | | | **Domain (❖)** |
| | | ❖ | | | | | | | | | | | Bladder |
| | ❖ | | | | | | | | | | | | Liver |
| | | ❖ | ❖ | | | | | | | | | | Heart |
| | ❖ | | | ❖ | | | | | | | | | Spleen |
| | ❖ | ❖ | ❖ | ❖ | | | | | | | | | Stomach |
| | | | | | | | | | | | | | |
| | | | | | | | | | | | | | |
| | | | | | | | | | | | | | **Flavour, nature (♦)** |
| | ♦ | | | | | | | | | | | | astringent |
| | ♦ | | | | | | | | | | | | bitter |
| | ♦ | | | | | | | | | | | | neutral |
| | | ♦ | ♦ | ♦ | | | | | | | | | sweet |
| | | | | ♦ | | | | | | | | | slightly warm |
| | | ♦ | ♦ | | | | | | | | | | cold |
| **Standard dosage range (g)** | 9–15 | 15–30 | see p.47 | 9–30 | | | | | | | | | |

## Hé Yè (Nelumbinis Folium) lotus leaf

**Preparation and usage** To dispel summerheat, the fresh leaf is best; for other internal Spleen problems, the dried leaf is used; for bleeding from heat in the blood, the fresh leaf is used; for bleeding in general, the charred leaf (*he ye tan* 荷叶炭) is preferred.

**Contraindications** None noted.

**Formulae** *Qing Luo Yin* (summerheat common cold); *Si Sheng Wan* (bleeding from heat in the blood); *Kai Jin San* (anorectic dysenteric disorder)

## Lǜ Dòu (Phaseoli radiati Semen) mung bean

**Preparation and usage** When used to counteract the toxicity of substances such as zhi fu zi (p.88), zhi chuan wu (p.94), cang er zi (p.90), and non herbal toxins such as pesticides and alcohol, 120 grams of freshly ground lu dou powder is mixed with cold water and taken. May also be combined with herbs such as gan cao (p.74) and huang lian (p.42) for this purpose.

**Contraindications** Middle burner yang deficiency with diarrhea.

**Formulae** *Lu Dou Yin*[1] (summerheat common cold); *Lu Dou Yin*[2] (antidote to poisoning by various substances)

## Xī Guā (Citrulli Fructus) watermelon

**Preparation and usage** The usual dose is one cup of fresh juice, although it can be taken as required. Not suitable for decoction.

**Contraindications** Caution in middle burner yang deficiency.

## Biǎn Dòu (Dolichos Semen) hyacinth bean

Also known as bái biǎn dòu 白扁豆.

**Preparation and usage** When taken directly as powder or in pills, the dose is 2–3 grams, two or three times daily. The unprocessed bean is used to dispel summerheat and counteract toxins; when stir fried (*chao bian dou* 炒扁豆) its ability to strengthen the Spleen is enhanced.

**Contraindications** Take caution when using unprocessed with patients with middle burner yang deficiency.

**Formulae** *Xiang Ru San* (summerdamp common cold); *Shen Ling Bai Zhu San* (diarrhea from Spleen qi deficiency); *Qing Luo Yin* (summerheat common cold); *Sha Shen Mai Dong Tang* (Lung and Stomach dryness and yin deficiency); *Shi Hu Qing Wei San* (vomiting from Stomach heat and yin deficiency)

### Substances from other groups

Other herbs that can dispel summerheat and summerdamp include huo xiang (p.16), pei lan (p.16), hua shi (p.20) and xiang ru (p.28).

---

1 *Jing Yue Quan Shu* (The Complete Works of Jing Yue)
2 *Zheng Zhi Zhun Sheng* (Standards of Patterns and Treatment)

| △ Indication / ▲ Strong Indication / E External Use / E Strong External Indication **INDICATIONS** | Shi Jue Ming 石决明 | Zhen Zhu Mu 珍珠母 | Mu Li 牡蛎 | Zi Bei Chi 紫贝齿 | Dai Zhe Shi 代赭石 | Ci Ji Li 刺蒺藜 | Jue Ming Zi 决明子 | Zhu Mao Cai 猪毛菜 | Lu Dou Yi 稆豆衣 | Luo Bu Ma Ye 罗布麻叶 | ○ Function / ● Strong Function **FUNCTIONS** |
|---|---|---|---|---|---|---|---|---|---|---|---|
| acid reflux, heartburn | △ | △ | △● | | △ | | | | | | astringes fluid leakage |
| belching, hiccup | ● | ○ | | ○ | △ | ○ | ○ | | | | brightens the eyes |
| bleeding – hematemesis | ○ | △○ | △○ | ○ | △○ | ● | ○ | ○ | ○ | ○ | calms the Liver |
| bleeding – hemoptysis, nose | | ○ | ○ | ○ | △ | | | | | | calms & sedates the shen |
| bleeding – traumatic | E | | E | | ○ | | ○ | | | | cools the blood |
| bleeding – uterine | ○ | ○ | △ | ○ | △ | | | | | ○ | cools the Liver |
| breast – abscess, mastitis | | | | | ● | △ | | | | | directs qi downward |
| breast – cysts & lumps | | | △ | | | △○ | | | | | dispels wind |
| breast – distension & pain | | | ● | | | ▲ | | | | | dissipates masses |
| constipation – heat, dryness | | | | | | ○ | △ | | | | dredges the Liver |
| convulsions – febrile in children | | △ | | △ | | | ○ | | | | moistens the Intestines |
| dizziness, vertigo | ▲ | △ | △ | △ | △ | ▲ | △ | △ | △○ | ▲ | nourishes yin & blood |
| ears – tinnitus; yin def., yang↑ | △● | △○ | △○ | ○ | △○ | △○ | △○ | △○ | ○ | ○ | pacifies ascendant yang |
| edema | | | | | | | | | △○ | | promotes urination |
| eyes – red, sore, blurring | ▲ | △ | ● | △ | | △ | ▲ | | | | softens hardness |
| eyes – excessive lacrimation | △ | △ | | | ○ | △ | △ | | | | stops bleeding |
| eyes – photophobia | △ | △ | | △ | | △● | △ | | | | stops itch |
| eyes – pterygia, corneal opacity | △ | | | △ | | △ | ▲ | | | | |
| eyes – vision, weakness of | △ | △ | | | | △ | △ | | | | |
| headache – yang↑, fire | △ | △ | △ | △ | △ | △ | △ | △ | △ | | |
| headache – wind heat | | | | | | △ | △ | | | | |
| hepatosplenomegaly | | △ | | | | | | | | | |
| hypercholesterolemia | | | | | | | △ | | | | |
| hypertension | △ | | | | | △ | △ | △ | | △ | |
| insomnia – yang↑, heat | △ | ▲ | △ | △ | | | | | | △ | |
| irritability, short temper | △ | △ | △ | | △ | △ | | | | △ | |
| masses – abdominal, phlegm | | | △ | | | | | | | | |
| menstruation – irregular | | | | | | △ | | | | | **Domain (✼)** |
| nodules & masses – phlegm | | | ▲ | | | | | ✼ | | | Large Intestine |
| pain – epigastric, & hyperacidity | △ | △ | △✼ | | | | | | | | Kidney |
| pain – hypochondriac | ✼ | ✼ | ✼ | ✼ | ✼ | △✼ | ✼ | ✼ | ✼ | ✼ | Liver |
| palpitations, anxiety | | ▲✼ | △ | △ | ✼ | | | | | △✼ | Heart |
| seizures, epilepsy | | △ | | | | | | | | | |
| skin – itching, urticaria, eczema | | | | | | ▲ | | | | | |
| skin – vitiligo | | | | | | △ | | | | | **Flavour, nature (◆)** |
| sweating – night sweats | | | △ | | | ◆ | | | △ | | acrid |
| sweating – spontaneous | | | ▲◆ | | | | | | | | astringent |
| thyroid – nodules, goitre | | | ▲ | ◆ | | ◆ | | | | ◆ | bitter |
| tremor & spasm – post febrile | ◆ | ◆ | △◆ | ◆ | | ◆ | | ◆ | | | salty |
| urination – frequent, nocturia | | | △ | | | | | ◆ | ◆ | ◆ | sweet |
| vomiting, nausea – severe | ◆ | ◆ | | | ▲◆ | | | ◆ | | | cold |
| wheezing – def. & excess types | | | ◆ | | △ | | ◆ | | | ◆ | cool |
| withdrawal mania (*dian kuang*) | | △ | △ | ◆ | | ◆ | | | ◆ | | neutral |
| **Standard dosage range (g)** | 15–30 | 15–30 | 15–30 | 9–15 | 9–30 | 6–15 | 9–15 | 15–30 | 6–15 | 3–15 | |

Functions and indications overlap between this group, the wind extinguishing group and the heavy shen calming substances. Some texts place the yang pacifying and wind extinguishing substances together, however I follow the authority of the *Zhong Yao Xue* (2000) in distinguishing between them. Although wind and ascendant yang share many features, the existence of wind is signified specifically by involuntary movement, tremor, spasm and sudden changes of consciousness.

### Shí Jué Míng (Haliotidis Concha) abalone shell

**Preparation and use** Break up the shell in a mortar and pestle and cook for 30 minutes[1] prior to the other herbs. To pacify ascendant yang, the unprocessed shell is used; calcining (*duan shi jue ming* 煅石决明) enhances its astringency and is preferred for visual problems, external use and hyperacidity.

**Contraindications** Middle burner yang deficiency with loss of appetite and loose stools.

**Formulae** *Shi Jue Ming Wan* (visual weakness and irritated eyes from Liver yin and blood deficiency); *E Jiao Ji Zi Huang Tang* (Liver yin deficiency with ascendant yang); *Tian Ma Gou Teng Yin* (insomnia, dizziness and headache from ascendant Liver yang)

### Zhēn Zhū Mǔ (Margaritiferae Concha usta) mother of pearl shell

**Preparation and use** Break up the shell in a mortar and pestle and cook for 30 minutes[2] prior to the other herbs.

**Contraindications** Caution during pregnancy, in patients with middle burner yang deficiency and sinking Spleen qi.

**Formulae** *Zhen Zhu Mu Wan* (insomnia and shen disturbances from Heart and Liver yin and blood deficiency with ascendant yang); *Jia Yi Gui Zang Tang* (headache and dizziness from Liver yin deficiency with ascendant yang); *An Shen Bu Xin Wan* (shen disturbances from Heart yin and blood deficiency)

### Mǔ Lì (Ostreae Concha) oyster shell

**Preparation and use** Break up the shell in a mortar and pestle and cook for 30 minutes[3] prior to the other herbs. Unprocessed mu li is best for pacifying ascendant yang, calming the shen and softening hard phlegm; calcining (*duan mu li* 煅牡蛎) enhances its astringency, ability to prevent leakage of fluids, and antacid action.

**Contraindications** Sweating or discharge from damp heat or other excess pathogens that should be expelled; gastric hyperacidity associated with middle burner yang deficiency.

**Formulae** *Zhen Gan Xi Feng Tang* (headache and hypertension from ascendant yang); *San Jia Fu Mai Tang* (post febrile yin deficiency with tremor and spasm); *Chai Hu Jia Long Gu Mu Li Tang* (shen disturbances from Liver fire and phlegm heat); *Xiao Luo Wan* (phlegm masses); *Mu Li San* (sweating from deficiency); *Gui Zhi Jia Long Gu Mu Li Tang* (post traumatic shen disturbance and sweating from disruption to the Heart Kidney axis); *Lai Fu Tang* (severe sweating from collapse of yang qi); *Jin Suo Gu Jing Wan* (frequent urination and loss of essence from Kidney deficiency); *Gao Lin Tang* (turbid urination from Kidney deficiency); *Gu Chong Tang* (uterine bleeding from *chōng mài / rèn mài* deficiency); *An Zhong San* (epigastric pain from cold)

### Zǐ Bèi Chǐ (Mauritiae/Cypraeae Concha) cowrie shell

**Preparation and use** Break up the shell in a mortar and pestle and cook for 30 minutes[4] prior to the other herbs.

**Contraindications** Caution in middle burner yang deficiency.

### Dài Zhě Shí (Haematitum) hematite, an iron oxide with the chemical composition $Fe_2O_3$

**Preparation and use** Break up the stone in a mortar and pestle and cook for 30 minutes[5] prior to the other herbs. When taken directly in pills or powder, the dose is 1–3 grams, two or three times daily. Unprocessed dai zhe shi is used to pacify ascendant yang and direct qi downwards; calcining (*duan dai zhe shi* 煅代赭石) enhances its ability to stop bleeding.

**Contraindications** Caution during pregnancy and in middle burner yang deficiency. Should not be used for more than a few weeks at a time. Avoid concurrent use of coffee and tea[6].

**Formulae** *Zhen Gan Xi Feng Tang* (headache and hypertension from ascendant yang); *Xuan Fu Dai Zhe Tang* (vomiting and nausea from rebellious Stomach qi); *Zhen Ni Tang* (vomiting from Liver fire invading the Stomach); *Han Jiang Tang* (vomiting blood from Stomach fire); *Zhen Ling Dan†* (persistent uterine bleeding from yang deficiency and blood stasis)

### Cì Jí Lí (Tribuli Fructus) tribulus fruit

Also known as *bái jí lí* 白蒺藜.

**Preparation and use** The unprocessed fruit is best to disperse wind heat, stop itch and improve vision; when stir fried (*chao ci ji li* 炒刺蒺藜) its acrid dispersing nature is reduced and its ability to dredge the Liver and pacify yang enhanced.

**Contraindications** Pregnancy[7]. Caution in patients with qi and blood deficiency.

**Formulae** *Ji Li Ju Hua Tang* (dizziness and headache from ascendant Liver yang); *Bai Ji Li San* (wind heat eye disorders); *Shi Hu Ye Guang Wan†* (visual weakness from Liver and Kidney yin deficiency); *Dang Gui Yin Zi* (chronic itchy skin disorder from blood deficiency)

### Jué Míng Zǐ (Cassiae Semen) cassia seed

**Preparation and use** The seeds are crushed before decoction. When taken directly in pills or powders the daily dose is 3–6 grams. When used for constipation, cook no longer than 15 minutes. Used to treat high blood cholesterol, doses of up to 30 grams per day can be used, but watch for loose stools. If loose stools occur, stir fried seeds can be used. Unprocessed seeds are better for clearing heat and pacifying ascendant yang. When stir fried (*chao jue ming zi* 炒决明子), the heat clearing and laxative action is reduced, while its Liver and Kidney tonic action is enhanced. The stir fried seeds are used for deficiency type eye conditions and patients with loose stools.

**Contraindications** Diarrhea from Spleen deficiency; low blood pressure. Caution during pregnancy.

**Formulae** *Ji Li Ju Hua Tang* (dizziness and headache from ascendant Liver yang); *Jue Ming Zi San* (wind heat eye disorders); *Jue Ming Wan* (color blindness from Liver and Kidney deficiency); *Ling Yang Jiao San*[8]*†* (eye pain and visual disorders from Liver fire)

### Zhū Máo Cài (Salsola collina Herba) tumbleweed; slender Russian thistle

**Contraindications** None noted.

### Lǔ Dòu Yī (Glycinis Testa) soybean skin

**Contraindications** None noted.

### Luó Bù Má Yè (Apocyni veneti Folium) dogbane leaf

**Preparation and use** Can be decocted as per usual, or simply steeped in hot water and sipped frequently as a tea for patients with hypertension.

**Contraindications** Long term use can deplete potassium, which may need to be supplemented.

### Substances from other groups

Substances from other groups that have an ability to pacify ascendant yang include sang ye (p.26), ju hua (p.26), long gu (p.72), long chi (p.72), ci shi (p.72), bai shao (p.78), gui ban (p.80), bie jia (p.80), tian ma (p.96), ling yang jiao (p.96) and shan yang jiao (p.96).

### Endnotes

† These formulae traditionally contain items from endangered animal species and/or obsolete toxic substances, and are unavailable in their original form.

---

1 Appendix 6, p.108
2 Ibid.
3 Ibid.
4 Ibid.
5 Ibid.

---

6 According to the *Zhong Yao Xue* (2000) these can react with the iron and cause a precipitate that interferes with digestion.
7 Chen (2004) is the only source to assert a contraindication.
8 *He Ji Ju Fang* (Imperial Grace Formulary of the Tai Ping Era)

| △ Indication / ▲ Strong Indication / E External Use / E Strong External Indication | | | | | | | | | |
|---|---|---|---|---|---|---|---|---|---|
| **INDICATIONS** | Ren Gong She Xiang 人工麝香 | Bing Pian 冰片 | Su He Xiang 苏合香 | An Xi Xiang 安息香 | Zhang Nao 樟脑 | Chan Su 蟾酥 | Shi Chang Pu 石菖蒲 | E Bu Shi Cao 鹅不食草 | **FUNCTIONS** (○ Function / ● Strong Function) |
| abscesses & sores – skin | △E | △E | | | E | ▲E | △E○ | △E | calms the shen |
| amenorrhea – blood stasis | △ | ○ | | | | | | | clears heat |
| angina | ▲ | △ | ▲ | △ | | | | ○ | dispels wind cold |
| anxiety, palpitations | ○ | | | ○ | | | ▲ | | invigorates blood |
| cancer – liver, blood, GIT, skin | | | | | ○ | △ | | | kills parasites |
| closed disorder – cold | △ | △ | ▲ | | | | | ● | opens the nose & sinuses |
| closed disorder – heat | △● | △○ | ● | △○ | △○ | △○ | ○ | | restores consciousness |
| concentration – poor | ○ | ○ | ○ | ○ | ○ | ● | ▲ | | stops pain |
| consciousness – loss of, coma | △ | △ | ▲ | △ | △ | △ | △○ | | transforms phlegm |
| convulsions – febrile | △ | | | | | ○ | | | treats tumours and sores |
| delirium – in high fever | △ | △ | | | △ | | △ | | |
| depression – phlegm | | | | | | | △ | | |
| dysenteric disorder – anorectic | | | | | | | △ | | |
| ears – tinnitus, hearing loss | △ | | | | | | △ | | |
| eyes – red & sore | | △ | | | | | | | |
| foggy head; mental cloudiness | | | | | | | ▲ | | |
| headache – blood stasis | △ | | | | | | | | |
| headache – wind cold; sinus | | | | | | | | △ | |
| insomnia | | | | | | | △ | | |
| masses – abdominal | △ | | | | | △ | | | |
| memory – poor | | | | | | | ▲ | | |
| nose – polyps in | | | | | | | | ▲ | |
| nasosinusitis (bi yuan) | | | | | | | | ▲ | |
| nodules & masses – phlegm | △ | | | | | △ | | | |
| pain – & injury, trauma | ▲E | | | | E | | | | |
| pain – abdominal, acute | △ | | △ | △ | △ | △ | | | |
| pain – cancer | | | | | | △ | | | **Domain (❖)** |
| pain – chest, acute | ▲ | △❖ | ▲ | △ | △ | | | ❖ | Lung |
| pain – joint, muscle | △E❖ | | | △ | | | △ | ❖ | Liver |
| painful obst. – wind damp | △E❖ | ❖ | ❖ | △❖ | ❖ | ❖ | △❖ | | Heart |
| paralytic ileus | △❖ | ❖ | ❖ | ❖ | ❖ | | | ❖ | Spleen |
| Pericardium – heat entering | △ | △ | | | | ❖ | | | Stomach |
| placenta, lochia – retention of | △ | | | | | | | | |
| rhinitis – hypertrophic | | | | | | | | ▲ | |
| seizures, epilepsy – phlegm | △ | | △ | | | | △ | | **Flavour, nature (♦)** |
| skin – itching of | | E | | | E♦ | ♦ | | | toxic |
| skin – scabies, tinea, ringworm | ♦ | E♦ | ♦ | ♦ | E♦ | ♦ | ♦ | ♦ | acrid |
| sudden turmoil disorder | | ♦ | | △♦ | △ | △ | △♦ | | bitter |
| summerheat – severe | | | | | △ | △♦ | | | sweet |
| throat – sore; acute, with pus | △ | △E♦ | | | | ▲ | △ | | cool |
| toothache | | E | | | E♦ | E | | | hot |
| ulcers – mouth | ♦ | △E | ♦ | | | ♦ | ♦ | ♦ | warm |
| wind stroke – acute phase | △ | | △ | △♦ | △ | | | | neutral |
| **Standard dosage range (g)** | see p.51 | see p.51 | 0.3–1 | 0.3–1 | see p.51 | see p.51 | 6–9 | 6–9 | |

These substances are mostly used for reviving consciousness in "closed disorder" (*bì zhèng* 闭证) and phlegm type seizures. They powerfully scatter qi and easily damage normal qi, therefore are suitable only for short term use. They are not suitable for treating "flaccid collapse" (*tuō zhèng* 脱证), a condition that requires herbs and techniques that rescue and consolidate dissipating yang. The last two herbs mentioned here are used to open blocked senses, the mind in the case of shi chang pu and the nose in the case of e bu shi cao.

### Rén Gōng Shè Xiāng (Synthetic muscone)
The synthetic version of shè xiāng (Moschus), the scent gland of the musk deer, has identical functions and strength. Musk deer are endangered, listed in Appendix 1 or 2 of CITES[1] depending on species. Although the animal is farmed in China for its valuable gland, extracting the musk is traumatic for the shy animal and often results in death. The practice should be condemned and the product avoided. The synthetic analogue is just as good and commonly used in prepared medicines. Most of the prepared medicine formulae noted below use synthetic muscone, but always check the label.

**Preparation and use** Not suitable for decoction. When taken internally the dose is 0.03–0.1 grams in pills or powders.

**Contraindications** Pregnancy. Caution in patients with qi or yin deficiency. Can cause photo reactive skin irritation in some patients, especially those with light skin, when used topically. Should not be taken at the same time as garlic.

**Formulae** *Zhi Bao Dan*† (impaired consciousness or coma); *Su He Xiang Wan*† (cold type closed disorder); *An Gong Niu Huang Wan*† (delirium, loss of consciousness and high fever from heat affecting the Pericardium); *Zi Xue Dan*† (febrile convulsions); *Qi Li San*† (traumatic injury); *Tong Qiao Huo Xue Tang*† (headache, tinnitus and hearing loss from blood stasis); *Bao Long Wan*† (seizures from phlegm heat); *Liu Shen Wan*† (sore swollen throat and boils from toxic heat); *Xing Jun San*† (severe sudden turmoil disorder)

### Bīng Piàn (Borneol) borneol, a crystalline extract of plants such as Artemesia, Dryoblanops or Blumea species[2]
**Preparation and use** Not suitable for decoction. When taken internally the dose is 0.03–0.1 grams in pills, powders or tinctures.

**Contraindications** Pregnancy. Do not expose to heat.

**Formulae** *Zhi Bao Dan*† (impaired consciousness or coma); *Su He Xiang Wan*† (sudden loss of consciousness from wind stroke; cold type closed disorder); *An Gong Niu Huang Wan*† (delirium, loss of consciousness and high fever from heat affecting the Pericardium); *Niu Huang Shang Qing Wan*† (ulceration and pain of the oral cavity, eyes and throat from fire); *Liu Shen Wan*† (sore swollen throat and boils from toxic heat); *Xing Jun San*† (severe sudden turmoil disorder); *Guan Xin Su He Xiang Wan*† (angina); *Jing Wan Hong* (ointment for burns and non healing sores); *Qing Yin Wan*† (hoarse voice, loss of voice and sore throat from Lung fire)

### Sū Hé Xiāng (Styrax Liquidis) liquidamber resin
**Preparation and use** Not suitable for decoction. Only used in pills, powders or tinctures.

**Contraindications** Closed syndrome from heat; flaccid collapse. Caution during pregnancy.

**Formulae** *Su He Xiang Wan*† (cold type closed disorder); *Guan Xin Su He Xiang Wan*† (angina)

### Ān Xī Xiāng (Benzoinum) benzoin, a resin derived from the Styrax tree
**Preparation and use** Not suitable for decoction. Only used in pills, powders or tinctures.

**Contraindications** Caution in patients with qi deficiency, and yin deficiency with heat.

**Formulae** *Su He Xiang Wan*† (cold type closed disorder); *Zhi Bao Dan*† (impaired consciousness or coma)

### Zhāng Nǎo (Camphora) camphor, a crystalline substance derived from the tree Cinnamonom camphora
Placed with the external use group in some texts.

**Preparation and use** Not suitable for decoction. Only used in powders or tinctures. When taken internally the dose is 0.1–0.2 grams. Not suitable for prolonged use (including external application) as toxic effects[3] can occur. The maximum dose should not be exceeded, nor should it be applied topically over large areas of the body.

**Contraindications** Pregnancy, infants, qi deficiency and yin deficiency with heat.

**Formulae** *Fu Fang Zhang Nao Ding* (tincture for abdominal pain and diarrhea); *Er Yan San* (topical powder for ear infection); *E Wei Hua Pi Gao*† (topical plaster for masses)

### Chán Sū (Bufonis Venenum) cane toad toxin
Placed with the external use group in some texts.

**Preparation and use** Not suitable for decoction. Only used in tiny pills (as in Liu Shen Wan) that enable tight dose regulation. When taken internally the dose is 0.015–0.03 grams. Not suitable for prolonged use as toxic effects[4] can occur. The maximum dose should not be exceeded.

**Contraindications** Pregnancy. Avoid contact with the eyes.

**Formulae** *Liu Shen Wan*† (sore swollen throat and boils from toxic heat); *Sha Qi Chan Su Wan*† (impaired consciousness, violent vomiting, diarrhea and abdominal pain in an acute summerheat attack); *Chan Su Gao* (topical paste for toxic sores and tumours)

### Shí Chāng Pú (Acori tatarinowii Rhizoma) acorus, sweetflag rhizome
**Preparation and use** If the fresh herb is available, 9–15 grams may be used.

**Contraindications** Caution in yin and blood deficiency.

**Formulae** *Chang Pu Yu Jin Tang* (delirium and fever from phlegm heat misting the Heart); *Di Tan Tang* (mental cloudiness, confusion and aphasia from wind stroke); *Ding Xian Wan*† (seizures from wind phlegm); *An Shen Ding Zhi Wan* (anxiety and insomnia from Heart qi deficiency); *Lian Po Yin* (vomiting and diarrhea from damp heat); *Chang Pu San* (wind cold damp painful obstruction); *Kai Jin San* (anorectic dysenteric disorder); *Bi Xie Fen Qing Yin* (turbid urine from Kidney deficiency); *Sang Piao Xiao San* (enuresis and nocturia from Heart and Kidney deficiency); *Wu Jing Jian Wan* (memory problems and debility from essence deficiency); *Er Long Zuo Ci Wan* (hearing deficit from Kidney yin deficiency)

### É Bù Shí Cǎo (Centipedae Herba) small centipeda herb
Placed in the acrid warm exterior releasing group in some texts.

**Preparation and use** This herb can be decocted, taken in pills or powdered and blown into the nose.

**Contraindications** Caution in patients with gastric ulcers and gastritis.

**Formulae** *Bi Yan Ning* (prepared medicine for chronic sinus congestion); *Bi Min Gan Wan* (prepared medicine for hay fever and rhinitis); *Bi Yun San* (inhaled powder for nasal congestion and frontal headache)

### Endnotes
† These formulae traditionally contain items from endangered animal species and/or obsolete toxic substances, and are unavailable in their original form.

---

1 Appendix 5, p.106
2 Much of the borneol presently available is synthetic. The synthetic version has the same activity, but is cheaper and considered inferior to the natural product.

---

3 Appendix 3.1, p.101
4 Ibid.

# 11. PARASITES – INTESTINAL, LIVER, SKIN

Legend:
- △ Indication
- ▲ Strong Indication
- E External Use
- **E** Strong External Indication
- ○ Function
- ● Strong Function
- Domain (❖)
- Flavour, nature (♦)

| INDICATIONS | Shi Jun Zi 使君子 | Ku Lian Pi 苦楝皮 | He Shi 鹤虱 | Bing Lang 槟榔 | Fei Zi 榧子 | Lei Wan 雷丸 | Wu Yi 芜荑 | Nan Gua Zi 南瓜子 | Da Suan 大蒜 | Guan Zhong 贯众 | He Cao Ya 鹤草芽 | FUNCTIONS |
|---|---|---|---|---|---|---|---|---|---|---|---|---|
| abscesses & sores – skin | | | | | | | | | △ E | ○ | | clears toxic heat |
| abdominal distension | △ | | | △ ● | | | | | | | | directs qi downward |
| accumulation disorder (gan ji) | △ ○ | ● | ○ | ○ | ○ | △ ○ | △ ○ | ○ | ○ | ○ | ○ | kills parasites |
| beriberi | | | | △ | ○ | | | | | | | moistens the Lungs |
| bleeding – hematemesis, rectal | | | | | ○ | | | | | △ | | moistens the Intestines |
| bleeding – uterine, from heat | | | | ○ | | | | | | ▲ | | promotes urination |
| common cold – wind heat | | | | | | | | | | △ ○ | | stops bleeding |
| constipation | △ | | | ▲ | △ ○ | | | | | | | stops cough |
| cough – dryness | ○ | | | | △ | | | | | | | strengthens the Spleen |
| cough – whooping | ○ | | | | | ○ | ○ | | △ | | | treats accumulation dis. |
| diarrhea | | | | | | | △ | | △ ○ | | | treats suppurative sores |
| dysenteric dis. – damp heat | | | | △ | | | | | △ | | | |
| edema – from excess | | | | △ | | | | | | | | |
| food stagnation | △ | | | △ | | | | | △ | | | |
| itch – genital, anal | | | E | | | | | | | | | |
| lactation – insufficient | | | | | | | | △ | | | | |
| leg qi – cold damp | | | | △ | | | | | | | | |
| malarial disorder | | | | △ | | | | | △ | | | |
| mumps | | | | | | | | | | △ | | |
| pain – abdominal, from worms | △ | △ | ▲ | △ | | △ | △ | | | | | |
| paralytic ileus – post surgical | | | | △ | | | | | | | | |
| parasites – blood flukes | | | | △ | | | | | △ | | | |
| parasites – fasciolopsis | | | | △ | △ | | | | | | | |
| parasites – hookworms | | △ | | △ | △ | △ | | | △ | △ | | **Domain (❖)** |
| parasites – intestinal flukes | | | △ | △ | △ ❖ | | | | ❖ | | | Lung |
| parasites – pinworms | △ | △ | △ | △ ❖ | △ ❖ | ❖ | | ❖ | △ | △ | ❖ | Large Intestine |
| parasites – roundworms | ▲ | ▲ ❖ | △ | △ | △ | △ | △ | △ | △ | △ ❖ | ❖ | Liver |
| parasites – schistosomiasis | | | | △ | | | | | △ | | ❖ | Small Intestine |
| parasites – tapeworms | ❖ | ❖ | △ ❖ | ▲ | ▲ | △ | △ ❖ | ▲ | ❖ | △ ❖ | △ | Spleen |
| skin – scabies | ❖ | E ❖ | ❖ | ❖ | ❖ | ❖ | ❖ | ❖ | ❖ | | | Stomach |
| skin – tinea, ringworm | | E | | | | | E | | E | | | |
| tenesmus | | | | ▲ | | | | | | | | |
| toothache, dental caries | E | E | | | | | | | | | | **Flavour, nature (♦)** |
| trichomonas vaginitis | | △ E ♦ | E | | | | | | | | E | toxic |
| warm diseases (wen bing) | ♦ | | ♦ | | | ♦ | | | | △ ♦ | | slightly toxic |
| | | | ♦ | ♦ | | | ♦ | | ♦ | | | acrid |
| | | | | | | | | | | | ♦ | astringent |
| | | ♦ | | | | | | | | ♦ | ♦ | bitter |
| | ♦ | | | | ♦ | | | ♦ | | | | sweet |
| | | ♦ | | | | ♦ | | | | | | cold |
| | | | | | | | | | | ♦ | ♦ | cool |
| | | | ♦ | | ♦ | | | ♦ | | | | neutral |
| | ♦ | | | ♦ | | | ♦ | | ♦ | | | warm |
| **Standard dosage range (g)** | 9–12 | 6–9 | 6–15 | 6–15 | 15–30 | 6–15 | 3–9 | 60–120 | *see p.53* | 9–15 | *see p.53* | |

### Shĭ Jūn Zĭ (Quisqualis Fructus) rangoon creeper fruit

**Preparation and use** For internal use the stir fried fruit (*chao shi jun zi* 炒 使君子) is preferred as this process reduces its toxicity[1], while enhancing its ability to kill parasites and strengthen the Spleen. The dose for children is 1–1.5 seeds for every year of age, taken on an empty stomach two or three times daily, for three consecutive days. The daily dose should not exceed 20 seeds. The seeds can simply be chewed and swallowed, powdered and eaten with porridge, or decocted. When decocted the seeds should be crushed first. Should not be taken with hot tea as the combination can increase the potential for unwanted effects.

**Contraindications** The maximum dose should not be exceeded.

**Formulae** *Fei Er Wan* (accumulation disorder with heat in infants); *Bu Dai Wan* (accumulation disorder from worms); *Lei Wan San* (accumulation disorder with worms)

### Kŭ Liàn Pí (Meliae Cortex) Chinaberry tree root bark

**Preparation and use** When fresh, 15–30 grams may be used. The active component is hard to extract so prolonged decoction over low heat is best. Can be used as a retention enema, over the course of 3–4 nights, for pinworms. Used as mouth wash for dental caries. Applied topically powdered and mixed with either vinegar or a carrier oil for parasitic skin disease.

**Contraindications** Pregnancy or in patients with impaired renal or hepatic function. Caution in middle burner yang deficiency, in debilitated patients or those with anemia. Not suitable for prolonged use as toxic effects[2] can occur. The maximum dose should not be exceeded.

**Formulae** *Hua Chong Wan*† (intestinal parasites); *Lian Pi Sha Chong Yin* (retention enema for pinworms)

### Hè Shī (Carpesii abrotanoidis Fructus) carpesium fruit

**Preparation and use** Can be used in decoction, pill or powder form. Should be decocted in a cloth bag[3].

**Contraindications** Pregnancy. Caution in debilitated patients. Not suitable for prolonged use as toxic effects[4] can occur. The maximum dose should not be exceeded.

**Formulae** *Hua Chong Wan*† (intestinal parasites); *Lei Wan San* (accumulation disorder with worms); *Bai Bu Gao* (ointment for itchy psoriasis)

### Bīng Láng (Arecae Semen) betel nut

**Preparation and use** Used for tapeworms and intestinal flukes (fasciolopsis), up to 120 grams in decoction can be used, in conjunction with nan gua zi (next column) and mang xiao (p.60). The newly picked nut is considered superior to the dried nut for killing parasites.

**Contraindications** Spleen qi deficiency with loose stools. Caution during pregnancy and in patients with qi deficiency type prolapses.

**Formulae** *Qu Tao Tang* (tapeworms); *Fei Zi Guan Zhong Tang* (hookworms); *Hua Chong Wan*† (intestinal parasites); *Mu Xiang Bing Lang Wan* (constipation and abdominal distension from severe food stagnation); *Liu Mo Tang* (abdominal pain from cold and qi stagnation); *Shao Yao Tang* (dysenteric disorder from damp heat); *Shu Zao Yin Zi* (yang edema; ascites); *Ji Ming San* (weakness, pain and swelling of the legs from cold damp); *Da Yuan Yin* (malarial disorder)

### Fĕi Zĭ (Torreyae Semen) torreya seeds

**Preparation and use** Generally considered most effective when stir fried (*chao fei zi* 炒榧子), or in pill or powder form. When taken directly the dose is 9–15 grams. Can also be decocted, in which case the unprocessed herb is used in doses of 15–30 grams.

**Contraindications** Loose stools or diarrhea; cough from Lung heat or phlegm heat. Antagonistic[5] to lu dou (p.46).

**Formulae** *Fei Zi Guan Zhong Tang* (hookworms)

### Léi Wán (Omphalia) fruiting body of omphalia fungus

**Preparation and use** Not suitable for decoction; only used in pill or powder form. When used for tapeworms, 12–18 grams can be taken three times daily after food, for three consecutive days.

**Contraindications** Caution in middle burner yang deficiency. This herb is traditionally designated as slightly toxic, however modern commentators[6] dispute this.

**Formulae** *Lei Wan San* (accumulation disorder with worms); *Wu Yi San* (abdominal pain from roundworms)

### Wú Yí (Ulmi Macrocarpae Fructus Preparatus) paste made from the fruit of the stinking elm

**Preparation and use** Taken directly in pill or powder form, the dose is 2–3 grams, two or three times daily. For external use the paste can be mixed with vinegar or honey.

**Contraindications** Middle burner deficiency.

**Formulae** *Wu Yi San* (abdominal pain from roundworms); *Bu Dai Wan* (accumulation disorder from worms)

### Nán Guā Zĭ (Curcubitae moschatae Semen) pumpkin seed

**Preparation and use** Can be eaten raw or, better, ground into a fine powder and mixed with cold water into a type of porridge. For tapeworms and intestinal flukes, 60–120 grams of ground nan gua zi is taken with cold water, followed 2 hours later by a decoction of 60–120 grams of bing lang (above), then finally 30 minutes later 15 grams of mang xiao (p.60) dissolved in water. Tapeworms, or parts thereof, should be observed in the resulting bowel motions. For schistosomiasis 120–200 grams of nan gua zi can be consumed daily over a prolonged period.

**Contraindications** None noted.

**Formulae** *Qu Tao Tang* (tapeworms)

### Dà Suàn (Alli sativi Bulbus) garlic

**Preparation and use** For internal use the dose is 3–5 cloves or 6–12 grams. Raw garlic is best, mixed with other food, porridge or sugar if preferred. The large purple skinned garlic is best. Can be taken orally and as a retention enema for dysentery. Useful prophylactically (raw garlic only) against gastrointestinal and respiratory infection.

**Contraindications** Pregnancy (as a retention enema); yin deficiency with heat, or in patients with disease of the oral cavity. Garlic is irritant to the skin and mucous membranes, and prolonged contact can cause blistering.

### Guàn Zhòng (Dryopteridis crassirhizomae Rhizoma) shield fern root

Also known as dōng bĕi guàn zhòng 东北贯众 and mián mă guàn zhòng 绵马贯众.

**Preparation and use** The unprocessed herb is used to kill worms and clear toxic heat; the charred herb (*guan zhong tan* 贯众炭) is used to stop bleeding.

**Contraindications** Pregnancy, infants, weak and debilitated patients and those with gastric ulcers or erosion; yin deficiency with heat; middle burner yang deficiency. Not suitable for prolonged use as toxic effects[7] can occur. The maximum dose should not be exceeded. Avoid concurrent consumption of fats and oils (including oily seeds and herbs) as this can potentiate toxicity.

**Formulae** *Fei Zi Guan Zhong Tang* (hookworms)

### Hè Căo Yá (Agrimonia pilosa Gemma) agrimony bud

**Preparation and use** Not suitable for decoction as the active component is degraded by heat; only used in powder. The dose for adults is 30–50 grams; for infants the dose is 0.7–.08 grams per kilogram of body weight.

**Contraindications** Can cause mild gastrointestinal upset, nausea, vomiting and diarrhea, in some patients.

### Substances from other groups

Other substances with an ability to kill parasites include chun pi (p.2), shi liu pi (p.4), gan qi (p.10), xian he cao (p.14), ban bian lian (p.20), bian xu (p.20), chang shan (p.22), hong teng (p.34), ya dan zi (p.36), ku shen (p.42), zhang nao (p.50), da huang (p.60), lu hui (p.60), qian niu zi (p.62), qian jin zi (p.62), bai bu (p.68), hua jiao (p.88) and hai tong pi (p.92). For parasitic skin conditions, see also pp.24/25.

---

1 Appendix 3.2, p.104
2 Appendix 3.1, p.101
3 Appendix 6, p.109
4 Appendix 3.2, p.103
5 Appendix 2, p.100

---

6 Bensky (2004) 3rd ed., p.1004
7 Appendix 3.2, p.103

| △ Indication<br>▲ Strong Indication<br>E External Use<br>E Strong External Indication<br><br>**INDICATIONS** | Zhi Ban Xia 制半夏 | Zhi Tian Nan Xing 制天南星 | Zhi Bai Fu Zi 制白附子 | Jie Geng 桔梗 | Bai Qian 白前 | Bai Jie Zi 白芥子 | Xuan Fu Hua 旋覆花 | Zao Jia 皂荚 | Zao Jiao Ci 皂角刺 | Mao Zhua Cao 猫爪草 | | | ○ Function<br>● Strong Function<br><br><br><br>**FUNCTIONS** |
|---|---|---|---|---|---|---|---|---|---|---|---|---|---|
| abscesses & sores – phlegm, yin | E | E | | ○ | | ▲ | | △ | ● | | | | aids discharge of pus |
| abscesses & sores – skin | E | E | | ○ | | | | | ▲ E | E | | | diffuses the Lungs |
| abscess – Lung | ○ | | | ▲ | ○ | | ● | | | | | | directs qi downward |
| belching, hiccup | | ○ | ● | | | | ▲ | ○ | | | | | dispels wind phlegm |
| cancer – lymphatic | ○ | ○ | ○ | | | ○ | | | | △ ○ | | | dissipates masses |
| cervical lymphadenitis (*luo li*) | ▲ ○ | △ ○ | E | | | △ | | ▲ | △ E | △ E | | | dries damp |
| chest – stifling sensation in | ▲ | △ | | △ ● | △ | △ | ▲ | | | | | | eases the throat |
| consciousness – loss of | | | | ○ | ○ | ○ | ○ | △ E ○ | ○ | | | | expels phlegm |
| constipation | | | | △ | | | | ▲ | ○ | | | | invigorates blood |
| cough – chronic; qi & yin def. | | | | | △ | | | ○ | | | | | opens the orifices |
| cough – phlegm damp | ▲ | △ ○ | ○ | ▲ | △ | △ | △ | △ | | | | | stops spasm |
| cough – phlegm heat | | | ○ | △ | △ | △ | ○ | △ | | | | | stops pain |
| cough – stubborn phlegm | ● | ▲ | | △ | △ | | △ ○ | ▲ | | | | | stops vomiting |
| cough – thin watery phlegm | △ ○ | △ ○ | ○ | | △ | ▲ | △ | | | ○ | | | transforms phlegm |
| cough – wind heat/wind cold | | | | △ | △ | ○ | | | | | | | warms the Lungs |
| dizziness & vertigo | ▲ | △ | △ | | | | | | | | | | |
| ears – blockage of; glue ear | | | | | | | | | △ | | | | |
| fallopian tube – blockage of | | | | | | | | | △ | | | | |
| headache – phlegm damp | △ | | | | | | | | | | | | |
| headache – migraine | | | ▲ | | | | | | | △ | | | |
| hemiplegia | | ▲ | ▲ | | | | | △ | | | | | |
| hydrothorax (*xuan yin*) | △ | | | | | △ | | | | | | | |
| itch – genital | | | △ E | | | | | | | | | | |
| morning sickness | ▲ | | | | | | △ | | | | | | |
| nausea, vomiting | ▲ | | | | | | △ | | | | | | |
| nodules & masses – phlegm | △ | △ | E | | | △ | | △ | | △ E | | | **Domain** (✧) |
| numbness – extremities | ✧ | △ ✧ | △ | ✧ | ✧ | △ ✧ | ✧ | ✧ | ✧ | ✧ | | | Lung |
| pain – facial, neuralgia | | | ▲ | | | | | ✧ | | | | | Large Intestine |
| pain – joints, from phlegm | | ✧ | ✧ | | | △ E | | | ✧ | ✧ | | | Liver |
| painful obst.. – phlegm, damp | ✧ | ✧ | △ | | | △ E | | | | | | | Spleen |
| paralysis – facial | ✧ | ▲ | ▲ ✧ | | | ✧ | ✧ | △ | ✧ | | | | Stomach |
| plum pit qi (globus hystericus) | △ | | | | | | | | | | | | |
| seizures, epilepsy | | △ | △ | | | | | △ | | | | | |
| skin – eczema, stubborn | | | △ E | | | | | | | | | | **Flavour, nature** (✦) |
| snakebite | E ✦ | E ✦ | E ✦ | | | | | | | E | | | toxic (unprocessed) |
| spasm – tetanic | | △ | △ | | | | | ✦ | | | | | slightly toxic |
| spasm & tremor | ✦ | ✦ | △ ✦ | ✦ | ✦ | ✦ | ✦ | ✦ | ✦ | ✦ | | | acrid |
| throat – sore, acute & chronic | | ✦ | | ▲ | ✦ | | | | | | | | bitter |
| thyroid – nodules, goitre | △ | | | | | △ | ✦ | ✦ | | △ | | | salty |
| ulcers – skin, chronic | | | ✦ | | | ▲ | | | | ✦ | | | sweet |
| urination – retention of | | | | △ ✦ | | | | | | | | | neutral |
| voice – hoarse, loss of | ✦ | ✦ | | ▲ | | ✦ | | ✦ | ✦ | | | | warm |
| wheezing – phlegm damp | | | | △ ✦ | ▲ | △ ✦ | △ | | | ✦ | | | slightly warm |
| **Standard dosage range (g)** | 3–12 | 3–9 | 3–5 | 3–9 | 3–9 | 3–6 | 3–9 | 1.5–5 | 3–9 | 9–15 | | | |

**Zhì Bàn Xià (Pinelliae Rhizoma preparata) processed pinellia rhizome**

**Preparation and use** For complete clarity, the processed form is always specified when writing a prescription for ingestion. The zhi here designates a general processing method to render ban xia safe. Unprocessed ban xia is toxic and not used internally but can be applied topically as a paste made from the powdered herb and vinegar to dissipate nodules, for phlegm and toxic heat type masses and swellings, and treat snake bite.

Other methods that render ban xia safe[1] for ingestion and enhance specific characteristics include processing with ginger (*jiang ban xia* 姜半夏) used for nausea, vomiting and watery cough; processing with lime and licorice root (*fa ban xia* 法半夏) used for drying damp; processing with dried bamboo sap (*zhu li ban xia* 竹沥半夏) used for phlegm heat and wind phlegm; processing with alum (*qing ban xia* 清半夏) used for weak patients and children with copious phlegm.

**Contraindications** Alone in deficiency patterns, dry cough, phlegm heat, dry phlegm and bleeding disorders. Caution when phlegm and mucus are enclosed in spaces such as the inner ear or sinus (where salty softening herbs should be employed), as it can dry and thicken the phlegm into a hard glue which is difficult to shift. Incompatible[2] with zhi fu zi (p.88), zhi chuan wu (p.94) and zhi cao wu (p.94).

**Formulae** *Er Chen Tang* (phlegm); *Wen Dan Tang* (phlegm heat); *Dao Tan Tang* (productive cough and chest oppression from stubborn phlegm damp); *Ban Xia Bai Zhu Tian Ma Tang* (dizziness and headache from wind phlegm); *Ban Xia Xie Xin Tang* (mixed heat and cold blocking the qi dynamic); *Xiao Xian Xiong Tang* (focal accumulation of phlegm heat in the chest); *Ban Xia Hou Po Tang* (plum pit qi); *Mai Men Dong Tang* (nausea and gnawing hunger from Stomach yin deficiency); *Xiao Chai Hu Tang* (shaoyang syndrome); *Gua Lou Xie Bai Ban Xia Tang* (chest pain and angina from phlegm accumulation); & 50+ more in Appendix 7.

**Zhì Tiān Nán Xīng (Arisaematis Rhizoma preparata) processed arisaema rhizome; jack in the pulpit**

**Preparation and use** For internal use, tian nan xing is always processed[3]. Processing with pig bile (*dan nan xing* 胆南星, p.58) moderates the harsh acrid nature, toxicity and dryness of the herb and is widely used for stubborn phlegm heat. Unprocessed tian nan xing is toxic and not used internally, but can be applied topically as a paste made from the powdered herb and vinegar to dissipate nodules, phlegm and toxic heat type masses and swellings, and treat snake bite.

**Contraindications** Pregnancy, dry or yin deficient cough, dry phlegm patterns and in spasms, seizures and internal wind resulting from heat, or yin and blood deficiency.

**Formulae** *Yu Zhen San* (rictus and tetanic spasm from wind phlegm); *Xiao Huo Luo Dan* (stubborn painful obstruction, loss of function and numbness from cold, phlegm and blood stasis)

**Zhì Bái Fù Zǐ (Typhonii Rhizoma preparata) processed typhonium rhizome**

**Preparation and use** For internal use, bai fu zi is always processed[4]. Unprocessed bai fu zi is toxic and not used internally, but can be applied topically as a paste made from the powdered herb and vinegar to dissipate nodules, for phlegm and toxic heat type masses and swellings, and snake bite.

**Contraindications** Pregnancy, and in spasms, seizures and internal wind resulting from heat, or yin and blood deficiency.

**Formulae** *Yu Zhen San* (rictus and tetanic spasm from wind phlegm); *Qian Zheng San* (facial paralysis from wind blocking the channels)

**Jié Gěng (Platycodi Radix) balloon flower root**

**Preparation and use** Mostly used unprocessed, but can be processed with honey (*zhi jie geng* 炙桔梗) to enhance its ability to moisten the Lungs and alleviate chronic dry cough. Stir frying (*chao jie geng* 炒桔梗) reduces its tendency to cause nausea, and is best for weak patients.

**Contraindications** Chronic cough from yin deficiency; hemoptysis.

**Formulae** *Jie Geng Tang* (Lung abscess); *Xuan Shen Gan Jie Tang* (chronic sore throat from yin deficiency); *Pu Ji Xiao Du Yin* (toxic heat in the throat and head); *Xing Su San* (wind cold common cold); *Sang Xing Tang* (dry wind heat common cold); *Shen Su Yin* (wind cold with qi deficiency); *Qing Yin Wan*† (hoarse voice, loss of voice and sore throat from Lung fire); *Zhi Sou San* (persistent cough in the aftermath of an external pathogenic invasion); *Bai He Gu Jin Tang* (cough and hemoptysis from Lung yin deficiency); *Sheng Xian Tang* (sinking da qi); *Xue Fu Zhu Yu Tang* (qi and blood stasis); & 20+ more in Appendix 7.

**Bái Qián (Cynanchi stauntonii Rhizoma) cynanchum root**

**Preparation and use** Stir frying with honey (*zhi bai qian* 炙白前) enhances its ability to moisten the Lungs, loosen sticky phlegm and treat chronic cough from yin deficiency; stir frying (*chao bai qian* 炒白前) reduces its acrid dispersing nature and is used for patients with weak qi.

**Contraindications** Chronic cough from Lung qi deficiency. Can irritate the Stomach and cause nausea and pain, and aggravate gastrointestinal bleeding in patients with weak middle burner qi.

**Formulae** *Bai Qian Tang* (wheezing and orthopnea from phlegm congestion in the Lungs); *Sang Pi Bai Qian Tang* (cough from Lung heat); *Er Qian Tang* (wind heat cough); *Zhi Sou San* (persistent cough in the aftermath of an external pathogenic invasion)

**Bái Jie Zǐ (Sinapsis Semen) white mustard seed**

**Preparation and use** For internal use, the stir fried herb is preferred (*chao bai jie zi* 炒白芥子); it should be cooked for no longer than 4–5 minutes to preserve its acrid nature. Unprocessed bai jie zi is reserved for external use as in the following examples: for chronic wheezing from cold phlegm in the Lungs, the seeds can be pounded to a paste and applied to the BL-13 (*fèi shū*), CV-17 (*dàn zhōng*) and N-BW-1 (*dìng chuǎn*) acupoints until a blister forms. Ground bai jie zi can be applied topically for cold damp type musculoskeletal pain (as in mustard plasters).

**Contraindications** Chronic cough from heat and dryness, qi or yin deficiency, heat in the Stomach, gastric and esophageal ulcers, bleeding disorders or allergic skin conditions.

**Formulae** *Bai Jie Zi San* (numbness and joint pain from phlegm blocking the channels and collaterals); *San Zi Yang Qin Tang* (chronic productive cough and wheezing from phlegm damp in the Lungs); *Kong Xian Dan* (thin mucus congesting the upper and middle burner); *Yang He Tang* (yin sores)

**Xuán Fù Huā (Inulae Flos) inula flower**

**Preparation and use** Cooked in a cloth bag[5] as the small hairs on the leaf can irritate the throat. Stir frying with honey (*zhi xuan fu hua* 炙旋覆花) enhances its ability to moisten the Lungs and moderates its acrid dispersing nature, being used for cough and wheezing from Lung qi and yin deficiency with sticky phlegm.

**Contraindications** Dry, yin deficient or wind heat type cough and wheezing, or for debilitated patients with loose stools.

**Formulae** *Xuan Fu Dai Zhe Tang* (vomiting and nausea from rebellious Stomach qi); *Xuan Fu Hua Tang* (wheezing and dyspnea from phlegm congestion in the chest); *Jin Fei Cao San* (wind cold common cold with cough and wheezing)

**Zào Jiá (Gleditsiae Fructus) Chinese honeylocust fruit**

Also commonly known as zào jiǎo 皂角.

**Preparation and use** For internal use, the baked form is used (*hei jiao zao jia* 焙焦皂荚). Taken directly as powder or pills, the dose is 0.6–1.5 grams. To restore consciousness, a small amount of powdered zao jia can be blown into the nose. The maximum dose should not be exceeded or toxic effects[6] may occur. Antagonistic[7] to ren shen (p.74).

**Contraindications** Pregnancy; qi and yin deficiency.

**Formulae** *Tong Guan San* (loss of consciousness from wind phlegm); *Zao Jia Wan* (chronic wheezing from stubborn phlegm)

---

1 Insufficient processing of the raw material may lead to toxic residues. Symptoms of toxicity can be found in Appendix 3.1, p.102
2 Appendix 2, p.100
3 See footnote 1
4 See footnote 1

---

5 Appendix 6, p.109
6 Appendix 3.2, p.104
7 Appendix 2, p.100

............continued on page 59

| INDICATIONS | Qian Hu 前胡 | Quan Gua Lou 全瓜楼 | Gua Lou Pi 瓜楼皮 | Gua Lou Ren 瓜楼仁 | Chuan Bei Mu 川贝母 | Zhe Bei Mu 浙贝母 | Zhu Ru 竹茹 | Zhu Li 竹沥 | Tian Zhu Huang 天竺黄 | Kun Bu 昆布 | Hai Zao 海藻 | Pang Da Hai 胖大海 | FUNCTIONS |
|---|---|---|---|---|---|---|---|---|---|---|---|---|---|
| abscess – breast, mastitis | | ▲ | △ | △ | | ▲ | | | | | | ○ | diffuses the Lungs |
| abscess – Intestinal | ○ | △ | | △ | | | | | | | | | directs qi downward |
| abscess – Lung | ○ | △ | △ | △ | △ | ▲ | | | | | | | dispels wind heat |
| abscesses & sores – skin | | | | △ | △ ○ | △ ● | | | | ○ | ○ | | dissipates masses |
| anxiety, irritability | | | | | | | ▲ | | △ | | | ○ | eases the throat |
| aphasia – after wind stroke | ○ | | | | | | | △ | ▲ | | | | expels phlegm |
| bleeding – hemoptysis | | | | ○ | △ | | △ | | | | | ○ | moistens the Intestines |
| breast – cysts & lumps | | △ | △ | | △ ● | ▲ | | | | | | | moistens the Lungs |
| cervical lymphadenitis (luo li) | | | | | △ | ▲ | | ○ | ● | △ | △ | | opens the orifices |
| chest – stifling sensation in | | ▲ | △ | △ | | | △ | | | ○ | ○ | | promotes urination |
| coma – phlegm obstruction | | | | | ○ | | | △ | ▲ | | | | stops cough |
| common cold – wind heat | △ | | | | | | | | ● | | | | stops spasm & tremor |
| constipation – dryness, heat | | | | ▲ | | | ● | | | | | △ | stops vomiting |
| convulsions – febrile | ○ | ● | ○ | ○ | ○ | ○ | ● | △ ○ | ▲ ● | ○ | ○ | ○ | transforms phlegm heat |
| convulsions – infantile | | ● | ○ | | | | | △ | ▲ | | | | unbinds the chest |
| cough – chronic, dry; def. | △ | | | △ | ▲ | | | | | | | | |
| cough – Lung heat | | △ | △ | △ | ▲ | △ | △ | | | | | △ | |
| cough – phlegm heat | △ | ▲ | △ | ▲ | ▲ | △ | | △ | △ | | | △ | |
| cough – stubborn phlegm | | ▲ | △ | △ | ▲ | △ | | △ | △ | | | | |
| cough – wind heat | △ | | | | △ | △ | | | | | | | |
| edema | | | | | | | | | | △ | △ | | |
| hemiplegia | | | | | | | | △ | △ | | | | |
| insomnia, restlessness | | | | | | | ▲ | | △ | | | | |
| liver – cirrhosis; hepatomegaly | | | | | | | | | | △ | △ | | |
| masses – abdominal | | | | | | △ | | | | △ | △ | | |
| morning sickness | | | | | | | ▲ | | | | | | |
| night terrors – phlegm heat | | | | | | | | | △ | | | | **Domain (❖)** |
| nodules & masses – phlegm | ❖ | ❖ | ❖ | ❖ | △ ❖ | ▲ ❖ | ❖ | ❖ | | △ | △ | ❖ | Lung |
| pain – chest, angina | | ▲ ❖ | △ ❖ | ❖ | | | | | | | | ❖ | Large Intestine |
| pain – chest; focal, pleuritic | | △ | ▲ | | | | | | | ❖ | ❖ | | Kidney |
| pain – testicular, with swelling | | | | | | | | | ❖ | △ ❖ | △ ❖ | | Liver |
| palpitations | | | | | | | △ ❖ | | ▲ ❖ | | | | Gallbladder |
| seizures, epilepsy | | | | | ❖ | ❖ | | △ ❖ | ▲ ❖ | | | | Heart |
| throat – sore & dry; chronic | | ❖ | ❖ | ❖ | | | ❖ | ❖ | | ❖ | ❖ | △ | Stomach |
| thyroid – benign nodules | | | | | | ▲ | | | | △ | △ | | |
| thyroid – goitre | | | | | | | | | | ▲ | ▲ | | |
| thyroid – hyperthyroidism | | | | | | | | | | ▲ | ▲ | | **Flavour, nature (♦)** |
| voice – hoarse, loss of | ♦ | | | | | | | | | | | ▲ | acrid |
| vomiting, nausea – phlegm heat | ♦ | | | ♦ | | ♦ | ▲ | | | | | | bitter |
| vomiting, nausea – St. def. | | | | | | | ▲ | | | ♦ | ♦ | △ | salty |
| wheezing – phlegm heat | △ | △ ♦ | △ ♦ | △ ♦ | △ ♦ | △ | ♦ | △ ♦ | ▲ ♦ | | | ♦ | sweet |
| wind stroke – sequelae of | ♦ | | | | ♦ | | ♦ | △ | △ | | | | cool |
| withdrawal mania (dian kuang) | | ♦ | ♦ | ♦ | | ♦ | | △ ♦ | ♦ | ♦ | | ♦ | cold |
| Standard dosage range (g) | 6–9 | 9–24 | 6–12 | 9–15 | 3–9 | 6–9 | 6–9 | 30–60 | 3–9 | 9–15 | 9–15 | see p.59 | |

△ Indication
▲ Strong Indication
E External Use
E Strong External Indication

○ Function
● Strong Function

## Zào Jiǎo Cì (Gleditsiae Spina) Chinese honeylocust thorn

**Contraindications** Pregnancy; ruptured lesions.

**Formulae** *Bai Ling Tiao Gan Tang* (infertility from blocked fallopian tubes or endometriosis); *Xian Fang Huo Ming Yin*† (toxic heat boils and sores); *Tou Nong San*† (yin sores); *Qin Jiao Bai Zhu Wan* (chronic constipation with bleeding, itchy hemorrhoids); *Nei Xiao San*† (suppurative skin lesions); *Gua Lou Niu Bang Tang* (acute mastitis and breast abscess)

## Māo Zhuǎ Cǎo (Ranunculus ternatus Radix) cat claw buttercup root

**Preparation and use** When used externally for phlegm nodules, the fresh herb can be mashed and applied topically.

**Contraindications** None noted.

### Substances from other groups

Other substances with some ability to transform phlegm include shi chang pu (p.50), chen pi (p.64), zhi shi (p.64), xie bai (p.64), xiang yuan (p.66), fo shou (p.66), yuan zhi (p.70), dong chong xia cao (p.82) and gan jiang (p.88).

### Endnotes

† These formulae traditionally contain items from endangered animal species and/or obsolete toxic substances, and are unavailable in their original form.

# 12.2 PHLEGM – PHLEGM HEAT

## Qián Hú (Peucedani Radix) hogfennel root

**Preparation and use** The unprocessed root is used for phlegm heat and wind heat cough; stir frying with honey (*mi zhi quan hu* 蜜炙前胡) enhances its warming and moistening properties, and is used for chronic dry cough from Lung deficiency.

**Contraindications** Cough from Lung yin deficiency (unprocessed) or cough and wheezing with thin watery phlegm.

**Formulae** *Qian Hu San* (cough from phlegm heat); *Er Qian Tang* (wind heat cough); *Xing Su San* (wind cold cough); *Shen Su Yin* (wind cold with qi deficiency); *Xuan Du Fa Biao Tang* (early stage of measles)

## Qúan Guā Lóu (Trichosanthis Fructus) trichosanthes fruit

Also known as guā lóu shí 瓜楼实. Gua lou 瓜楼 is also written as 栝楼.

**Contraindications** Spleen qi deficiency with diarrhea and thin or cold phlegm. Incompatible[1] with zhi fu zi (p.88), zhi chuan wu (p.94) and zhi cao wu (p.94).

**Formulae** *Gua Lou Xie Bai Ban Xia Tang* (chest pain and angina from phlegm accumulation); *Bei Mu Gua Lou San* (cough with sticky phlegm); *Si Sheng San* (breast, Lung and Intestinal abscesses); *Xiao Ru Tang*† (early stage of breast abscess and mastitis); *Bai Ling Tiao Gan Tang* (infertility from blocked fallopian tubes or endometriosis)

## Guā Lóu Pí (Trichosanthis Pericarpium) trichosanthes peel

**Preparation and use** In severe cases up to 30 grams can be used. Stir frying (*chao gua lou pi* 炒瓜楼皮) moderates its coldness and makes it better for productive cough without heat, and for patients with loose stools; stir frying with honey (*mi gua lou pi* 蜜瓜楼皮) enhances its ability to moisten the Lungs and alleviate dry cough from yin deficiency.

**Contraindications** Spleen qi deficiency with diarrhea and thin watery or cold phlegm. Incompatible[2] with zhi fu zi (p.88), zhi chuan wu (p.94) and zhi cao wu (p.94).

**Formulae** *Xiao Xian Xiong Tang* (focal chest wall and pleuritic pain from phlegm heat)

## Guā Lóu Rén (Trichosanthis Semen) trichosanthes seed

**Preparation and use** Should be broken up in a mortar and pestle before decoction. Stir frying (*chao gua lou ren* 炒瓜楼仁) reduces the tendency of the oily seeds to cause nausea and vomiting, while retaining an ability to moisten and transform phlegm; removing the oil altogether (*lou ren shuang* 楼仁霜) diminishes the seeds ability to moisten the Intestines, but is better for Spleen deficient patients with productive cough.

**Contraindications** Spleen qi deficiency with diarrhea and nausea. Incompatible[3] with zhi fu zi (p.88), zhi chuan wu (p.94) and zhi cao wu (p.94).

**Formulae** *Qing Qi Hua Tan Wan* (phlegm heat in the Lungs); *Ke Xue Fang* (hemoptysis from Liver fire invading the Lungs); *Gua Lou Niu Bang Tang* (acute mastitis and breast abscess); *Er Mu Ning Sou Wan* (phlegm heat in the Lungs)

## Chuān Bèi Mǔ (Fritillariae cirrhosae Bulbus) Sichuan fritillaria bulb

**Preparation and use** Can be decocted, but more often ground to a fine powder and taken directly[4], or followed by an appropriate decoction. When taken directly as powder, the dose is 1–1.5 grams, two or three times daily.

**Contraindications** Middle burner yang deficiency, thin cold or watery phlegm. Incompatible[5] with zhi fu zi (p.88), zhi chuan wu (p.94) and zhi cao wu (p.94).

**Formulae** *She Dan Chuan Bei Mo* (prepared powder for phlegm heat cough); *Er Mu San* (cough from Lung dryness or heat); *Er Mu Ning Sou Wan* (phlegm heat in the Lungs); *Qing Ge Jian* (cough from phlegm heat with particularly viscous phlegm); *Bai He Gu Jin Tang* (chronic dry cough from Lung yin deficiency)

## Zhè Bèi Mǔ (Fritillariae thunbergii Bulbus) Zhejiang fritillaria

**Contraindications** Middle burner yang deficiency, thin cold or watery phlegm. Incompatible[6] with zhi fu zi (p.88), zhi chuan wu (p.94) and zhi cao wu (p.94).

**Formulae** *Bei Mu Gua Lou San* (cough with sticky phlegm); *Xiao Luo Wan* (phlegm and phlegm heat type masses and nodules); *Hai Zao Yu Hu Tang* (goitre); *Xian Fang Huo Ming Yin*† (toxic heat boils and sores); *Nei Xiao San*† (suppurative skin lesions)

## Zhú Rú (Bambusae Caulis in taeniam) bamboo shavings

**Preparation and use** The unprocessed herb is used to transform phlegm heat; processing with ginger juice (*jiang zhu ru* 姜竹茹) moderates its coldness and enhances its ability to stop nausea and vomiting.

**Contraindications** Nausea and vomiting from cold in the Stomach (unprocessed), cough with thin watery phlegm.

**Formulae** *Wen Dan Tang* (insomnia, anxiety, bitter taste and nausea from Gallbladder and Stomach disharmony and phlegm heat); *Ju Pi Zhu Ru Tang* (nausea and vomiting from Stomach deficiency); *Huang Lian Zhu Ru Ju Pi Ban Xia Tang* (vomiting from phlegm heat)

## Zhú Lì (Bambusae Succus) dried bamboo sap

**Preparation and use** Should not be cooked. Dissolve in the warm strained decoction[7]. For disturbances or loss of consciousness, zhi li can be blown into the nose or given via enema.

**Contraindications** Cough from cold or deficiency, and middle burner deficiency with loose stools.

**Formulae** *Zhu Li Hua Tan Wan* (hemiplegia following wind stroke); *Zhu Li Da Tan Wan* (mania and mental disorders from phlegm fire); *Ding Xian Wan*† (seizures from wind phlegm)

---

1 Appendix 2, p.100
2 Ibid.
3 Ibid.

4 Appendix 6, p.109
5 Appendix 2, p.100
6 Appendix 2, p.100
7 Appendix 6, p.108

**Legend**

△ Indication
▲ Strong Indication
E External Use
E Strong External Indication

○ Function
● Strong Function

| INDICATIONS | Dan Nan Xing 胆南星 | Zhu Dan Zhi 猪胆汁 | Han Cai 蕹菜 | Ming Dang Shen 明党参 | Bi Qi 荸荠 | Luo Han Guo 罗汉果 | Hai Ge Qiao 海蛤壳 | Fu Hai Shi 浮海石 | Qing Meng Shi 青礞石 | | | | FUNCTIONS |
|---|---|---|---|---|---|---|---|---|---|---|---|---|---|
| abscesses & sores – skin | | E | E | | | | ○ | | | | | | alleviates gastric acidity |
| acid reflux, heartburn | | | ○ | | | | △ | | | | | | alleviates jaundice |
| bleeding – hemoptysis | | | | | ○ | △ | | △ | | | | | brightens the eyes |
| burns & scalds | | E | | | | | E | ○ | | | | | calms the Liver |
| cervical lymphadenitis (luo li) | | ○ | ○ | | △ | | ▲ | △ | | | | | clears toxic heat |
| chest – stifling sensation in | △ | △ | | | | | △ | ○ | | | | | directs qi downward |
| constipation – heat, dryness | | △ | | | △ | △ | ● | ○ | △ | | | | dissipates masses |
| convulsions – chronic childhood | ▲ | | | | | | | | △ ● | | | | drives out phlegm |
| cough – dry phlegm; yin def. | ○ | | | △ | △ | △ | | | | | | | extinguishes wind |
| cough – Lung heat | △ | △ | △ | △ | ○ | △ ● | △ | △ | | | | | generates fluids |
| cough – phlegm damp | | | ○ | △ | | | | | | | | | harmonizes the Stomach |
| cough – phlegm heat | △ | △ | △ | | △ | ○ | ▲ | ▲ | △ | | | | moistens the Lungs |
| cough – stubborn, chronic | ▲ ○ | △ | | △ | | | ▲ | ▲ | △ ○ | | | | stops spasm & tremor |
| cough – whooping | △ ● | △ ○ | ○ | ○ | ○ | ○ | ● | ○ | ○ | | | | transforms phlegm heat |
| dysenteric disorder | | △ | | | | | | | | | | | |
| dysuria – blood, stone | | | | | | | | △ | | | | | |
| dysuria – damp heat | | | | | | | | △ | | | | | |
| ears – otitis, acute & chronic | △ | △ | | | | | | | | | | | |
| ears – glue ear | △ | △ | | | | | | | | | | | |
| edema – damp heat | | | | | | | △ | | | | | | |
| eyes – cataract, pterygia | | | | | △ | | | | | | | | |
| eyes – red, sore | | | △ | | △ | | | | | | | | |
| food stagnation – severe | | | | | | | | △ | | | | | |
| gallstones | | △ | | | | | | | | | | | |
| hemiplegia | △ | | | | | | | | | | | | **Domain (❖)** |
| jaundice – damp heat | ❖ | △ ❖ | △ ❖ | ❖ | ❖ | ❖ | ❖ | ❖ | ❖ | | | | Lung |
| nasosinusitis (bi yuan) | ▲ | ▲ ❖ | | | ❖ | ❖ | | | | | | | Large Intestine |
| nodules & masses – phlegm | ❖ | ❖ | ❖ | ❖ | | | ▲ | △ | ❖ | | | | Liver |
| pain – epigastric, & hyperacidity | | ❖ | | | | | △ | | | | | | Gallbladder |
| palpitations | ❖ | | | | | | | ▲ | | | | | Spleen |
| paralysis – facial | △ | | | | ❖ | | ❖ | | | | | | Stomach |
| seizures, epilepsy | △ | | | | | | | △ | | | | | |
| skin – damp rashes; nappy rash | | | | | | | E | | | | | | |
| thirst – in warm disease | | | | △ | △ | △ | | | | | | | **Flavour, nature (◆)** |
| throat – sore; acute | △ | △ | △ ◆ | | | △ | | | | | | | acrid |
| thyroid – nodules, goitre | ◆ | | | | | | ▲ | △ | | | | | slightly acrid |
| tonsils – chronic swelling of | ▲ ◆ | ◆ | △ ◆ | | | △ | ◆ | | | | | | bitter |
| tremors – wind phlegm | △ | | | ◆ | | | | | △ | | | | slightly bitter |
| ulcers – gastric | | | | | | | △ ◆ | ◆ | ◆ | | | | salty |
| ulcers – skin, chronic | | | | ◆ | ◆ | ◆ | E | ◆ | | | | | sweet |
| wheezing – phlegm damp | | ◆ | △ | | | | ◆ | ◆ | | | | | cold |
| wheezing – phlegm heat | △ ◆ | | △ | △ ◆ | ◆ | ◆ | △ | △ | ▲ | | | | cool |
| withdrawal mania (dian kuang) | | | ◆ | | | | | | △ ◆ | | | | neutral |
| **Standard dosage range (g)** | 3–6 | 3–6 | 9–30 | 6–12 | 30–90 | see p.59 | 9–15 | 6–9 | 6–9 | | | | |

**Tiān Zhú Huáng (Bambusae Concretio silicea)** crystalline secretion of bamboo, composed largely of silica; also known as tabasheer or bamboo sugar

**Preparation and use** Taken directly as powder, the dose is 0.6–1 gram.

**Contraindications** Cough from cold or deficiency. Caution in patients with middle burner deficiency.

**Formulae** *Tian Zhu Huang San* (night terrors and infantile convulsions from phlegm heat); *Bao Long Wan*† (seizures from phlegm heat); *Qing Fei Hua Tan Wan* (cough from phlegm heat)

**Kūn Bù (Eckloniae Thallus)** kelp

**Preparation and use** When used to treat relatively severe hyperthyroidism, doses of up to 60 grams may be used for a week or two.

**Contraindications** Incompatible[1] with gan cao (p.74).

**Formulae** *Hai Zao Yu Hu Tang* (goitre); *Ju He Wan* (testicular swelling and pain from cold damp); *Xia Ku Cao Gao* (phlegm nodules)

**Hǎi Zǎo (Sargassum)** sargassum seaweed

**Preparation and use** When used to treat relatively severe hyperthyroidism, doses of up to 60 grams may be used for a week or two.

**Contraindications** Incompatible[2] with gan cao (p.74).

**Formulae** *Hai Zao Yu Hu Tang* (goitre); *Nei Xiao Luo Li Wan* (neck lumps and scrofula from phlegm); *Ju He Wan* (testicular swelling and pain from cold damp)

**Pàng Dà Hǎi (Sterculiae lychnophorae Semen)** sterculia seed

**Preparation and use** The dose is 3–5 seeds. Can be taken as tea (several seeds steeped in boiling water) and sipped throughout the day for those using their voices to excess.

**Contraindications** Middle burner yang deficiency; cold type cough.

**Dǎn Nán Xīng (Arisaema cum Bile)** bile processed arisaema

This is tian nan xing processed with cow, pig or goat bile. While normally considered a variant of the parent herb and listed in the same category, its action is sufficiently distinct for inclusion in this section. The harsh acrid, drying and toxic nature of the parent herb (zhi tian nan xing, p.54) is reduced, and it becomes bitter and cool. Dan nan xing is not considered toxic (but see appendix 3.2, p.103), and is more widely applicable than the parent herb.

**Preparation and use** Mostly used in pills and powders. Quite unpleasant in decoction and easily causes nausea.

**Contraindications** Pregnancy. Caution in patients with middle burner yang deficiency or cold phlegm problems.

**Formulae** *Hui Chun Dan*† (childhood febrile convulsions); *Qian Jin San*† (chronic childhood convulsions from phlegm heat); *Bao Long Wan*† (seizures from phlegm heat); *Ding Xian Wan*† (seizures from wind phlegm); *Qing Qi Hua Tan Wan* (phlegm heat in the Lungs); *Qing Ge Jian* (cough from phlegm heat with particularly viscous phlegm); *Sheng Tie Luo Yin*† (mania from phlegm fire); *Zhu Li Hua Tan Wan* (hemiplegia following wind stroke); *Di Tan Tang* (mental cloudiness, confusion and aphasia from wind stroke); *Cang Fu Dao Tan Tang* (amenorrhea from phlegm damp)

**Zhū Dǎn Zhī (Suis Fel)** pig bile

**Preparation and use** Used primarily in prepared medicines as concentrated syrup, in pills, or powder packed in capsules. The dose of concentrated extract is 1–1.5 grams, two or three times daily. For severe heat type constipation, 30–60 milliliters of bile can be inserted in the rectum with a commercial enema device.

**Contraindications** Caution in middle burner yang deficiency and cold phlegm problems.

**Formulae** *Bai Ri Ke Ke Li Ji* (whooping cough); *Dan Bai Zhi Ke Pian* (chronic bronchitis); *Huo Dan Wan* (chronic sinus congestion); *Bi Yan Ning* (prepared medicine for chronic sinus congestion); *Er Yan San* (topical powder for ear infection)

**Hǎn Cài (Rorippa montana Herba)** yellow cress

**Preparation and use** The fresh herb can be crushed and applied topically.

**Contraindications** None noted.

**Míng Dǎng Shēn (Changii Radix)** changium root

**Contraindications** Pregnancy and middle burner deficiency.

**Bí Qí (Eleocharitis Rhizoma)** water chestnut

**Preparation and use** Can be crushed into a powder and taken as porridge for Stomach heat and dryness problems. If the juice extracted from the fresh corms is used, the dose is 30–60 milliliters.

**Contraindications** Middle burner yang deficiency, blood deficiency.

**Luó Hàn Guǒ (Momordicae Fructus)** momordica fruit

**Preparation and use** The usual dose is 1–2 fruit (or 15–30 grams) at a time. This fruit is processed into a variety of widely available prepared forms.

**Contraindications** None noted.

**Hǎi Gé Qiào (Meretricis/Cyclinae)** clam shell

**Preparation and use** The shell should be crushed and decocted in a cloth bag for 30 minutes[3] prior to the other herbs. Can be taken directly as a fine powder. For transforming hot phlegm and softening hardness the unprocessed shell is used; for topical use and to counteract gastric hyperacidity the calcined shell is used (*duan ge qiao* 煅蛤壳).

**Contraindications** Cough from Lung deficiency with cold and for patients with middle burner yang deficiency.

**Formulae** *Dai Ge San* (cough and hemoptysis from Liver fire invading the Lungs); *Han Hua Wan* (phlegm type benign thyroid nodules and cervical lymphadenopathy); *Zhu Gen San* (rectal or uterine bleeding from heat); *Nei Xiao Luo Li Wan* (neck lumps and scrofula from phlegm)

**Fú Hǎi Shí (Costaziae Os)** costazia (bryozoan) skeleton; largely composed of calcium carbonate

Also known as hǎi fú shí 海浮石.

**Preparation and use** Should be crushed and decocted in a cloth bag for 30 minutes[4] prior to the other herbs.

**Contraindications** Cough from Lung deficiency with cold and middle burner yang deficiency.

**Formulae** *Qing Dai Hai Shi Wan* (phlegm heat in the Lungs); *Qing Ge Jian* (cough from phlegm heat with viscous phlegm); *Ke Xue Fang* (hemoptysis from Liver fire invading the Lungs)

**Qīng Méng Shí (Chloriti Lapis)** chlorite

**Preparation and use** Should be crushed and decocted in a cloth bag for 30 minutes[5] prior to the other herbs. When taken directly in pills or powder the dose is 1.5–3 grams. The calcined form (*duan meng shi* 煅礞石) is preferred for internal use.

**Contraindications** Pregnancy, chronic childhood convulsions, the absence of phlegm heat, and middle burner deficiency.

**Formulae** *Meng Shi Gun Tang Wan* (phlegm fire type mental disorders, mania, severe palpitations or seizures); *Zhu Li Da Tan Wan* (mania and mental disorders from phlegm fire)

**Substances from other groups**

Other substances with an ability to transform phlegm heat include yu jin (p.8), wa leng zi (p.10), che qian zi (p.18), dong gua zi (p.18), huang yao zi (p.86) and niu huang (p.96).

**Endnotes**

† These formulae traditionally contain items from endangered animal species and/or obsolete toxic substances, and are unavailable in their original form.

---

1 Appendix 2, p.100. This incompatibility is not adhered to, and both kun bu and hai zao appear in prescriptions with gan cao, without discernible consequences. The prohibition, while still cited in many contemporary texts, was removed from the official pharmacopoeia in 1977.
2 Ibid.

---

3 Appendix 6, p.108
4 Ibid.
5 Ibid.

| △ Indication / ▲ Strong Indication / E External Use / E Strong External Indication — INDICATIONS | Da Huang 大黄 | Mang Xiao 芒硝 | Fan Xie Ye 番泻叶 | Lu Hui 芦荟 | Huo Ma Ren 火麻仁 | Yu Li Ren 郁李仁 | Song Zi Ren 松子仁 | ○ Function / ● Strong Function — FUNCTIONS |
|---|---|---|---|---|---|---|---|---|
| abscesses & sores – skin | △E○ | E | | E | | | | clears damp heat |
| abscess – breast, mastitis | ● | E○ | ○ | ○ | | | | clears heat |
| abscess – Intestinal | ▲● | ○ | | | | | | clears toxic heat |
| accumulation disorder (*gan ji*) | ○ | | | △ | | | | cools the blood |
| alopecia | | | | ○ | E | | | cools the Liver |
| amenorrhea – bld. stasis, heat | ▲○ | | | | | | | invigorates blood |
| ascites | △○ | | △ | ○ | | | | kills parasites |
| bleeding – epistaxis, Lu. heat | △ | | | | ○ | ○ | ○ | moistens the Intestines |
| bleeding – hematemesis, heat | △ | | | | | | ○ | moistens the Lungs |
| burns & scalds | E | | ○ | | | ○ | | promotes urination |
| constipation – dryness, chronic | ● | ○ | ○ | ○ | ▲ | ▲ | △ | purges the Intestines |
| constipation – excess heat | ▲ | ▲○ | △ | △ | | | | softens hardness |
| constipation – Liver heat | | | | ▲ | | | ○ | stops cough |
| constipation – qi stagnation | | | | | △ | △ | | |
| constipation – yin, blood def. | | | | | ▲ | ▲ | △ | |
| convulsions – febrile in children | | | | △ | | | | |
| cough – dry, unproductive | | | | | | △ | | |
| cough – stubborn phlegm heat | △ | △ | | | | | | |
| delirium – in high fever | △ | | | | | | | |
| dizziness, vertigo – Liver fire | | | | △ | | | | |
| dysentery – early stage of | ▲ | | | | | | | |
| dysuria – damp heat | △ | | | | | | | |
| edema – mild, superficial | | | | | | △ | | |
| edema – pulmonary, pleural | △ | | | | | | | |
| erysipelas | | E | | | | | | **Domain (❖)** |
| eyes – red & sore | △ | E❖ | | △ | | | ❖ | Lung |
| gallstones; cholecystitis | ▲❖ | ❖ | ❖ | ❖ | ❖ | ❖ | ❖ | Large Intestine |
| headache – Liver fire | ❖ | | | △❖ | | | ❖ | Liver |
| hemorrhoids – heat, damp heat | ❖ | | | E | | | | Heart |
| jaundice – damp heat | ▲ | | | | | ❖ | | Small Intestine |
| mania – phlegm fire | △❖ | | | | ❖ | ❖ | | Spleen |
| masses – abdominal; bld. stasis | △❖ | ❖ | | | ❖ | | | Stomach |
| pain – hypochondriac | | | | △ | | | | |
| parasites – intestinal | △ | | | △ | | | | |
| parasites – candidiasis | △ | | | | | | | **Flavour, nature (♦)** |
| skin – eczema | ♦ | E | ♦ | ♦ | | | | slightly toxic |
| skin – scabies | | | E | | | ♦ | | acrid |
| skin – tinea, ringworm | E♦ | ♦ | ♦ | E♦ | | ♦ | | bitter |
| seizures – phlegm heat, fire | △ | △♦ | | | | | | salty |
| throat – sore; acute | △ | E | ♦ | | ♦ | | ♦ | sweet |
| traumatic injury | △E♦ | ♦ | ♦ | ♦ | | | | cold |
| ulcers – mouth | △ | △E | | | ♦ | ♦ | | neutral |
| yang ming organ syndrome | ▲ | ▲ | △ | △ | | | ♦ | warm |
| **Standard dosage range (g)** | 3–15 | 9–15 | 1–6 | 1–2 | 9–15 | 6–12 | 6–9 | |

## PURGATIVES

### Dà Huáng (Rhei Radix et Rhizoma) rhubarb root

**Preparation and use** For purgation, large doses are used in decoction, up to 15 grams in *yang ming* syndrome with high fever. To break up blood stasis, smaller doses, 3–6 grams are used. As a purge, da huang should be added 3–5 minutes before the end[1] of cooking time – the shorter the cooking the stronger the purge. It can take 6–12 hours to open the bowel. To enhance its ability to invigorate blood it is cooked longer, at least 20 minutes. When used in pill form reduce the dose by half. Unprocessed da huang is a stronger purge than processed. Processing with wine (*jiu da huang* 酒大黄) enhances its ability to clear heat from the upper body; processing with vinegar (*cu da huang* 醋大黄) enhances its ability to break up blood stasis; and can be charred (*da huang tan* 大黄炭) to stop bleeding.

**Contraindications** Pregnancy, during menstruation, postpartum and while breast–feeding, in acute surface syndromes or middle burner yang deficiency. Caution in patients with qi and blood deficiency. Not suitable for prolonged use as habituation and toxic effects[2] may occur.

**Formulae** *Da Cheng Qi Tang* (*yang ming* organ syndrome); *Ma Zi Ren Wan* (chronic dry constipation); *Wen Pi Tang* (constipation from Spleen yang deficiency); *Zeng Ye Cheng Qi Tang* (constipation following a febrile disease); *Liang Ge Tang* (fire flaring to the head); *Xie Xin Tang* (bleeding from heat in the blood); *Jin Huang San* (topical treatment for boils and burns); *Da Huang Mu Dan Tang* (Intestinal abscess); *Tao He Cheng Qi Tang* (blood stasis and heat in the lower burner); *Fu Yuan Huo Xue Tang*† (traumatic blood stasis); *Da Huang Zhe Chong Wan* (severe blood stasis); *Yin Chen Hao Tang* (damp heat jaundice); *Bi Huo Dan* (topical ointment for burns and scalds); & 30+ more in Appendix 7.

### Máng Xiāo (Natrii Sulfas) sodium sulphate; Glauber's salts

**Preparation and use** Dissolved[3] into the warm strained decoction. When used topically it is dissolved in water and used to soak a cloth that is applied warm to the affected area, or mixed with a neutral carrier, such as sorbolene, to hold it in place.

**Contraindications** Pregnancy, if used internally during breast feeding, and in middle burner yang deficiency.

**Formulae** *Da Cheng Qi Tang* (*yang ming* organ syndrome); *Liang Ge Tang* (fire flaring to the head); *She Gan Tang* (sore throat from Lung heat)

### Fān Xiè Yè (Senna Folium) senna leaf

**Preparation and use** For a mild laxative effect 1–2 grams is sufficient; for a stronger purge 3–9 grams can be used. Most frequently steeped as tea. If decocted with other herbs, it should be added about 5 minutes[4] before the end of cooking. If used in powder or pill form the effect is milder. Not suitable for prolonged use as habituation can occur.

**Contraindications** Pregnancy, during menstruation or while breast feeding, in chronic constipation and in weak or debilitated patients. Repeated large doses (over 6 grams) can cause toxic symptoms[5].

### Lú Huì (Aloe) dried latex of Aloe barbadensis or A. ferox.

❋ Aloes are listed in Appendix 2 of CITES[6] which permits limited trade with appropriate documentation.

**Preparation and use** Not suitable for decoction. Use in pill, capsule or powder form only.

**Contraindications** Pregnancy and middle burner yang deficiency. Caution during breast feeding. Not suitable for prolonged use as habituation is common and toxic effects[7] may occur.

**Formulae** *Dang Gui Long Hui Wan* (Liver fire with constipation); *Fei Er Wan* (accumulation disorder with fever and heat in infants)

### Endnotes

† These formulae traditionally contain items from endangered animal species and/or obsolete toxic substances, and are unavailable in their original form.

## MOIST LAXATIVES

### Huǒ Má Rén (Cannabis Semen) cannabis seed

**Preparation and use** Crush before decoction to break the husk and release the oils. Crushed cannabis seeds are commonly cooked with rice porridge (*zhou* 粥) for chronic constipation in the elderly. For alopecia in adults and cradle cap in infants the oil derived from the crushed seeds can be massaged into the scalp.

**Contraindications** None noted when used within the normal dosage range. Excessive or chronic consumption (with food for example) may lead to gastrointestinal upset, numbness of the limbs and clouding of consciousness.

**Formulae** *Ma Zi Ren Wan* (chronic dry constipation); *Ma Ren Cong Rong Tang* (constipation in postpartum women with blood deficiency); *Run Chang Wan* (chronic constipation from blood dryness); *Zhi Gan Cao Tang* (arrhythmia from qi and blood deficiency); *Da Ding Feng Zhu* (spasms and tremors from yin and blood deficiency)

### Yù Lǐ Rén (Pruni Semen) bush cherry seed

**Preparation and use** Crush before decoction.

**Contraindications** Pregnancy.

**Formulae** *Wu Ren Wan* (chronic constipation from dryness or blood deficiency); *Yu Li Ren Tang* (edema)

### Sōng Zǐ Rén (Pinus Semen) pine nut

**Preparation and use** Crushed pine nuts are commonly cooked with rice porridge (*zhou* 粥) or other appropriate foods for chronic dry constipation.

**Contraindications** Caution in patients with phlegm damp and Spleen qi deficiency.

### Substances from other groups

Herbs from other groups that can purge the bowel include qian niu zi (p.62) and ba dou shuang (p.62).

Herbs from other groups with some lubricating effect on the bowel include tao ren (p.6), dong kui zi (p.20), niu bang zi (p.26), xuan shen (p.40), sheng di huang (p.40), jue ming zi (p.48), fei zi (p.52), gua lou ren (p.56), luo han guo (p.58), zhu dan zhi (p.58) xing ren (p.68), bai zi ren (p.70), feng mi (p.74), dang gui (p.78), sang shen (p.78), he shou wu (p.78), sha shen (p.80), mai dong (p.80), hei zhi ma (p.80), hu tao ren (p.82) and qin jiao (p.92).

Herbs from other groups that can encourage bowel movement by stimulating peristalsis include hou po (p.16), liu huang (p.24), lai fu zi (p.30), bing lang (p.52), jie geng (p.54), zao jia (p.54), da fu pi (p.64), zhi shi (p.64), su zi (p,.68), rou cong rong (p.82) and suo yang (p.82).

---

1 Appendix 6, p.108
2 Appendix 3.2, p.103
3 Appendix 6, p.108
4 Ibid.
5 Appendix 3.2, p.103
6 Appendix 4, p.105
7 Appendix 3.2, p.103

| △ Indication<br>▲ Strong Indication<br>E External Use<br>**E** Strong External Indication<br><br>**INDICATIONS** | Qian Niu Zi 牵牛子 | Gan Sui 甘遂 | Hong Da Ji 红大戟 | Yuan Hua 芫花 | Shang Lu 商陆 | Ba Dou Shuang 巴豆霜 | Qian Jin Zi 千金子 | | | | | | ○ *Function*<br>● *Strong Function*<br><br><br><br>**FUNCTIONS** |
|---|---|---|---|---|---|---|---|---|---|---|---|---|---|
| abdominal distension – drum like | △ | ▲ | ▲ | △ | ▲ | △ | △ ○ | | | | | | breaks up blood stasis |
| abscess – Lung | | | ○ | | ○ | △ | ○ | | | | | | dissipates masses |
| abscesses & sores – skin | ○ | E ○ | △ E | E ○ | E | E ○ | E | | | | | | drives out phlegm |
| amenorrhea – blood stasis | ○ | | | ○ | | ○ | △ ○ | | | | | | kills parasites |
| ascites | △ ○ | ▲ ○ | ▲ ○ | △ ○ | ▲ ○ | △ ○ | △ ○ | | | | | | purges fluids |
| bronchitis – chronic | △ ○ | | | △ | | ○ | | | | | | | purges the Intestines |
| cervical lymphadenitis (*luo li*) | | | △ E | | | ○ | | | | | | | warms the Intestines |
| constipation – cold | | | | | | △ | | | | | | | |
| cough – phlegm damp | △ | | | △ | | | | | | | | | |
| diarrhea – chronic cold, spurious | | | | | | △ | | | | | | | |
| edema – generalized, severe | ▲ | △ | △ | △ | △ | △ | △ | | | | | | |
| edema – pulmonary | △ | | | | | | | | | | | | |
| edema – schistosomiasis | | | | | | △ | | | | | | | |
| epilepsy, seizures – wind phlegm | | △ | | | | △ | | | | | | | |
| food stagnation – severe | △ | | | | | | | | | | | | |
| hydrothorax (*xuan yin*) | △ | △ | ▲ | △ | △ | | | | | | | | |
| intestinal obstruction (simple) | △ | | | | | ▲ | | | | | | | |
| mania – phlegm fire | | △ | | | | | | | | | | | |
| masses – abdominal | | | | | | △ | | | | | | | |
| pain – abdominal, from worms | △ | | | | | | | | | | | | |
| parasites – pinworms | △ | | | | | | | | | | | | |
| parasites – roundworms | △ | | | | | | | | | | | | |
| parasites – tapeworms | △ | | | | | | | | | | | | |
| skin – scabies | | | | E | | E | | | | | | | |
| skin – ringworm, tinea | | | | E | | | E | | | | | | |
| skin – tinea capitis | | | | E | | | | | | | | | **Domain** (❖) |
| throat – phlegm blockage of | ❖ | ❖ | | ❖ | ❖ | △ | | | | | | | Lung |
| urination – difficult, retention of | △ ❖ | △ ❖ | △ ❖ | △ ❖ | ▲ ❖ | △ ❖ | ❖ | | | | | | Large Intestine |
| wheezing – phlegm damp, severe | △ ❖ | ❖ | ❖ | △ ❖ | ❖ | | ❖ | | | | | | Kidney |
| *yang ming* organ syndrome | △ | | | | | △ | ❖ | | | | | | Liver |
| | | ❖ | | | | | | | | | | | Spleen |
| | | | | | | ❖ | | | | | | | Stomach |
| | | | | | | | | | | | | | |
| | | | | | | | | | | | | | |
| | | | | | | | | | | | | | **Flavour, nature** (♦) |
| | | ♦ | | ♦ | ♦ | ♦ | ♦ | | | | | | toxic |
| | ♦ | | ♦ | | | | | | | | | | slightly toxic |
| | ♦ | | | | | ♦ | ♦ | | | | | | acrid |
| | ♦ | ♦ | ♦ | ♦ | ♦ | | | | | | | | bitter |
| | | ♦ | | | | | | | | | | | sweet |
| | ♦ | ♦ | ♦ | | ♦ | | | | | | | | cold |
| | | | | ♦ | | | ♦ | | | | | | warm |
| | | | | | | ♦ | | | | | | | hot |
| **Standard dosage range (g)** | 3–6 | 0.5–1 | 1.5–3 | 1.5–3 | 3–9 | 0.1–0.3 | 0.5–1 | | | | | | |

The primary action of these herbs is to eliminate accumulated fluids from within body cavities. By forcefully expelling fluid through the urine and bowels, they treat pathological fluid accumulation in the abdomen (ascites), pleura (pleural effusion), pericardium (cardiac tamponade) and lungs (pulmonary edema). Their action is powerful and iatrogenesis likely, so they are only used for short periods of time, a few days at most, until fluids are moving and the patient out of danger. All are toxic to some degree. The maximum recommended dose should not be exceeded or toxic effects[1] may occur.

## Qiān Niú Zǐ (Pharbitidis Semen) morning glory seed
Also known as hēi chǒu 黑丑 (the black seeds) or bái chǒu 白丑 (the white seeds).

**Preparation and use** Crush before decoction. Taken directly in pill or powder form the dose is 1.5–3 grams per day. Stir frying (*chao qian niu zi* 炒牵牛子) reduces its violent nature somewhat.

**Contraindications** Pregnancy. Caution in weak and deficient patients. Should not be combined with ba dou shuang (this page).

**Formulae** *Zhou Che Wan*† (ascites and severe excess type edema); *Mu Xiang Bing Lang Wan* (constipation and abdominal distension from severe food stagnation)

## Gān Suì (Kansui Radix) euphorbia kansui root
❀ Euphorbia species are listed in Appendix 2 of CITES[2] which permits limited trade with appropriate documentation.

**Preparation and use** Used in pill or powder form only. For internal use, the root is processed with vinegar (*cu gan sui* 醋甘遂) to mitigate its toxicity and harsh cathartic nature somewhat. The unprocessed root can be used externally.

**Contraindications** Pregnancy, and in weak or deficient patients. Only used in relatively robust patients with excess conditions. Incompatible[3] with gan cao (p.74).

**Formulae** *Da Xian Xiong Wang* (fluids and heat accumulating in the chest and pleura); *Gan Sui Tong Jie Tang* (intestinal obstruction); *Shi Zao Tang* (ascites); *Zhou Che Wan*† (ascites and severe excess type edema); *Kong Xian Dan* (thin mucus congesting the upper and middle burner)

## Hóng Dà Jǐ (Knoxiae Radix) knoxia root
Traditionally there were two plants known as da ji – hong da ji, the root of *Knoxia valerianoides* and jīng dà jǐ 京大戟, the root of *Euphorbia pekinensis*. Their therapeutic action is very similar, but jing da ji is more toxic and cathartic. Hong da ji is much less toxic, better tolerated and currently the preferred species.

**Preparation and use** For internal use, the root is processed with vinegar (*cu da ji* 醋大戟) to mitigate its toxicity and harsh cathartic nature somewhat.

**Contraindications** Pregnancy and in weak or deficient patients. Incompatible[4] with gan cao (p.74)

**Formulae** *Shi Zao Tang* (ascites); *Zhou Che Wan*† (ascites and severe excess type edema); *Kong Xian Dan* (thin mucus congesting the upper and middle burner); *Zi Jin Ding*† (toxic lesions and summerheat stroke); *Bai Qian Tang* (wheezing and orthopnea from phlegm congestion in the Lungs)

## Yuán Huā (Genkwa Flos) lilac daphne flower
**Preparation and use** For internal use, processing with vinegar (*cu yuan hua* 醋芫花) reduces its toxicity while retaining its cathartic effects. The unprocessed flower is reserved for external use.

**Contraindications** Pregnancy and in weak or deficient patients. Only used in relatively robust patients with excess conditions. Incompatible[5] with gan cao (p.74).

**Formulae** *Shi Zao Tang* (ascites and pleural effusion); *Zhou Che Wan*† (ascites and severe excess type edema)

## Shāng Lù (Phytolaccae Radix) poke root
**Preparation and use** For internal use, processing with vinegar (*cu shang lu* 醋商路) reduces its toxicity while enhancing its cathartic effects. Mostly used in decoction. The unprocessed root is reserved for external use.

**Contraindications** Pregnancy. Caution in weak and deficient patients.

**Formulae** *Shu Zao Yin Zi* (yang edema; ascites)

## Bā Dòu Shuāng (Crotonis Fructus Pulveratum) defatted croton seed
**Preparation and use** This is the form of croton seed from which the oil, the most toxic component, has been removed. Unprocessed seeds are highly toxic and not used internally. For internal use, ba dou shuang is used in pills or enteric capsules.

**Contraindications** Pregnancy, and in weak or deficient patients. Only used in relatively robust patients with excess conditions. Should not be combined with qian niu zi (this page).

**Formulae** *San Wu Bei Ji Wan* (severe disruption to the qi dynamic by cold; intestinal obstruction); *San Wu Bai San* (Lung abscess); *Chan Su Gao* (topical paste for toxic sores and tumours)

## Qiān Jīn Zǐ (Euphorbia lathyris Semen) caper spurge seed
Also known as xù súi zǐ 续随子.

❀ Euphorbia species are listed in Appendix 2 of CITES[6] which permits limited trade with appropriate documentation.

**Preparation and use** The unprocessed seeds are reserved for external use. For internal use, the defatted seeds (*qian jin zi shuang* 千金子霜) are ground and packed in pills or enteric capsules.

**Contraindications** Pregnancy, in weak or deficient patients. Only used in relatively robust patients with excess conditions.

**Formulae** *Xu Sui Zi Wan*[7] (yang edema); *Xu Sui Zi Wan*[8]† (abdominal masses); *Zi Jin Ding*† (toxic lesions and summerheat stroke)

## Endnotes
† These formulae traditionally contain items from endangered animal species and/or obsolete toxic substances, and are unavailable in their original form.

1 Appendix 3, pp.101–104
2 Appendix 4, p.105
3 Appendix 2, p.100
4 Ibid.
5 Ibid.
6 Appendix 4, p.105
7 *Yi Xue Fa Ming* (Medical Innovations)
8 *Sheng Ji Zong Lu* (Comprehensive Recording of the Sages' Benefits)

| Legend | | |
|---|---|---|
| △ Indication | ○ Function | |
| ▲ Strong Indication | ● Strong Function | |
| E External Use | | |
| E Strong External Indication | | |

| INDICATIONS | Chen Pi 陈皮 | Qing Pi 青皮 | Zhi Shi 枳实 | Zhi Ke 枳壳 | Xiang Fu 香附 | Mu Xiang 木香 | Wu Yao 乌药 | Chuan Lian Zi 川楝子 | Xie Bai 薤白 | Da Fu Pi 大腹皮 | Chen Xiang 沉香 | Tan Xiang 檀香 | FUNCTIONS |
|---|---|---|---|---|---|---|---|---|---|---|---|---|---|
| abdominal distension | ▲ | ▲○ | ▲○ | △ | △ | ▲ | △ | | | △ | △ | | alleviates food stagnation |
| abscess – breast, mastitis | | △○ | ○ | | | | | | | | | | breaks up stagnant qi |
| angina | | | ● | | | | ○ | | ▲○ | ○ | ○ | △ | directs qi downward |
| appetite – loss of | △ | | △ | △ | ○ | △ | | ○ | | | | | dredges the Liver |
| breast – cysts & lumps | ○ | ▲ | | | △ | | | | | | | | dries damp |
| breast – distension & pain | ○ | ▲ | | | ▲ | ○ | | | | | ○ | ○ | harmonizes the middle |
| chest – stifling sensation in | △ | △ | ▲ | △ | | △ | △ | | ▲ | ○ | △ | △ | promotes urination |
| constipation | | | ▲ | | | ● | | | | △ | △ | | regulates menstruation |
| cough – phlegm damp | ▲○ | △ | | ○ | | ○ | ○ | | △ | | ○ | ○ | regulates qi |
| damp blocking middle burner | ▲ | △ | △ | △ | ○ | ○ | ○ | ● | | △ | ○ | ○ | stops pain |
| depression | ○ | △ | ○ | | △ | | | | ○ | | | | transforms phlegm |
| diarrhea – chronic | △ | | | | | ▲ | ○ | | | △ | ○ | | warms the Kidneys |
| dysenteric disorder – chronic | | | △ | | | △ | | | | △ | ○ | ○ | warms the middle burner |
| dysmenorrhea | | | | | ▲ | | △ | △ | ● | | △ | | unblocks chest yang |
| dysuria – qi constraint | | | | | | | | ▲ | | | △ | | |
| edema | | | | | | | | | | △ | | | |
| epigastric distension | ▲ | ▲ | ▲ | △ | △ | △ | △ | | | △ | △ | | |
| flatulence, belching | △ | △ | △ | △ | | △ | | | | △ | △ | | |
| food stagnation | △ | ▲ | ▲ | △ | | △ | | | | △ | | | |
| hepatosplenomegaly | | △ | | | | | | | | | | | **Domain (❖)** |
| hiccup | △❖ | | △ | △ | | | ❖ | | ❖ | | △ | ❖ | Lung |
| menstruation – irregular | | | ❖ | ❖ | ▲ | ❖ | | | ❖ | ❖ | | | Large Intestine |
| morning sickness | △ | | | | | | ❖ | | | | △❖ | | Kidney |
| nausea, vomiting | ▲ | | | | △ | △ | ❖ | ❖ | | | ▲ | △ | Bladder |
| nodules, masses – qi, bld. stasis | | △❖ | | | ❖ | | | ❖ | | | | | Liver |
| pain – abdominal, qi constraint | △ | △❖ | △ | | △ | △❖ | ▲ | ▲ | | | △ | △ | Gallbladder |
| pain – abdominal, cold damp | △ | △ | | | | △ | △ | ❖ | | ❖ | △ | △ | Small Intestine |
| pain – abdominal, from worms | | | | | | ❖ | | ▲ | | | | | Triple Burner |
| pain – chest; phlegm, qi const. | ❖ | | △❖ | ❖ | | ❖ | △❖ | △ | ▲ | ❖ | ❖ | ▲❖ | Spleen |
| pain – epigastric; cold; qi const. | △ | △❖ | △❖ | ❖ | △ | ▲❖ | △ | ❖ | ❖ | ❖ | △❖ | △❖ | Stomach |
| pain – epigastric; heat, qi const. | | | △ | | △ | | | ▲ | | | | | |
| pain – hypochondriac | | ▲ | △ | | △ | △ | △ | | | | | | |
| pain – testicular; cold; qi const. | | △ | | | △ | | ▲ | △ | | | △ | | **Flavour, nature (♦)** |
| prolapse – rectal, uterine | | | △ | △ | | | | ♦ | | | | | slightly toxic |
| qi dynamic – blockage of | ▲♦ | △♦ | ▲♦ | ♦ | △♦ | △♦ | ♦ | | ♦ | ♦ | ♦ | ♦ | acrid |
| spasm & cramp – smooth mm. | ▲♦ | △♦ | △♦ | ♦ | △ | ▲♦ | △ | △♦ | ♦ | | △♦ | △ | bitter |
| tenesmus | | | △ | | | ♦ | ▲ | | | △ | | | slightly bitter |
| urination – difficult | | | | | | ♦ | | | | △ | △ | | slightly sweet |
| urination – frequent; yang def. | | ♦ | ♦ | | | | ▲ | | | | | | cool |
| urination – incontinence of | | | | | | | △ | ♦ | | | | | cold |
| wheezing – Kidney deficiency | | | | ♦ | | | | | | | ▲ | | neutral |
| wheezing – phlegm damp | △♦ | ♦ | | | | | ♦ | ♦ | | △♦ | ♦ | ♦ | warm |
| | | | | | | | | | | | ♦ | | slightly warm |
| **Standard dosage range (g)** | 3–9 | 3–9 | 3–9 | 3–9 | 6–12 | 3–9 | 3–9 | 3–9 | 6–9 | 6–12 | 1–1.5 | 1–3 | |

## Chén Pí (Citri reticulatae Pericarpium) aged tangerine peel

Also known as jú pí 橘皮. A commonly specified variant seen in some formulae is jú hóng 橘红 (Citri reticulatae Exocarpium rubrum), the dried peel of the red tangerine, interchangeable with chen pi. The seeds of the tangerine, jú hé 橘核 (Citri reticulatae Semen) regulate qi and dissipate masses, and are used for testicular swellings.

**Preparation and use** Mostly used unprocessed, but stir frying (*chao chen pi* 炒陈皮) moderates its acrid dispersing nature, while enhancing its ability to dry damp in patients with Spleen qi deficiency.

**Contraindications** Dry cough from qi deficiency, yin deficiency and/or fluid damage. Caution in patients with internal excess heat, or vomiting or spitting blood. Prolonged use can damage source qi.

**Formulae** *Ping Wei San* (abdominal bloating and reflux from phlegm damp blocking the middle burner); *Er Chen Tang* (phlegm); *Wen Dan Tang* (nausea and shen disturbance from phlegm heat); *Dao Tan Tang* (fainting or vertigo from phlegm blocking the senses); *Di Tan Tang* (mental cloudiness, confusion and aphasia from wind stroke); *Tong Xie Yao Fang* (colicky abdominal pain and diarrhea from Liver Spleen disharmony); *Ju Pi Tang* (nausea and morning sickness); *Ju Pi Zhu Ru Tang* (nausea and dry retching from Stomach yin deficiency); *Bao He Wan* (food stagnation); *Huo Xiang Zheng Qi San* (summerdamp common cold); *Qing Qi Hua Tan Tang* (phlegm heat in the Lungs); *Chai Hu Shu Gan San* (Liver qi constraint); & 60+ more in Appendix 7.

## Qīng Pí (Citri reticulatae viride Pericarpium) green tangerine peel

**Preparation and use** Can be stir fried (*chao qing pi* 炒青皮) to moderate its dispersing nature and render it better for harmonizing the Liver and Spleen; processing with vinegar (*cu qing pi* 醋青皮) enhances its ability to dredge the Liver and stop pain; processing with wine (*jiu qing pi* 酒青皮) enhances its ability to dissipate masses.

**Contraindications** Caution in patients with internal heat and in cases with yin deficiency, qi deficiency, and/or fluid damage. Contraindicated in patients who sweat heavily. Prolonged use can damage source qi.

**Formulae** *Qing Pi Wan* (abdominal pain, distension and indigestion from qi and food stagnation); *Mu Xiang Shun Qi San* (abdominal pain from qi constraint); *Tian Tai Wu Yao San* (cold type testicular pain); *Bie Jia Wan* (abdominal masses); *Gua Lou Niu Bang Tang* (acute mastitis and breast abscess); *Bai Ling Tiao Gan Tang* (infertility from blocked fallopian tubes or endometriosis); *Jie Nüe Qi Bao Yin* (malarial disorder; true malaria)

## Zhǐ Shí (Aurantii Fructus immaturus) unripe bitter orange

**Preparation and use** In severe cases up to 15 grams can be used. Mostly used unprocessed, but can be stir fried (*chao zhi shi* 炒枳实) to warm it and moderate its strong dispersing nature.

**Contraindications** Caution during pregnancy and in patients with significant Spleen qi deficiency (used alone).

**Formulae** *Zhi Shi Dao Zhi Wan* (damp heat blockage in the middle burner); *Zhi Shi Xiao Pi Wan* (epigastric blockage with Spleen deficiency); *Zhi Shi Xie Bai Gui Zhi Tang* (cold phlegm blocking chest yang; angina); *Zhi Zhu Wan* (food stagnation); *Si Ni San* (Liver qi constraint); *Ju He Wan* (testicular swelling and pain from cold damp); *Xiao Cheng Qi Tang* (heat blocking the Intestines); *Ma Zi Ren Wan* (constipation from dryness and heat); *Wen Dan Tang* (nausea and shen disturbance from phlegm heat); *Dao Tan Tang* (fainting or vertigo from phlegm blocking the senses); *Di Tan Tang* (mental cloudiness, confusion and aphasia from wind stroke); *Qing Qi Hua Tan Tang* (phlegm heat in the Lungs)

## Zhǐ Ké (Aurantii Fructus) bitter orange

**Preparation and use** Can be stir fried (*chao zhi ke* 炒枳壳) to moderate its dispersing nature. For prolapse, large doses, to 24 grams, are used.

**Contraindications** Caution during pregnancy.

**Formulae** *Ji Chuan Jian* (chronic constipation from yang deficiency); *Mu Xiang Shun Qi San* (abdominal pain from qi constraint); *Chai Hu Shu Gan San* (Liver qi constraint); *Xue Fu Zhu Yu Tang* (qi and blood stasis); *Qin Jiao Bai Zhu Wan* (chronic constipation with bleeding, itchy hemorrhoids); & 20+ more in Appendix 7.

## Xiāng Fù (Cyperi Rhizoma) nut grass rhizome

**Preparation and use** Processing with vinegar (*cu xiang fu* 醋香附) enhances its ability to stop pain; processing with wine (*jiu xiang fu* 酒香附) enhances its ability to regulate menstruation; processing with ginger jiuce (*jiang chao xiang fu* 姜炒香附) enhances its ability to transform phlegm; stir frying until charred on the outside (*hei xiang fu* 黑香附) enhances its ability to stop abnormal menstrual bleeding.

**Contraindications** Qi deficiency without stagnation, menstrual problems from yin deficiency with heat or heat in the blood.

**Formulae** *Ai Fu Nuan Gong Wan* (infertility, dysmenorrhea and irregular menses from Kidney deficiency); *Cang Fu Dao Tan Tang* (amenorrhea from phlegm damp); *Yue Ju Wan* (abdominal bloating and reflux from the 'six stagnations')[1]; *Chai Hu Shu Gan San* (Liver qi constraint); *Xiang Su San* (wind cold common cold with abdominal distension from qi constraint); *Yi Mu Sheng Jin Dan* (irregular menses and dysmenorrhea from blood deficiency with blood stasis); *Tong Jing Wan* (amenorrhea and dysmenorrhea from blood stasis); & 20+ more in Appendix 7.

## Mù Xiāng (Aucklandiae Radix) aucklandia root

✿ Listed in Appendix 1 of CITES[2], with trade in wild plants prohibited. Limited exemptions exist for farmed product where certification is available. See Appendix 4, p.105.

**Preparation and use** Should not be cooked longer than 15 minutes[3]. Used unprocessed to regulate qi; when roasted (*wei mu xiang* 煨木香) its qi regulating action is reduced and its ability to stop diarrhea enhanced.

**Contraindications** Caution in patients with yin deficiency and damaged fluids, and those with problems due to fire.

**Formulae** *Mu Xiang Shun Qi San* (abdominal pain from Liver qi constraint); *Mu Xiang Bing Lang Wan* (dysenteric disorder from damp heat and blockage of the qi dynamic); *Jian Pi Wan* (food stagnation and Spleen deficiency); *Xiang Sha Liu Jun Zi Tang* (qi deficiency with phlegm damp); *Xiang Lian Wan* (tenesmus in dysenteric disorder); & 30+ more in Appendix 7.

## Wū Yào (Linderae Radix) lindera root

**Preparation and use** Mostly used unprocessed, but stir frying (*chao wu yao* 炒乌药) moderates its acrid dispersing nature, and enhances its ability to warm cold and stop pain.

**Contraindications** Qi and blood deficiency; internal heat.

**Formulae** *Suo Quan Wan* (Kidney deficiency type frequent urination; *Tian Tai Wu Yao San* (cold type testicular pain); *Wu Yao Tang* (qi and blood stasis dysmenorrhea); *Nuan Gan Jian* (hypochondriac and groin pain from cold in the Liver channel or Liver yang deficiency); *Bi Xie Fen Qing Yin* (turbid urine from Kidney deficiency); *Liu Mo Tang* (abdominal pain from cold and qi stagnation)

## Chuān Liàn Zǐ (Toosendan Fructus) Sichuan pagoda tree

Also known as jīn líng zǐ 金铃子.

**Preparation and use** Usually used unprocessed, but stir frying (*chao chuan lian zi* 炒川楝子) moderates its coldness and makes it easier on the Spleen; processing with salt (*yan chuan lian zi* 盐川楝子) helps direct its action to the Kidneys for alleviating testicular pain. For external use, grind to a fine powder and mix with lard or sesame oil.

**Contraindications** Middle burner yang deficiency. Do not exceed dosage range or use for prolonged periods.

**Formulae** *Jin Ling Zi San* (pain from qi constraint with heat); *Yi Guan Jian* (hypochondriac pain from Liver yin deficiency); *Dao Qi Tang* (testicular pain from cold in the Liver channel); *Zhen Gan Xi Feng Tang* (headache and hypertension from ascendant Liver yang)

## Xiè Bái (Allii macrostemi Bulbus) Chinese garlic chive

**Contraindications** Qi deficiency without significant stagnation, Stomach deficiency or in patients intolerant of onions and garlic.

**Formulae** *Guo Luo Xie Bai Bai Jiu Tang* (phlegm blocking chest yang; angina); *Zhi Shi Xie Bai Gui Zhi Tang* (angina from cold phlegm blocking chest yang)

---

1 qi, blood, fire, food, damp, phlegm
2 Appendix 4, p.105
3 Appendix 6, p.108

# 14. QI REGULATING

| △ Indication / ▲ Strong Indication / E External Use / E Strong External Indication | Gan Song 甘松 | Xiang Yuan 香橼 | Fo Shou 佛手 | Shi Di 柿蒂 | Li Zhi He 荔枝核 | Mei Gui Hua 玫瑰花 | Suo Luo Zi 娑罗子 | Ba Yue Zha 八月扎 | Dao Dou 刀豆 | Jiu Xiang Chong 九香虫 | Zi Su Geng 紫苏梗 | Tu Mu Xiang 土木香 | ○ Function / ● Strong Function |
|---|---|---|---|---|---|---|---|---|---|---|---|---|---|
| **INDICATIONS** | | | | | | | | | | | | | **FUNCTIONS** |
| abdominal distension | △ | △ | ▲ | | | △ | △ | | | △ | △ ● | △ | calms restless fetus |
| acid reflux, heartburn | | △ | △ | ○ | | | | | ○ | | | | directs qi downward |
| appetite – loss of | ▲ | △ | △ | | ○ | △ | | | | | | | disperses cold |
| belching, flatulence | | △ | △ | △ | | △ | | | ○ | △ | | | dissipates masses |
| breast – cysts & lumps | | ○ | ○ | | | ○ | ○ | ▲ ○ | | | | | dredges the Liver |
| breast – distension & pain | | ○ | ● | | | ▲ | △ ○ | △ | | | ○ | ○ | harmonizes the middle |
| cervical lymphadenitis (*luo li*) | | | | | | ○ | | △ | | | | | invigorates blood |
| chest – stifling sensation in | △ ○ | △ ○ | △ ○ | | ○ | △ ○ | △ ○ | △ ○ | | ○ | △ ○ | △ ○ | regulates qi |
| cough – phlegm damp | ○ | △ | △ | | | | | | | | | | stimulates the appetite |
| depression | | △ | △ | ● | | ▲ | | △ | ○ | | | | stops hiccup |
| diarrhea – chronic | ○ | | | ○ | | | | | | ○ | | △ ○ | stops pain |
| dysenteric disorder – chronic | | ○ | ○ | | | | | | | | | △ | transforms phlegm |
| dysmenorrhea | | | | | △ | ▲ | | | ○ | ○ | | | warms the Kidneys |
| dysuria – qi stag.; stone | | | | | | | | △ | | | | | |
| epigastric distension | △ | △ | ▲ | | | △ | △ | | | △ | △ | △ | |
| food stagnation | | △ | △ | | | | | | | | | | |
| hiccup | | | | ▲ | | | | | ▲ | | | | |
| impotence – Kidney yang def. | | | | | | | | | | △ | | | |
| Liver & Spleen disharmony | △ | △ | △ | | | △ | △ | △ | | △ | △ | △ | |
| malarial disorder | | | | | | | | | | | △ | | |
| menstruation – irregular | | | | | | ▲ | | | | | | | |
| miscarriage – threatened | | | | | | | | | | | △ | | |
| morning sickness | | △ | | | | | | | | | ▲ | | |
| nausea | | △ | △ | △ | | | | | △ | | △ | △ | |
| nodules & masses – qi, phlegm | | | | | | | | △ | | | | | **Domain (❖)** |
| pain – & injury, trauma | | ❖ | ❖ | | | △ | | | | | ❖ | ❖ | Lung |
| pain – abdominal | ▲ | △ | △ | | △ | △ | △ | | ❖ | △ ❖ | △ | ▲ | Kidney |
| pain – chest | | ❖ | ❖ | | ❖ | | △ ❖ | △ ❖ | | ❖ | | ❖ | Liver |
| pain – epigastric | ▲ ❖ | △ ❖ | △ ❖ | | △ | △ ❖ | ▲ | | | △ ❖ | △ ❖ | ▲ ❖ | Spleen |
| pain – hypochondriac | ❖ | △ | △ ❖ | ❖ | ❖ | △ | △ ❖ | △ ❖ | ❖ | △ | △ ❖ | △ | Stomach |
| pain – inguinal | | | | | ▲ | | | | | | | | |
| pain – lower back, leg, knee | | | | | | | | | △ | ▲ | | | |
| pain – postpartum, abdominal | | | | | △ | | | | | | | | **Flavour, nature (◆)** |
| pain – testicular, cold, qi stag. | ◆ | ◆ | ◆ | | ▲ ◆ | | | △ | | | ◆ | ◆ | acrid |
| rumination – excessive | △ | △ | | ◆ | | | | | | | | | astringent |
| spasm & cramp – smooth mm. | ▲ | △ | △ ◆ | | △ | △ | △ | △ ◆ | | △ | △ | △ ◆ | bitter |
| tenesmus | | ◆ | | | ◆ | ◆ | | | | | | △ | slightly bitter |
| toothache – Kidney deficiency | E | | | | | | | | | ◆ | | | salty |
| tumours – breast, digestive | | ◆ | | | | | | △ | | | | | sour |
| urination – frequent, nocturia | ◆ | | | | | ◆ | ◆ | | ◆ | △ | ◆ | | sweet |
| vomiting – phlegm, qi stag. | | △ | ▲ | △ ◆ | | | | | ◆ | △ | ▲ | △ | neutral |
| | ◆ | ◆ | ◆ | | ◆ | ◆ | ◆ | | | ◆ | | ◆ | warm |
| | | | | | | | | | | | ◆ | | slightly warm |
| **Standard dosage range (g)** | 3–6 | 3–9 | 3–9 | 3–12 | 9–15 | 3–6 | 3–9 | 6–12 | 3–9 | 3–9 | 6–9 | 3–9 | |

**Dà Fù Pí** (Arecae Pericarpium) betel nut husk

**Contraindications** Caution during pregnancy and in patients with edema from qi deficiency.

**Formulae** *Jia Jian Zheng Qi San* (damp and qi stagnation blocking the upper and middle burner); *Da Fu Pi San* (edema of the legs); *Wu Pi Yin* (lower body edema); *Shi Pi Yin* (edema and watery diarrhea from Spleen yang deficiency); *Shu Zao Yin Zi* (yang edema; ascites); *Huang Qin Hua Shi Tang* (damp heat febrile disease; heat greater than damp)

**Chén Xiāng** (Aquilariae Lignum resinatum) aloeswood ~ p.64

☸ Listed in Appendix 2 of CITES[1] which permits limited trade with appropriate documentation.

**Preparation and use** Mostly used in pills and powders. Not suitable for decoction, but can be ground into a powder and added to the warm strained decoction just before ingestion.

**Contraindications** Caution in patients with yin deficiency and heat, and in qi deficiency prolapse and sinking qi.

**Formulae** *Chen Xiang Jiang Qi San* (irregular menstruation and dysmenorrhea from Liver Spleen disharmony); *Chen Ding Er Xiang San* (vomiting and hiccup from cold in the Stomach); *Chen Xiang Hua Qi Wan* (nausea, vomiting and constipation from phlegm and qi constraint blocking the qi dynamic); *Liu Mo Tang* (abdominal pain from cold and qi stagnation); *Nuan Gan Jian* (hypochondriac and groin pain from cold in the Liver channel or Liver yang deficiency)

**Tán Xiāng** (Santali albi Lignum) sandalwood ~ p.64

**Contraindications** Yin deficiency with heat, and patterns of bleeding or chest pain from heat.

**Formulae** *Dan Shen Yin* (chest and epigastric pain from Heart and Stomach qi and blood stasis); *Guan Xin Su He Xiang Wan*† (angina); *Chang Pu San* (vomiting from cold in the Stomach)

**Gān Sōng** (Nardostachydis Radix seu Rhizoma) nardostachys root

**Contraindications** Contraindicated in cases with heat in the blood and qi deficiency.

**Formulae** *Da Qi Xiang Wan* (abdominal pain from cold and qi constraint)

**Xiāng Yuán** (Citri Fructus) citron

**Contraindications** Caution in pregnant patients with qi deficiency, and in patients with yin and blood deficiency.

**Fó Shǒu** (Citri sarcodacylis Fructus) finger citron fruit

**Contraindications** Caution in patients with yin deficiency and heat, and in the absence of stagnation.

**Shì Dì** (Kaki Calyx) persimmon calyx

**Contraindications** None noted.

**Formulae** *Shi Di Tang* (Stomach cold type hiccups); *Ding Xiang Shi Di Tang* (hiccups from yang deficiency)

**Lì Zhī Hé** (Litchi Semen) lychee seed

**Preparation and use** Crush in a mortar and pestle before decoction. Can be processed with salt (*yan li zhi he* 盐荔枝核) to enhance its ability to enter the Kidneys and stop pain.

**Contraindications** Caution in patients without cold pathology.

**Formulae** *Shan Qi Nei Xiao Wan* (groin and testicular pain from cold in the Liver channel); *Juan Tong San* (dysmenorrhea and postpartum abdominal pain from qi and blood stasis)

**Méi Guī Huā** (Rosae rugosae Flos) Chinese rose bud

**Preparation and use** Can be decocted, but commonly prepared by steeping in wine, either alone or with other qi and blood regulating herbs. Wine extract is especially good for breast pain, dysmenorrhea and irregular menses, and taken in 10–20 milliliter doses.

**Contraindications** None noted.

**Suō Luó Zǐ** (Aesculi Semen) horse chestnut

**Preparation and use** Crush in a mortar and pestle before decoction.

**Contraindications** Caution in patients with qi or yin deficiency.

**Bā Yuè Zhá** (Akebiae Fructus) akebia fruit

**Preparation and use** Crush in a mortar and pestle before decoction.

**Contraindications** Caution during pregnancy.

**Dāo Dòu** (Canavaliae Semen) sword bean

**Preparation and use** Can be decocted, roasted, ground to a powder and taken directly.

**Contraindications** Caution in patients with Stomach heat.

**Jiǔ Xiāng Chóng** (Aspongopus) stinkbug; citrus shield bug

Some texts place this insect in the yang tonic group.

**Preparation and use** Usually stir fried (*chao jiu xiang chong* 炒九香虫), to reduce the unpleasant odor and enhance the ability of the bug to mobilize qi and warm yang. When ground and taken directly as powder or in pills, the dose is 1.5–3 grams.

**Contraindications** Yin deficiency with heat.

**Zǐ Sū Gěng** (Perillae Caulis) perilla stem

**Preparation and use** Not to be cooked longer than 5–8 minutes.

**Contraindications** None noted.

**Tǔ Mù Xiāng** (Inulae Radix) inula root

**Preparation and use** Used unprocessed to stop pain; when roasted (*wei tu mu xiang* 煨土木香) its qi regulating action is reduced, and nausea and the diarrhea alleviating action is enhanced.

**Contraindications** Caution in patients with yin deficiency and damaged fluids, or those with problems due to fire.

Substances from other groups

Herbs from other groups with some qi regulating, mobilizing or descending effect include chuan xiong (p.6), yan hu suo (p.6), yu jin (p.8), lu lu tong (p.8), jiang huang (p.8), san leng (p.10), e zhu (p.10), hou po (p.16), sha ren (p.16), bai dou kou (p.16), zi su ye (p.28), lai fu zi (p.30), dai zhe shi (p.48), bing lang (p.52), xuan fu hua (p.54), qian hu (p.56), qing meng shi (p.58), xing ren (p.68), sang bai pi (p.68), su zi (p.68), zi wan (p.68), kuan dong hua (p.68), pi pa ye (p.68), he huan pi (p.70), he huan hua (p.70), xie cao (p.70), xiao hui xiang (p.88), ba jiao hui xiang (p.88), wu zhu yu (p.88) and ding xiang (p.88).

---

1 Appendix 4, p.105

**Legend:**
△ Indication
▲ Strong Indication
E External Use
**E** Strong External Indication
○ Function
● Strong Function

| INDICATIONS | Xing Ren 杏仁 | Sang Bai Pi 桑白皮 | Su Zi 苏子 | Zi Wan 紫菀 | Kuan Dong Hua 款冬花 | Pi Pa Ye 枇杷叶 | Bai Bu 百部 | Bai Guo 白果 | Ting Li Zi 葶苈子 | Ai Di Cha 矮地茶 | Zhong Ru Shi 钟乳石 | Man Shan Hong 满山红 | FUNCTIONS |
|---|---|---|---|---|---|---|---|---|---|---|---|---|---|
| ascites | ○ | ○ | ● | | | | | ● | ▲○ | ○ | ○ | ○ | alleviates wheezing |
| amenorrhea – blood stasis | | | | | | | | ○ | | △ | | | astringes the Lungs |
| painful obstruction – wind damp | | ○ | | | | ○ | | | | △ | | | cools the lungs |
| belching – Stomach heat | | | ● | | ○ | △● | | | | | | | directs qi downward |
| bleeding – hemoptysis | | △ | | △ | | | | | ○ | △ | | | drains fluid from Lungs |
| constipation – dryness | ▲ | | △○ | ○ | ○ | | | | | ○ | | ○ | expels phlegm |
| cough – chronic dry | ▲ | | | ▲ | △ | △○ | ▲ | △ | | | | | harmonizes the Stomach |
| cough – Lung heat; phlegm heat | △ | ▲ | | △ | △ | ▲ | | △ | △ | △○ | | | invigorates blood |
| cough – phlegm damp | | | ▲ | △ | △ | | ○ | △ | △ | △ | | △ | kills parasites |
| cough – whooping | ○ | | ○ | | | | ▲ | △ | | | | | moistens the intestines |
| cough – wind cold | ▲ | | | △○ | △○ | | △○ | | | | | | moistens the Lungs |
| cough – wind heat | △ | ▲ | | △ | △ | △ | | | | | ○ | | promotes lactation |
| cough – yin deficiency | △ | ○ | | △ | △ | △ | ▲ | △ | ● | ○ | | | promotes urination |
| dysuria – turbid | | | | | | | | △○ | | | | | restrains urine |
| edema – face, limbs; excess, heat | ● | ▲○ | ○ | ○ | ● | ○ | ○ | | △ | △○ | | ○ | stops cough |
| edema – pulmonary | | | | | | | | ○ | ▲ | | | | stops leukorrhea |
| hiccup – Stomach heat | | | | | | △ | | | | | ○ | | warms the Kidneys |
| hydrothorax (xuan yin) | | | | | | | | | ▲ | | ○ | ○ | warms the Lungs |
| hypertension – yang ↑ | | △ | | | | | | | | | | | |
| impotence – Kidney yang def. | | | | | | | | | | | △ | | |
| jaundice – damp heat | | | | | | | | | | △ | | | |
| lactation – insufficient | | | | | | | | | | | △ | | |
| leukorrhea – damp heat | | | | | | | | △ | | | | | |
| leukorrhea – Sp. qi def., damp | | | | | | | | △ | | | | | **Domain (❖)** |
| orthopnea | ❖ | ❖ | ❖ | ❖ | ❖ | ❖ | ❖ | ❖ | ▲❖ | ❖ | ❖ | ❖ | Lung |
| pain – & injury, trauma | ❖ | | ❖ | | | | | | | △ | | | Large Intestine |
| pain – abdominal, blood stasis | | | | | | | | ❖ | | △ | ❖ | | Kidney |
| pain – lower back, leg, knee | | | | | | | | | ❖ | | △ | | Bladder |
| parasites – head & body lice | | | | | | | E | | | ❖ | | | Liver |
| parasites – pinworms | | | | | | ❖ | △ | | | | ❖ | | Stomach |
| skin – itchy wind rash; urticaria | | | | | | | E | | | | | | |
| skin – scabies, tinea, ringworm | | | | | | | E | E | | | | | |
| sperm – involuntary loss of | | | | | | | | △ | | | △ | | **Flavour, nature (♦)** |
| urination – difficult | ♦ | △ | | | | | | ♦ | △ | △ | | ♦ | slightly toxic |
| urination – frequent | | | ♦ | ♦ | ♦ | | | △ | ♦ | ♦ | | ♦ | acrid |
| urination – turbid | | | | | | | | △♦ | | | | | astringent |
| vomiting, nausea – St. heat | ♦ | | ♦ | | | ▲♦ | ♦ | ♦ | ♦ | ♦ | | ♦ | bitter |
| wheezing – external pathogen | △ | △♦ | ▲ | | △ | | | ♦ | ♦ | | ♦ | | sweet |
| wheezing – cold in the Lungs | △ | ♦ | | △ | | | | △ | | | | ▲ | cold |
| wheezing – Lung & Kidney def. | | | | | | | | ▲ | ♦ | △ | ▲ | | very cold |
| wheezing – phlegm damp | △ | | ▲ | | △ | ♦ | | △♦ | ▲ | △♦ | △ | △ | neutral |
| wheezing – phlegm heat | △ | △ | ♦ | | △♦ | | | ▲ | | △ | ♦ | ♦ | warm |
| | ♦ | | ♦ | | | | ♦ | | | | | | slightly warm |
| **Standard dosage range (g)** | 3–9 | 9–15 | 3–9 | 6–9 | 6–9 | 9–15 | 6–9 | 6–9 | 3–9 | 9–30 | 9–15 | 6–15 | |

### Xìng Rén (Armeniacae Semen) apricot seed

**Preparation and use** Unprocessed seeds moisten the bowels and are better for cough accompanied by constipation; stir frying (chao xing ren 炒杏仁) reduces the bitterness and laxative effect while retaining the antitussive action, being preferred for patients with Spleen deficiency and a tendency to loose stools; the defatted seeds (xing ren shuang 杏仁霜) have no laxative effect but still stop cough and wheezing. Crush before decoction and add towards the end[1] of cooking. When used in pill or powder form the skin around the seed should be removed by blanching. Peeled seeds are less toxic than un–peeled seeds, and decoction is safer than direct ingestion.

**Contraindications** Cough from yin and qi deficiency, in infants and debilitated patients. Caution in patients with diarrhea. The dosage range should not be exceeded to avoid toxic effects[2] from the amygdalin content, common to all seeds of the Prunus genus (apricot, almond, cherry, plum and peach [tao ren p.6]).

**Formulae** Xing Su San (wind cold cough); Sang Ju Yin (wind heat cough); Ma Huang Tang (wind cold common cold with wheezing); Ma Xing Shi Gan Tang (Lung heat wheezing and cough); Ding Chuan Tang (wheezing from phlegm heat); Ma Zi Ren Wan (constipation from dry Intestines); San Ren Tang (damp heat in the qi level); Huo Po Xia Ling Tang (lingering damp in the qi level); & 20+ more in Appendix 7.

### Sāng Bái Pí (Mori Cortex) mulberry tree root bark

**Preparation and use** Use unprocessed for Lung heat conditions, edema and hypertension; stir frying with honey (zhi sang bai pi 炙桑白皮) moderates its coldness and enhances its ability to moisten the Lungs, support qi, treat cough and wheezing from deficiency, and alleviate cough with sticky, hard to expectorate phlegm.

**Contraindications** Cough and wheezing from cold in the Lungs (unprocessed).

**Formulae** Xie Bai San (cough from Lung heat); Ding Chuan Tang (wheezing from phlegm heat); Bu Fei Tang (chronic cough and dyspnea from Lung qi deficiency); Jiu Xian San† (chronic cough from qi and yin deficiency); Ren Shen Ge Jie San (wheezing from Lung and Kidney deficiency); Wu Pi Yin (superficial upper body edema); Shi Wei San[3] (stone dysuria); & 12+ more in Appendix 7.

### Sū Zǐ (Perillae Fructus) perilla fruit

**Preparation and use** Unprocessed seeds are strongest in particular at alleviating wheezing and moistening the Intestines, preferred when wheezing and cough are accompanied by constipation; stir frying (chao su zi 炒苏子) moderates its pungency, reduces its laxative effect and is the preferred form for wheezing from cold phlegm in patients with normal or loose stools; stir frying with honey (zhi su zi 炙苏子) enhances its ability to moisten the Lungs, and is used for wheezing and cough with sticky phlegm.

**Contraindications** Caution (unprocessed) in patients with wheezing and cough from Lung qi or yin deficiency, and in Spleen qi deficiency with loose stools.

**Formulae** Su Zi Jiang Qi Tang (wheezing from thin phlegm damp); San Zi Yang Qin Tang (thin phlegm congestion in the Lungs and middle burner); Ding Chuan Tang (wheezing from phlegm heat); Ma Ren Cong Rong Tang (constipation in postpartum women with blood deficiency)

### Zǐ Wǎn (Asteris Radix) aster root

**Preparation and use** Unprocessed zi wan is used for externally contracted, excess type, and productive cough; stir frying with honey (zhi zi wan 炙紫菀) is preferred for chronic or dry cough from deficiency.

**Contraindications** Used alone in cough from yin deficiency with heat, excess heat and dryness and hemoptysis.

**Formulae** Zi Wan Tang (chronic cough from Lung qi deficiency); Zhi Sou San (persistent cough in the aftermath of an external pathogenic invasion); Bai Ri Ke Ke Li Ji (whooping cough); She Gan Ma Huang Tang (wheezing from cold phlegm in the Lungs); Bu Fei Tang (chronic cough and dyspnea from Lung qi deficiency)

### Kuǎn Dōng Huā (Farfarae Flos) coltsfoot

**Preparation and use** Unprocessed kuan dong hua is used for externally contracted and cold phlegm type cough; stir frying with honey (zhi kuan dong hua 炙款冬花) is preferred for chronic cough from deficiency.

**Contraindications** Caution when used alone in patients with hemoptysis and cough from Lung abscess.

**Formulae** Kuan Dong Hua Tang (cough from phlegm heat); Ding Chuan Tang (wheezing from phlegm heat); She Gan Ma Huang Tang (wheezing from cold phlegm in the Lungs); Jiu Xian San† (chronic cough from qi and yin deficiency); Bai Hua Gao (syrup for chronic dry cough from Lung yin deficiency)

### Pí Pa Yè (Eriobotryae Folium) loquat leaf

**Preparation and use** Use unprocessed for nausea and vomiting; stir frying with honey (zhi pi pa ye 炙枇杷叶) is best for cough. Should be cooked in a cloth bag[4] to stop the small hairs on the leaf from irritating the throat.

**Contraindications** Alone for Lung cold type cough and Stomach cold type vomiting.

**Formulae** Pi Pa Qing Fei Yin (Lung heat cough); Qing Zao Jiu Fei Tang (dry cough from Lung yin and fluid damage); Bai Ji Pi Pa Wan (hemoptysis from Lung yin deficiency); Pi Pa Ye Yin (vomiting from Stomach heat); She Dan Chuan Bei Pi Pa Gao (syrup for dry cough)

### Bǎi Bù (Stemonae Radix) stemona root

**Preparation and use** Unprocessed bai bu irritates the digestive tract and mucous membranes, and is therefore reserved for external use in tinctures and washes. For internal use, bai bu is always processed. Stir frying with honey (zhi bai bu 炙百部) enhances its ability to moisten the Lungs and stop cough, it is used for chronic dry and deficient cough, and cough in infants and children; steaming (zheng bai bu 蒸百部) alleviates its irritating tendency while retaining its antitussive and antiparasitic properties and can be used for both acute and chronic cough, or as a retention enema for pinworms.

**Contraindications** Spleen qi deficiency with loose stools.

**Formulae** Bai Bu Tang (chronic cough from Lung qi and yin deficiency); Bai Ri Ke Ke Li Ji (whooping cough); Zhi Sou San (persistent cough in the aftermath of an external pathogenic invasion); Bai Bu Ding (tincture for head and body lice); Bai Bu Gao (ointment for itchy psoriasis); She Chuang Zi San (a wash for itching from numerous causes)

### Bái Guǒ (Ginkgo Semen) ginkgo nut

This herb appears in the astringent group in other texts.

**Preparation and use** The unprocessed seeds are slightly toxic[5] in the raw state, but decocting or heating the seeds denatures the toxic component. When decocted, unprocessed seed can be used, and should be crushed first. When used in pill or powder form, the seeds are stir fried (chao bai guo 炒白果) or roasted (wei bai guo 煨白果).

**Contraindications** Wheezing and cough from acute common cold. Not suitable for use in children or for prolonged or excessive use.

**Formulae** Ding Chuan Tang (wheezing from phlegm heat); Yi Huang Tang (chronic leukorrhea from Spleen deficiency and damp heat)

### Tíng Lì Zǐ (Lepidii/Descurainiae Semen) lepidium seed or descurainia seed

**Preparation and use** Unprocessed seeds are very cold and easily damage the middle burner. Stir frying (chao ting li zi 炒葶苈子) moderates their coldness while retaining the ability to drain the Lungs and alleviate wheezing.

**Contraindications** Cough and wheezing from Lung deficiency, and alone for edema or urinary dysfunction from Lung, Spleen or Kidney deficiency.

**Formulae** Ting Li Da Zao Xie Fei Tang (wheezing from fluid congestion in the Lungs); Da Xian Xiong Wan (painful cough from heat and pathogenic fluids accumulating in the chest); Ji Jiao Li Huang Wan (fluid accumulation in the Stomach and Intestines, ascites)

---

1 Appendix 6, p.108
2 Appendix 3.2, p.104
3 Pu Ji Ben Shen Fang (Formulas of Universal Benefit from My Practice)

4 Appendix 6, p.109
5 Appendix 3.2, p.103

| △ Indication<br>▲ Strong Indication<br>E External Use<br>E Strong External Indication<br><br>**INDICATIONS** | Suan Zao Ren 酸枣仁 | Bai Zi Ren 柏子仁 | Yuan Zhi 远志 | He Huan Pi 合欢皮 | He Huan Hua 合欢花 | Ye Jiao Teng 夜交藤 | Xiao Mai 小麦 | Ling Zhi 灵芝 | Xie Cao 缬草 | | | ○ Function<br>● Strong Function<br><br>**FUNCTIONS** |
|---|---|---|---|---|---|---|---|---|---|---|---|---|
| abscess – Lung | ● | ○ | ○ | △○ | ○ | ● | ○ | ○ | ○ | | | calms the shen |
| abscesses & sores – skin | | | △ E | △ | | ○ | | | | | | dispels wind |
| altitude sickness | | | ○ | | | | | △ | | | | dissipates masses |
| amenorrhea – blood stasis | | | | | ○ | | | △ | | | | harmonizes the Stomach |
| anxiety, palpitations | ▲ | △ | △ | | ○ | ▲ | | △ | △○ | | | invigorates blood |
| appetite – loss of | | ○ | | | △ | | | ▲ | | | | moistens the Intestines |
| bleeding – hemorrhoids | ○ | △○ | | | | ○ | ○ | ○ | | | | nourishes the Heart |
| bones – poor healing of broken | | | | △○ | ○ | | | | | | | regulates Liver qi |
| breast – distension & pain | ○ | | △ | | | | | | | | | stops sweating |
| breast – cysts & lumps | | | △ | | | | | ○ | | | | stops cough & wheeze |
| constipation – dry, chronic | | △ | | | | | | ○ | | | | tonifies qi & blood |
| constipation – postpartum | | △ | ○ | | | | | | | | | transforms phlegm |
| cough – phlegm damp | | | △ | | | ○ | | △ | | | | unblocks collaterals |
| debility – generalized chronic | | | | | | | | △ | | | | |
| depression – deficiency | △ | △ | | | | △ | △ | | | | | |
| depression – excess | | | △ | ▲ | △ | | | | | | | |
| diarrhea – Spleen qi deficiency | | | | | | | | △ | | | | |
| disorientation – phlegm | | | △ | | | | | | | | | |
| dysmenorrhea – blood stasis | | | | | | | | △ | | | | |
| dysuria – cloudy | | | △ | | | | | | | | | |
| foggy head; mental cloudiness | | | ▲ | | | | | | | | | |
| insomnia – blood & yin def. | ▲ | △ | △ | △ | △ | △ | | △ | | | | |
| insomnia – Liver qi constraint | | | | ▲ | △ | | | △ | | | | |
| irritability | ▲ | △ | | ▲ | △ | △ | | | | | | |
| leukopenia | | | | | | | | △ | | | | |
| memory – poor | △ | △ | ▲ | △ | △ | | | △ | | | | **Domain (❖)** |
| night terrors in children | | △ | ❖ | | | | | ❖ | | | | Lung |
| nightmare disturbed sleep | △ | ❖ | | ▲ | | ▲ | | | | | | Large Intestine |
| numbness – blood deficiency | | ❖ | | | | △ | | | | | | Kidney |
| pain – & injury, trauma | ❖ | | | △❖ | ❖ | ❖ | ❖ | ❖ | △❖ | | | Liver |
| pain – abdominal, blood stasis | ❖ | ❖ | ❖ | ❖ | | ❖ | ❖ | ❖ | △❖ | | | Heart |
| pain – chest, phlegm | | | △ | | ❖ | | | | | | | Stomach |
| pain – muscle; blood deficiency | | | | | | ▲ | | | | | | |
| painful obst. – blood def. | | | | | | ▲ | | | | | | |
| painful obst. – wind damp | | | | | | △ | | △ | | | | **Flavour, nature (♦)** |
| restless organs (*zang zao*) | | | ♦ | | | | △ | ♦ | | | | acrid |
| rumination, obsessive thinking | | | △♦ | | | | | | | | | bitter |
| seizures, epilepsy – phlegm | ♦ | | △ | | | | | △ | | | | sour |
| skin – itchy & dry; eczema | ♦ | ♦ | | ♦ | ♦ | △E♦ | ♦ | ♦ | ♦ | | | sweet |
| sweating – night sweats | ▲ | △ | | | | | ♦ | | | | | cool |
| sweating – spontaneous | △♦ | ♦ | | ♦ | ♦ | ♦ | | ♦ | | | | neutral |
| tonsils – chronic swelling of | | | △ | | | | | ♦ | | | | warm |
| wheezing – phlegm, chronic | | | △♦ | | | | | ▲ | | | | slightly warm |
| **Standard dosage range (g)** | 9–18 | 9–18 | 6–15 | 9–15 | 6–9 | 15–30 | 30–60 | 3–15 | 3–6 | | | |

**Ǎi Dì Chá (Ardisia japonicae Herba) Japanese ardisia**
Also known as zǐ jīn niú 紫金牛.
**Contraindications** None noted.
**Formulae** *Fu Fang Ai Di Cha Pian* (prepared medicine for phlegm heat in the Lungs)

**Zhōng Rǔ Shí (Stalactitum) stalactite**
Placed with the yang tonics in some texts.
**Preparation and use** Calcining (*duan zhong ru shi* 煅钟乳石) enhances its ability to warm Kidney yang and assist the Kidneys in grasping qi. This form is most commonly used.
**Contraindications** Acute patterns of cough and wheezing from heat, and in cases with hemoptysis. Not suitable for prolonged or excessive use as calculi can form in the stomach.
**Formulae** *Zhong Ru Wan* (chronic wheezing from cold phlegm); *Zhong Ru Bu Fei Tang* (chronic wheezing from Lung yang qi deficiency); *Zhong Ru Tang* (insufficient lactation from Stomach heat or yin deficiency)

**Mǎn Shān Hóng (Rhododendron daurici Folium) rhododendron leaf**
**Preparation and use** Commonly prepared as alcohol extract for chronic bronchitis, with 100 grams of powdered leaf steeped in one litre of grain alcohol (vodka will do) for one week. Discard the dregs and take 5–15 milliliters three times daily.
**Contraindications** Not suitable for prolonged use. Caution in patients with liver disease. The maximum recommended dose should not be exceeded. Symptoms of toxicity[1] may occur with high doses or long use.
**Formulae** *Fu Fang Man Shan Hong Jiao Nang* (prepared medicine for chronic bronchitis)

## Substances from other groups
Other herbs with some ability to alleviate cough and/or wheezing (the most important in bold) include **wu wei zi** (p.4), ce bai ye (p.12), shi wei (p.20), sang ye (p.26), **ma huang** (p.28), xi xin (p.28), zhi ban xia (p.54), **jie geng** (p.54), bai qian (p.54), chuan bei mu (p.56), **qian hu** (p.56), han cai (p.58), luo han guo (p.58), song zi ren (p.60), ling zhi (p.70), ge jie (p.82), dong chong xia cao (p.82), zi he che (p.82) and chuan shan long (p.92).

## Endnotes
† These formulae traditionally contain items from endangered animal species and/or obsolete toxic substances, and are unavailable in their original form.

---

1 Appendix 3.2, p.104

# 16.1 SEDATIVE, SHEN CALMING – NOURISHING

**Suān Zǎo Rén (Ziziphi spinosae Semen) sour jujube seed**
**Preparation and use** Crush in a mortar and pestle before decoction. Can be ground into a fine powder and taken before bed, at a dose of 1.5–3 grams. Unprocessed seeds are best for insomnia and shen disturbances from yin deficiency and heat; stir fried seeds (*chao suan zao ren* 炒酸枣仁) are best for shen problems from qi and blood deficiency, and excessive sweating.
**Contraindications** Shen disturbances from excess heat, fire, phlegm damp or phlegm heat. Caution during pregnancy[1] and in patients with diarrhea.
**Formulae** *Suan Zao Ren Tang* (insomnia from Liver yin and blood deficiency); *Gui Pi Tang* (shen disturbance and bleeding from Heart blood and Spleen qi deficiency); *Tian Wang Bu Xin Dan* (Heart and Kidney yin deficiency); *Zhen Zhu Mu Wan* (insomnia and shen disturbances from Heart and Liver yin and blood deficiency with ascendant yang)

**Bǎi Zǐ Rén (Platycladi Semen) Chinese arborvitae seed**
**Preparation and use** Crush in a mortar and pestle before decoction. For patients with nausea or loose stools from qi deficiency, the stir fried seeds (*chao bai zi ren* 炒柏子仁) or defatted seeds (*bai zi ren shuang* 柏子仁霜) can be used.
**Contraindications** Caution (unprocessed) in patients with loose stools, nausea and phlegm problems.
**Formulae** *Yang Xin Tang* (Heart qi and blood deficiency); *Bai Zi Yang Xin Tang* (Heart and Kidney not communicating); *Tian Wang Bu Xin Dan* (Heart and Kidney yin deficiency); *Wu Ren Wan* (chronic constipation from dryness and blood deficiency)

**Yuǎn Zhì (Polygalae Radix) polygala root**
**Preparation and use** Unprocessed yuan zhi is best for clearing the mind and enhancing memory, but can irritate the digestive tract; processing with licorice root (*zhi yuan zhi* 制远志 or *qing yuan zhi* 清远志) reduces its drying nature and tendency to irritate the gut; it is therefore better for calming the shen; stir frying with honey (*mi yuan zhi* 蜜远志) enhances its ability to transform phlegm and stop coughing.
**Contraindications** Shen disturbances from Heart fire or phlegm heat. Caution (unprocessed) in patients with gastritis and peptic ulcers.
**Formulae** *Kai Xin San* (memory problems from qi and blood deficiency); *Gui Pi Tang* (shen disturbance and bleeding from Heart blood and Spleen qi deficiency); *An Shen Ding Zhi Wan* (insomnia and memory problems from Heart qi deficiency); *Ding Xian Wan*† (seizures from wind phlegm); *Tian Wang Bu Xin Dan* (Heart and Kidney yin deficiency); *Sang Piao Xiao San* (enuresis and nocturia from Heart and Kidney deficiency)

**Hé Huān Pí (Albiziae Cortex) Persian silk tree bark**
**Contraindications** Caution during pregnancy.
**Formulae** *An Shen Bu Xin Wan* (shen disturbances from Heart yin and blood deficiency)

**Hé Huān Huā (Albiziae Flos) Persian silk tree flower**
**Contraindications** None noted.
**Formulae** *An Shen Wan* (insomnia and dream disturbed sleep from blood deficiency); *Jia Yi Gui Zang Tang* (headache and dizziness from Liver yin deficiency with ascendant yang)

**Yè Jiāo Téng (Polygoni multiflori Caulis) fleeceflower vine**
Also commonly known as shǒu wū téng 首乌藤.
**Contraindications** None noted.
**Formulae** *An Shen Bu Xin Wan* (shen disturbances from Heart yin and blood deficiency); *Tian Ma Gou Teng Yin* (insomnia, dizziness and headache from ascendant Liver yang); *Jia Yi Gui Zang Tang* (headache and dizziness from Liver yin deficiency with ascendant yang)

**Xiǎo Mài (Tritici Fructus) wheat**
**Contraindications** None noted.
**Formulae** *Gan Mai Da Zao Tang* ('dry organ' syndrome; menopausal shen disturbances)

**Líng Zhī (Ganoderma) reishi mushroom**
**Preparation and use** Taken directly in pill or powder form, the dose is 1.5–3 grams, two or three times daily.
**Contraindications** Caution in patients without deficiency.
**Formulae** *Zi Ling Wan* (chronic debility; convalescence)

**Xié Cǎo (Valeriana officinalis Rhizoma) valerian root**
**Preparation and use** Best taken an hour or so before bed. Commonly used in alcohol extract.
**Contraindications** None noted.

## Substances from other groups
Herbs from other groups with some shen calming effects include lian zi (p.2), wu wei zi (p.4), dan shen (p.6), fu ling (p.18), shi chang pu (p.50), ren shen (p.74), da zao (p.74), long yan rou (p.78) and bai he (p.80).

## Endnotes
† These formulae traditionally contain items from endangered animal species and/or obsolete toxic substances, and are unavailable in their original form.

---

1 Chen (2004) is the only source to make this claim.

| △ Indication<br>▲ Strong Indication<br>E External Use<br>E Strong External Indication<br>**INDICATIONS** | Long Gu 龙骨 | Long Chi 龙齿 | Ci Shi 磁石 | Hu Po 琥珀 | Zi Shi Ying 紫石英 | Sheng Tie Luo 生铁落 | | | | | | ○ Function<br>● Strong Function<br><br>**FUNCTIONS** |
|---|---|---|---|---|---|---|---|---|---|---|---|---|
| amenorrhea – blood stasis | | | ○ | △ | | | | | | | | aids Kidney in grasping qi |
| anxiety, easily startled | △ | ▲ | △ | △ ○ | △ | △ | | | | | | alleviates dysuria |
| bleeding – hematemesis, rectal | △ ● | | | | | | | | | | | astringes fluid leakage |
| bleeding – hematuria | | | ○ | △ | | | | | | | | benefits hearing |
| bleeding – uterine, menorrhagia | △ | | ○ | | △ | | | | | | | brightens the eyes |
| convulsions – chronic childhood | △ ○ | △ | | ▲ | △ | ○ | | | | | | calms the Liver |
| cough – chronic; Lung qi def. | ○ | ● | ○ | ○ | △ ○ | ○ | | | | | | calms & sedates the shen |
| diarrhea – chronic | △ | | | ○ | | | | | | | | invigorates blood |
| dizziness, vertigo – yang↑, wind | △ ● | ○ | ▲ ○ | | | | | | | | | pacifies ascendant yang |
| dysenteric disorder – chronic | △ | | | | ○ | | | | | | | warms Kidneys & Uterus |
| dysuria – damp heat; stone | | | | △ | ○ | | | | | | | warms the Lungs |
| dysuria – blood | | | | ▲ | | | | | | | | |
| ears – hearing loss | | | ▲ | | | | | | | | | |
| ears – tinnitus | △ | | ▲ | | | | | | | | | |
| eyes – blurring vision, sporadic | △ | | △ | | | | | | | | | |
| eyes – corneal opacity, cataract | | | △ | | | | | | | | | |
| eyes – weak vision; yin def. | | | △ | | | | | | | | | |
| fibroids, endometriosis | | | | △ | | | | | | | | |
| headache – ascendant yang | △ | | △ | | | | | | | | | |
| hematocele | | | | △ | | | | | | | | |
| infertility – Kidney yang def. | | | | | ▲ | | | | | | | |
| insomnia; dream disturbed sleep | △ | ▲ | △ | △ | △ | △ | | | | | | |
| irritability, restlessness | ▲ | △ | △ | △ | △ | ▲ | | | | | | |
| leukorrhea – Sp. & Kid. def. | △ | | | | | | | | | | | |
| masses – abdominal | | | | △ | | | | | | | | |
| nightmares, night terrors | △ | ▲ | | △ | | | | | | | | |
| pain – & injury, trauma | | | | △ | | | | | | | | **Domain (❖)** |
| pain – abdominal; bld. stasis | | | | △ | ❖ | | | | | | | Lung |
| pain – chest, angina; bld. stasis | | | ❖ | △ | ❖ | | | | | | | Kidney |
| pain – testicular; bld. stasis | | | | △ ❖ | | | | | | | | Bladder |
| palpitations | △ ❖ | ▲ ❖ | △ ❖ | ▲ ❖ | △ ❖ | △ ❖ | | | | | | Liver |
| seizures, epilepsy | △ ❖ | △ ❖ | △ ❖ | ▲ ❖ | △ ❖ | ❖ | | | | | | Heart |
| sweating – night sweats | △ | | | | | | | | | | | |
| sweating – profuse, in shock | △ | | | | | | | | | | | |
| sweating – spontaneous | △ | | | | | | | | | | | **Flavour, nature (♦)** |
| tremor | △ | | △ ♦ | ▲ | △ | ♦ | | | | | | acrid |
| ulcers – skin, chronic | E ♦ | ♦ | | E | | | | | | | | astringent |
| urination – frequent, nocturia | ▲ | | ♦ | | | | | | | | | salty |
| urination – painful | ♦ | ♦ | | △ ♦ | ♦ | | | | | | | sweet |
| urination – urinary calculi | | | ♦ | △ | | | | | | | | cold |
| wheezing – Kidney deficiency | ♦ | ♦ | △ | | | ♦ | | | | | | cool |
| wheezing – Lung cold | | | | ♦ | △ | | | | | | | neutral |
| withdrawal mania (*dian kuang*) | ▲ | △ | ▲ | | △ ♦ | ▲ | | | | | | warm |
| **Standard dosage range (g)** | 15–30 | 15–30 | 15–30 | 1.5–3 | 9–15 | 30–60 | | | | | | |

These mineral substances weigh down and sedate a chaotic, unstable shen. They can be hard on the Spleen and Stomach, and may upset digestion, thus are usually combined with other herbs to protect the middle burner. Considerable overlap exists between the sedative shen calming group and the wind extinguishing group, with different texts emphasizing some aspects over others and classifying substances accordingly.

### Lóng Gǔ (Fossilia Ossis Mastodi) fossilized bone

**Preparation and use** Crush and cook for 30 minutes[1] before the other herbs. Unprocessed long gu is used to calm the Heart and Liver; calcined long gu (*duan long gu* 煅龙骨) is used to prevent leakage of fluids and promote healing. Finely powdered calcined long gu is applied externally.

**Contraindications** Damp heat patterns and when any acute or lingering pathogen is present.

**Formulae** *Chai Hu Jia Long Gu Mu Li Tang* (shen disturbance from ascendant Liver yang, phlegm and heat); *Zhen Gan Xi Feng Tang* (headache and hypertension from ascendant Liver yang); *Jin Suo Gu Jing Wan* (frequent urination and loss of essence from Kidney deficiency); *Gu Chong Tang* (uterine bleeding from *chōng mài / rèn mài* deficiency); *Gui Zhi Jia Long Gu Mu Li Tang* (post traumatic shen disturbance and sweating from disruption to the Heart Kidney axis); *Sang Piao Xiao San* (enuresis and nocturia from Heart and Kidney deficiency)

### Lóng Chǐ (Fossilia Dentis Mastodi) fossilized teeth

**Preparation and use** Crush and cook for 30 minutes[2] before the other herbs. Unprocessed long chi is better for calming a shen disturbed by heat; when calcined (*duan long chi* 煅龙齿) its cooling nature is reduced, and astringency enhanced. The calcined form is better able to bind and tranquilize a restless shen, and is used for shen disturbances and fright from causes other than heat.

**Contraindications** Damp heat patterns and when any acute or lingering pathogen is present.

**Formulae** *Long Chi San* (infantile night terrors from heat); *An Shen Ding Zhi Wan* (anxiety and insomnia from Heart qi deficiency); *Zhen Zhu Mu Wan* (insomnia and shen disturbances from Heart and Liver yin and blood deficiency with ascendant yang); *Jia Yi Gui Zang Tang* (headache and dizziness from Liver yin deficiency with ascendant yang)

### Cí Shí (Magnetitum) magnetite; $Fe_3O_4$ ferrous–ferric oxide

**Preparation and use** Crush and cook for 30 minutes[3] before the other herbs. Calcining facilitates pulverization and absorption, and is the form used in pills or powders. In pill and powder form the dose is 1–3 grams, two to three times daily. Unprocessed ci shi is best for calming the shen, pacifying the Liver and anchoring yang; when calcined (*duan ci shi* 煅磁石), its ability to treat hearing and vision and to assist the Kidneys in grasping qi and alleviate wheezing is enhanced.

**Contraindications** Caution in patients with middle burner deficiency, especially when taken directly in pill or powder form. Not suitable for prolonged use.

**Formulae** *Er Long Zuo Ci Wan* (hearing deficit from Kidney yin deficiency); *Ci Shi Liu Wei Wan* (chronic wheezing from Kidney deficiency); *Ci Zhu Wan*† (insomnia and palpitations from disruption to the Heart Kidney axis)

### Hǔ Pò (Succinum) amber

**Preparation and use** Not suitable for decoction. Amber is finely pulverized (*hu po mo* 琥珀末), and used as pills, powder or mixed with honey.

**Contraindications** Yin deficiency with heat.

**Formulae** *Hu Po Ding Zhi Wan*† (insomnia, forgetfulness and easy fright from disruption to the Heart Kidney [shen and zhi] axis); *Hu Po Bao Long Wan*† (childhood convulsions, epilepsy and shen disturbances from phlegm heat); *Ding Xian Wan*† (seizures from wind phlegm); *Hu Po San* (hematuria and urinary calculi); *Tong Jing Wan* (amenorrhea and dysmenorrhea from blood stasis)

### Zǐ Shí Yīng (Fluoritum) fluorite, a mineral largely composed of calcium fluoride, with the chemical composition $CaF_2$
Placed in the yang tonic section of other texts.

**Preparation and use** Crush and cook for 30 minutes[4] before the other herbs.

**Contraindications** Infertility and impotence from yin deficiency with heat; wheezing from Lung heat.

**Formulae** *Feng Yin Tang* (seizures and tremors from phlegm heat affecting the Heart); *Zi Shi Ying Wan* (infertility and impotence from yang deficiency); *Zhong Ru Bu Fei Tang* (chronic wheezing from Lung yang qi deficiency); *Zhen Ling Dan*† (persistent uterine bleeding from yang deficiency and blood stasis)

### Shēng Tiě Luò (Ferri Frusta) iron oxide, oxidized iron filings
Placed in the wind extinguishing section of other texts.

**Preparation and use** Cook for 30 minutes[5] before the other herbs.

**Contraindications** Liver and Heart qi and blood deficiency type shen disturbances; middle burner yang qi deficiency.

**Formulae** *Sheng Tie Luo Yin*† (mania from phlegm fire)

### Substances from other groups
Substances from other groups with some shen sedating effect include mu li (p.48), zi bei chi (p.48), zhen zhu mu (p.48) and zhen zhu (p.96).

### Endnotes
† These formulae traditionally contain items from endangered animal species and/or obsolete toxic substances, and are unavailable in their original form.

---

1 Appendix 6, p.108
2 Ibid.
3 Ibid.

4 Ibid.
5 Ibid.

△ Indication
▲ Strong Indication
E External Use
**E** Strong External Indication

○ Function
● Strong Function

| INDICATIONS | Ren Shen 人参 | Dang Shen 党参 | Tai Zi Shen 太子参 | Xi Yang Shen 西洋参 | Huang Qi 黄芪 | Bai Zhu 白术 | Shan Yao 山药 | Huang Jing 黄精 | Da Zao 大枣 | Gan Cao 甘草 | Yi Tang 饴糖 | Feng Mi 蜂蜜 | FUNCTIONS |
|---|---|---|---|---|---|---|---|---|---|---|---|---|---|
| abdominal distension | | | | | | △ | | | | ○ | ○ | ○ | alleviates spasm & pain |
| abscesses – chronic, yin type | | | | | △ | | | | ○ | △ E | | | alleviates toxicity |
| abscesses & sores – skin | | | | | | | ○ | | | △ | | E | augments the Kidneys |
| appetite – loss of | ▲ | ▲ | △ | | △ | ▲○ | △ | △ | △ | △ | △ | | calms restless fetus |
| arrhythmia – qi & blood def. | ○ | | | | | | | | ○ | ▲ | | | calms the shen |
| bleeding – Lung, Intestine; heat | | | | △ | | | | | | ○ | | | clears toxic heat |
| bleeding – uterine; qi def. | | | | | △ | ○ | | | | | | | dries damp |
| blood deficiency | △ | △ | | | ▲○ | | | | ▲ | | | | fortifies the exterior |
| constipation – heat, dryness | ○ | ○ | ○ | △○ | | | | | | | | △ | generates fluids |
| constipation – qi def., atonic | | | | | | △ | | ○ | | ○ | ○ | ○ | moistens the Lungs |
| cough – excess (wind, heat, etc.) | | | | ○ | | | | ○ | ○ | ▲ | | | nourishes yin |
| cough – Lung qi deficiency | ▲ | ▲ | △ | △ | ● | | | △ | △ | △ | △ | △ | promotes healing |
| cough – Lung yin def., dry | | △ | △ | △ | ○ | ○ | △ | ▲ | | | | ▲ | promotes urination |
| diarrhea – Spleen qi deficiency | △ | △ | | | △● | ▲ | ▲ | | △ | | | | raises yang & sinking qi |
| diabetes (*xiao ke*) | ▲ | | | △ | ▲● | ○ | ▲ | ▲ | | | | | stops sweating |
| edema – during pregnancy | ● | ○ | ○ | ○ | ● | ▲○ | ○ | ○ | ○ | ○ | ○ | ○ | tonifies qi |
| edema – qi deficiency | ● | △ | | | ▲ | △ | | | | | | | tonifies source qi |
| fever – chronic; qi, yin def. | | | ▲ | △ | ▲ | | | | | | | | |
| hemiplegia; paralysis; numbness | | | | | ▲ | | | | | | | | |
| immunity low – defensive qi def. | △ | △ | △ | | ▲ | △ | | | | | | | |
| impotence – Kidney yang def. | ▲ | | | | | | | | | | | | |
| insomnia, dream disturbed sleep | △ | | | △ | | | | | △ | | | | |
| leukorrhea – Sp. qi def., damp | | | | | | △ | ▲ | | | | | | |
| Lung & Kidney yin deficiency | | | | △ | | | △ | | | | | | |
| memory – poor | ▲ | | △ | △ | | | | ▲ | △ | | | | |
| miscarriage – threatened | | | | | | △ | | | | | | | **Domain (❖)** |
| pain – epigastric & abdominal | ❖ | ❖ | ❖ | ❖ | ❖ | | ❖ | ❖ | | ▲❖ | △❖ | △❖ | Lung |
| pain – lower back, leg, knee | | | | | | | ❖ | △ | | | | ❖ | Large Intestine |
| painful obst. – wind damp | | | | ❖ | △ | △ | ❖ | ❖ | | | | | Kidney |
| palpitations, anxiety | ▲ | | △ | ❖ | | | | | △ | ▲❖ | | | Heart |
| prolapse – uterus, rectal, ptosis | △❖ | △❖ | ❖ | | ▲❖ | ❖ | ❖ | ❖ | ❖ | ❖ | ❖ | ❖ | Spleen |
| radio/chemotherapy – side effects | | | | | ▲ | ❖ | | | | ❖ | ❖ | ❖ | Stomach |
| restless organs (*zang zao*) | | | | | | | | | △ | △ | | | |
| shock – collapse from | ▲ | | | | | | | | | | | | |
| spasm & cramp – all muscles | | | | | | | | | | △ | | | **Flavour, nature (♦)** |
| sweating – spontaneous | △ | △ | △ | ♦ | ▲ | △♦ | △ | | △ | △ | | | bitter |
| thin mucus disorder (*tan yin*) | ♦ | | ♦ | | | △ | | | | | | | slightly bitter |
| thirst, dryness – post febrile | ▲♦ | △♦ | ▲♦ | ▲ | ♦ | | △♦ | △♦ | ♦ | ♦ | ♦ | ♦ | sweet |
| throat – sore; acute & chronic | | | | ♦ | | | | | | ▲ | | E | slightly sweet |
| thrombocytopenia | | | | ♦ | | | | | △ | | | | cold |
| ulcers, wounds – non-healing | | ♦ | ♦ | | ▲ | | ♦ | ♦ | | ♦ | | E♦ | neutral |
| urination – frequent, qi def. | △ | | | | | | ♦ | ▲ | ♦ | | ♦ | | warm |
| wheezing – Lung qi deficiency | ▲♦ | ▲ | | | ♦ | | | △ | | △ | | | slightly warm |
| **Standard dosage range (g)** | 6–9 | 9–30 | 9–30 | 3–6 | 9–15 | 6–15 | 9–30 | 9–15 | 9–30 | 3–9 | 15–60 | 15–30 | |

Qi tonic herbs improve the function of the Lungs and Spleen, and thus harvesting and transformation of raw materials of food and air into the form of qi the body can use. The fundamental features of qi deficiency – fatigue and weakness that are worse with exertion, breathlessness and pallor – are implicit indications of all the qi tonic herbs.

### Rén Shēn (Ginseng Radix) ginseng root

Wild ginseng is listed in Appendix 2 of CITES[1]. All ginseng available on the open market is cultivated.

**Preparation and use** Traditionally double boiled[2] in a special vessel and taken separately. Due to the expense of good quality ginseng, the most convenient and cost effective delivery method is powder, either directly or in capsules, with a dose of 1–2 grams, two or three times daily. For emergency use in cases of shock and hemorrhagic shock, a large dose (15–30 grams) of the best quality processed ren shen (*hong shen* 红参 [red ginseng]) is required. If unable to ingest the liquid, it can be delivered via the rectum. The ginseng from China is generally considered milder than Korean ginseng. Korean ginseng is generally warmer than the Chinese varieties, is steamed before drying and becomes red (*hong shen* 红参). Being warm, it should be used cautiously in conditions where there is any heat. Where there is mild heat, unprocessed or white ginseng (*bai ren shen* 白人参) can be specified.

**Contraindications** All internal excess heat patterns, bleeding due to heat in the blood, yin deficiency with ascendant yang, bone steaming fever, phlegm heat in the Lungs, ascendant Liver yang and the presence of pathogenic influences without concurrent qi deficiency. Inappropriate use or overdose can lead to side effects[3]. Normal doses can compound the adrenergic effects of coffee and other stimulants. Caution in patients with hypertension and peptic ulcer disease. Incompatible[4] with li lu (p.22), and antagonistic[5] to zao jia[6] (p.54), wu ling zhi (p.6) and lai fu zi (p.30). Avoid consumption of radish, daikon and tea when using ginseng, as these are thought to reduce its effectiveness[7].

**Formulae** *Si Jun Zi Tang* (Spleen qi deficiency); *Li Zhong Wan* (Spleen yang deficiency); *Bu Zhong Yi Qi Tang* (sinking Spleen qi); *Shen Ling Bai Zhu San* (Spleen qi deficiency with dampness and diarrhea); *Shen Fu Tang* (collapse of yang qi; shock); *Sheng Mai San* (Lung qi and yin deficiency); *Ren Shen Ge Jie San* (wheezing from Lung and Kidney deficiency); *Gui Pi Tang* (shen disturbance and bleeding from Heart blood and Spleen qi deficiency); *Tian Wang Bu Xin Dan* (Heart and Kidney yin deficiency shen disturbance); *Ba Zhen Tang* (qi and blood deficiency); *Ren Shen Lu Rong Wan* (impotence from Kidney yang deficiency); *Shen Su Yin* (wind cold with qi deficiency); *Bai Hu Jia Ren Shen Tang* (heat in the qi level with fluid damage); *Xiao Chai Hu Tang* (shao yang syndrome); *Yu Quan Wan* (diabetes); *Ren Shen Bai Du San* (wind cold common cold with qi deficiency); & 70+ more in Appendix 7.

### Dǎng Shēn (Codonopsis Radix) codonopsis root

**Preparation and use** Dang shen is commonly used as a cost effective substitute for ren shen for qi deficiency. Its action is similar to, although not as strong as, ren shen. The rule of thumb is that dang shen can substitute for ren shen in chronic diseases but not acute, severe problems, such as sudden bleeding and shock.

**Contraindications** Qi stagnation in the middle burner, Liver fire and the presence of pathogenic influences without concurrent qi deficiency. Incompatible[8] with li lu (p.22) and antagonistic[9] to wu ling zhi (p.6).

### Tài Zǐ Shēn (Pseudostellariae Radix) pseudostellaria root
Also known as *hái ér shēn* 孩儿参 (childrens root).

**Preparation and use** Commonly used instead of ren shen for children, and when there is concurrent yin deficiency.

**Contraindications** Lingering pathogens in patients without significant underlying deficiency.

### Xī Yáng Shēn (Panacis quinquefolii Radix) American ginseng

Wild american ginseng is listed in Appendix 2 of CITES[10]. The majority of american ginseng available on the open market is cultivated.

**Preparation and use** Traditionally double boiled[11] in a special vessel and taken separately. Commonly used instead of ren shen when there is concurrent yin deficiency and fluid damage from chronic heat.

**Contraindications** Middle burner yang deficiency; cold damp blocking the middle burner; Liver qi constraint with heat; excess heat conditions.

**Formulae** *Qing Shu Yi Qi Tang* (qi and yin damage in the aftermath of a summerheat common cold)

### Huáng Qí (Astragali Radix) astragalus root

**Preparation and use** In severe or resistent cases of hemiplegia, paralysis and chronic ulceration, doses of 30–120 grams may be used. Unprocessed huang qi is used to stop sweating, promote urination and reduce edema, and promote healing; stir frying with honey (*zhi huang qi* 炙黄芪) enhances its ability to tonify qi and raise sinking qi.

**Contraindications** Acute common cold patterns, when any external pathogen remains on the surface or in patterns of yin deficiency with ascendant yang. Huang qi must be used cautiously when qi and damp obstruct the middle burner or during the early stages of superficial suppurative sores. Long term use of huang qi can generate internal heat, but this can be offset by combining it with small amounts of moistening, heat clearing herbs, such as xuan shen (p.40) and zhi mu (p.32).

**Formulae** *Bu Zhong Yi Qi Tang* (sinking Spleen qi); *Yu Ping Feng San* (defensive qi deficiency); *Gui Pi Tang* (shen disturbance and bleeding from Heart blood and Spleen qi deficiency); *Dang Gui Bu Xue Tang* (blood deficiency following hemorrhage); *Shi Quan Da Bu Tang* (qi and blood deficiency with cold; chronic ulceration); *Fang Ji Huang Qi Tang* (wind damp pain and edema with qi deficiency); *Bu Yang Huan Wu Tang* (hemiplegia from qi deficiency with blood stasis); *Mu Li San* (sweating from deficiency); *Juan Bi Tang* (wind damp pain); *Huang Qi Gui Zhi Wu Wu Tang* (numbness from qi and blood deficiency); *Tou Nong San*† (yin sores); *Huang Qi Tang* (diabetes from qi deficiency); *Yu Ye Tang* (diabetes from qi and yin deficiency); *Dang Gui Liu Huang Tang* (severe night sweats from yin deficiency); *Gu Chong Tang* (uterine bleeding from *chōng mài / rèn mài* deficiency)

### Bái Zhú (Atractylodis macrocephalae Rhizoma) white atractylodes rhizome

**Preparation and use** Unprocessed bai zhu is used to promote urination, reduce edema, consolidate the exterior, stop sweating, activate peristalsis, and ease wind damp painful obstruction. For stubborn atonic constipation, up to 120 grams of unprocessed bai zhu can be used until the bowels are moving, then tapered off to a maintenance dose. Stir frying (*chao bai zhu* 炒白术) enhances its ability to strengthen the Spleen, tonify qi and calm fetal restlessness; processing with earth (*tu bai zhu* 土白术) or charring (*jiao bai zhu* 焦白术) enhances its ability to strengthen the Spleen and stop diarrhea.

**Contraindications** Yin deficiency patterns with internal heat and fluid damage; constipation from excess heat.

**Formulae** *Si Jun Zi Tang* (Spleen qi deficiency); *Li Zhong Wan* (Spleen yang deficiency); *Shen Ling Bai Zhu San* (chronic diarrhea from Spleen qi deficiency with damp); *Yu Ping Feng San* (defensive qi deficiency); *Tong Xie Yao Fang* (diarrhea and abdominal pain from Liver and Spleen disharmony); *Wan Dai Tang* (leukorrhea from Spleen deficiency with dampness); *Wu Ling San* (generalized edema; edema in tai yang syndrome); *Zhen Wu Tang* (edema from Spleen and Kidney yang deficiency); *Ling Gui Zhu Gan Tang* (phlegm damp [thin mucus] in the Intestines); *Ban Xia Bai Zhu Tian Ma Tang* (dizziness and headache from wind phlegm); *An Tai Yin* (threatened miscarriage from qi deficiency with heat); *Qin Jiao Bai Zhu Wan* (chronic constipation with bleeding, itchy hemorrhoids)

---

1 Appendix 4, p.105
2 Appendix 6, p.109
3 Appendix 3.2, p.104
4 Appendix 2, p.100
5 Ibid.
6 *Zhong Yao Xue* (2000)
7 *Zhong Yao Xue* (2000)
8 Appendix 2, p.100
9 Ibid.

10 Appendix 4, p.105
11 Appendix 6, p.109

## Shān Yào (Dioscoreae Rhizoma) Chinese yam

**Preparation and use** Unprocessed shan yao nourishes yin and generates fluids; stir frying (*chao shan yao* 炒山药) enhances its ability to strengthen the Spleen, stop diarrhea and leukorrhea. The stir fried herb is preferred for use in pill or powder form. To assist in regulating blood sugar levels in prediabetes, 120–250 grams can be used per day. Can be eaten (or added to oats) as a porridge.

**Contraindications** Excess heat patterns. Can aggravate bloating when there is damp or food stagnation obstructing the middle burner.

**Formulae** *Shen Ling Bai Zhu San* (chronic diarrhea from Spleen qi deficiency with damp); *Wan Dai Tang* (leukorrhea from Spleen deficiency with dampness); *Fu Tu Dan* (leukorrhea and seminal emission from Kidney deficiency); *Yi Huang Tang* (leukorrhea from Spleen deficiency with damp heat); *Yu Ye Tang* (diabetes from qi and yin deficiency); *Liu Wei Di Huang Wan* (Kidney yin deficiency); *Suo Quan Wan* (nocturia and urinary frequency from Kidney deficiency); *Gao Lin Tang* (turbid urination from Kidney deficiency)

## Huáng Jīng (Polygonati Rhizoma) Siberian solomons seal rhizome

Placed in the yin tonic group in some texts.

**Preparation and use** Processing with wine (*jiu huang jing* 酒黄精) tempers its richness, makes it easier on digestion and improves its ability to alleviate lower back and knee pain. When repeatedly steamed and dried (*shu huang jing* 熟黄精) its ability to tonify qi is enhanced. If the fresh herb is available, 30–60 grams can be used. Generally needs to be taken for a long time for optimal effect.

**Contraindications** Excess heat patterns, damp heat and phlegm heat. This herb is quite cloying to the digestion and should be used cautiously in those with middle burner qi stagnation, phlegm damp or abdominal distension.

**Formulae** *Er Jing Wan* (general debility, visual and reproductive weakness from Liver and Kidney yin deficiency); *Wu Jing Jian Wan* (memory problems and profound debility from essence deficiency)

## Dà Zǎo (Jujubae Fructus) jujube, Chinese date

**Preparation and use** Usually dispensed by pieces of fruit, in which case 3–8 dates are typically used. Da zao is often used as a binding agent for tonic pills or, with the pip removed, as a casing for harsh or irritant herbs.

**Contraindications** Da zao can be quite cloying to the digestion and is contraindicated in those with qi stagnation, significant phlegm and damp, internal excess heat patterns, phlegm heat, damp heat and abdominal bloating.

**Formulae** *Gan Mai Da Zao Tang* (restless organ syndrome); *Yi Pi Bing* (loss of appetite and diarrhea from Spleen deficiency); *Ting Li Da Zao Xie Fei Tang* (pulmonary edema; moderates the harshness of ting li zi)

## Gān Cǎo (Glycyrrhizae Radix) licorice root

**Preparation and use** When used as the principal herb in a formula, 15–30 grams can be used. Unprocessed gan cao is neutral in temperature and used to treat suppurating skin disorders and Lung heat; when stir fried with honey (*zhi gan cao* 炙甘草) it becomes warm and better for tonifying Spleen and Heart qi. To promote urination and treat painful urination syndrome from heat, the rootlets of the licorice root (*gan cao shao* 甘草梢) are preferred.

**Contraindications** Components of gan cao exhibit a mineralocorticoid like effect with prolonged use or high doses, leading to electrolyte imbalances from increased reabsorption of sodium and increased excretion of potassium. This can contribute to edema and hypertension. Gan cao should not be used in large doses or for prolonged periods in patients with chronic renal insufficiency, congestive cardiac failure, hypertension, hypokalemia and edema. Caution in patients with abdominal bloating, nausea and vomiting from damp. Incompatible[1] with hong da ji (p.62), yuan hua (p.62) and gan sui (p.62).

**Formulae** *Zhi Gan Cao Tang* (arrhythmia from qi and blood deficiency); *Si Jun Zi Tang* (Spleen qi deficiency); *Gan Mai Da Zao Tang* (restless organ syndrome); *Bai Tou Weng Jia Gan Cao E Jiao Tang* (postpartum blood deficient type dysenteric disorder); *Ma Xing Shi Gan Tang* (wheezing from Lung heat); *Ma Huang Tang* (wind cold common cold); *Shao Yao Gan Cao Tang* (muscle spasm and cramp); *Xiao Yao San* (Liver qi constraint); *Gan Jie Tang* (sore throat from heat); *Shao Yao Tang* (damp heat dysenteric disorder with abdominal pain); *Di Yu Gan Cao Tang* (rectal bleeding with abdominal pain); *Yang He Tang* (yin sores); *Xian Fang Huo Ming Yin*† (toxic heat boils and sores); *Dao Chi San* (Heart fire type dysuria); & 200+ more in Appendix 7.

## Yí Táng (Maltosum) malt sugar

**Preparation and use** Dissolve in the warm strained decoction[2].

**Contraindications** Damp heat patterns, phlegm heat cough, middle burner qi stagnation, abdominal bloating and children with accumulation disorder (gan ji).

**Formulae** *Xiao Jian Zhong Tang* (abdominal pain from Spleen yang deficiency); *Da Jian Zhong Tang* (abdominal pain from cold); *Du Sheng San* (dysmenorrhea and postpartum abdominal pain from blood stasis); *Yi Wei Tang* (Stomach yin deficiency)

## Fēng Mì (Mel) honey

**Preparation and use** Dissolve in the warm strained decoction[3]. Often used to bind laxative, tonic or antitussive pills. When used topically on open lesions, a good quality sterilized medical honey, such as Manuka[4], should be used.

**Contraindications** Caution in patients with damp and phlegm blocking the middle burner, damp heat patterns, middle burner qi stagnation, abdominal bloating, nausea and vomiting, loose stools or diarrhea.

**Formulae** *Zao Jia Wan* (chronic wheezing from stubborn phlegm); *Qing Yin Wan*† (hoarse voice, loss of voice and sore throat from Lung fire); *Wu Ren Wan* (chronic constipation from dryness or blood deficiency)

## Substances from other groups

Other herbs with some qi tonic effect include bian dou (p.46), ling zhi (p.70), ge jie (p.82), dong chong xia cao (p.82), zi he che (p.82) and hu tao ren (p.82).

## Endnotes

† These formulae traditionally contain items from endangered animal species and/or obsolete toxic substances, and are unavailable in their original form.

---

1 Appendix 2, p.100.
2 Appendix 6, p.108
3 Ibid.
4 A product of bees collecting pollen from the Manuka bush, a plant that has antibiotic properties.

Blood tonic herbs generate blood. They provide the building blocks for blood manufacture, but require a strong Spleen to transform their nutrients into blood. When the Spleen is weak, qi tonics must also be given to ensure that adequate transformation takes place. Most of these herbs are rich and cloying, can upset the digestion and are combined with digestion improving and qi regulating herbs to offset this.

### Shú Dì Huáng (Rehmanniae Radix preparata) rehmannia root

**Preparation and use** In severe cases 30–60 grams may be used. To offset its richness for those with weak digestion, the root can be stir fried (*chao shu di* 炒熟地); this can also be mitigated by combining with sha ren (p.16) or chen pi (p.64). Charring (*shu di tan* 熟地炭) enhances its ability to stop bleeding.

**Contraindications** Phlegm and damp, middle burner qi stagnation, abdominal bloating, loss of appetite or diarrhea.

**Formulae** *Si Wu Tang* (blood deficiency); *Ba Zhen Tang* (qi and blood deficiency); *Liu Wei Di Huang Wan* (Kidney yin deficiency); *Da Bu Yin Wan* (bone steaming fever from Kidney yin deficiency); *Jin Gui Shen Qi Wan* (Kidney yang deficiency); *Jiao Ai Tang* (chronic uterine bleeding from cold and deficiency); *Zhen Yuan Yin* (chronic wheezing and breathlessness from Liver and Kidney deficiency); *Dang Gui Liu Huang Tang* (severe night sweats from yin deficiency); *Gu Zhi Zeng Sheng Wan* (bony proliferation, osteophytes); *Hu Qian Wan†* (weakness and atrophy of the legs from Liver and Kidney deficiency); *Qin Jiao Ji Sheng Tang* (postpartum joint pain from blood deficiency with wind); *Rou Cong Rong Wan* (infertility and impotence from Kidney yang deficiency); *Wu Ji Bai Feng Wan* (menstrual disorders from qi and blood deficiency); & 25+ more in Appendix 7.

### Dāng Guī (Angelicae sinensis Radix) Chinese angelica root

**Preparation and use** When used to tonify blood, during pregnancy and for threatened miscarriage, the main body of the root (*dang gui shen* 当归身) is preferred; to invigorate blood the tips of the root (*dang gui wei* 当归尾) are used; to harmonize (i.e. both tonify and invigorate) blood, the whole root (*quan dang gui* 全当归) is specified. Unprocessed dang gui is best when moistening the Intestines to treat dry constipation; processing with wine (*jiu dang gui* 酒当归) enhances its ability to invigorate blood and promote menstruation.

**Contraindications** Caution in Spleen deficiency, and phlegm damp patterns with abdominal bloating, loss of appetite or diarrhea.

**Formulae** *Dang Gui Bu Xue Tang* (blood deficiency following hemorrhage); *Dang Gui Shao Yao San* (dysmenorrhea and premenstrual edema); *Dang Gui Si Ni San* (numbness and pain in the extremities from cold in the channels); *Dang Gui Nian Tong Tang* (leg pain and swelling from damp heat); *Dang Gui Sheng Jiang Yang Rou Tang* (postpartum weakness); *Dang Gui Yin Zi* (chronic itchy skin disorder from blood deficiency); *Dang Gui Hong Hua Yin* (skin rash from heat and blood stasis); *Dang Gui San* (threatened miscarriage from heat); *Dang Gui Long Hui Wan* (Liver fire with constipation); *Dang Gui Liu Huang Tang* (severe night sweats from yin deficiency); *Si Wu Tang* (blood deficiency); *Gui Pi Tang* (shen disturbance and bleeding from Heart blood and Spleen qi deficiency); *Xiao Yao San* (Liver qi constraint with blood deficiency); *Tao Hong Si Wu Tang* (blood deficiency with blood stasis); *Wen Jing Tang* (infertility and dysmenorrhea from cold and deficient *chōng mài / rèn mài*); *Sheng Hua Tang* (postpartum blood stasis); *Jiao Ai Tang* (chronic uterine bleeding from cold and deficiency); *Er Xian Tang* (hypertension and menopausal symptoms from Kidney yin and yang deficiency); *Si Miao Yong An Tang* (peripheral ulcers and gangrene from toxic heat and blood stasis); *Xian Fang Huo Ming Yin†* (toxic heat boils and sores); *Tou Nong San†* (chronic yin sores); *Su Zi Jiang Qi Tang* (chronic wheezing from phlegm congestion); *Ji Chuan Jian* (chronic constipation from yang deficiency); *Juan Bi Tang* (wind damp painful obstruction); & 100+ more in Appendix 7.

### Bái Sháo (Paeoniae Radix alba) white peony root

**Preparation and use** For severe cramping and colicky pain, up to 30 grams can be used. Unprocessed bai shao is used to protect and nourish yin, calm the Liver and treat dysenteric disorder with cramping abdominal pain; stir frying (*chao bai shao* 炒白芍) reduces its coldness and enhances its ability to soften the Liver, harmonize the Liver and Spleen and stop pain. Stir frying also makes it easier on a weak Spleen. Processing with vinegar (*cu bai shao* 醋白芍) enhances its ability to target the Liver and stop bleeding; processing with wine (*jiu bai shao* 酒白芍) enhances its warmth and ability to both nourish and gently invigorate blood, and makes it better for cold type abdominal pain, menstrual and postpartum disorders.

**Contraindications** Should not be used alone or unprocessed in yang deficiency and cold conditions. Incompatible[1] with li lu (p.22).

**Formulae** *Shao Yao Tang* (dysenteric disorder with abdominal pain from damp heat); *Shao Yao Gan Cao Tang* (muscle spasm and cramp); *Dang Gui Shao Yao San* (dysmenorrhea and premenstrual edema); *Si Wu Tang* (blood deficiency); *Tong Xie Yao Fang* (colicky abdominal pain and diarrhea from Liver and Spleen disharmony); *Si Ni San* (Liver qi constraint); *Xiao Jian Zhong Tang* (abdominal pain from Spleen yang deficiency); *Gui Zhi Tang* (nutritive defensive qi disharmony); *San Jia Fu Mai Tang* (post febrile yin deficiency with tremor and spasm); *Huang Qi Gui Zhi Wu Wu Tang* (numbness from qi and blood deficiency); *Zhen Gan Xi Feng Tang* (dizziness and headaches from ascendant Liver yang); *Fu Zi Tang* (cold damp painful obstruction); *San Bi Tang* (qi and blood deficiency type painful obstruction); & 70+ more in Appendix 7.

### Ē Jiāo (Asini Corii Colla) donkey skin gelatin

**Preparation and use** This comes in hard resinous blocks, and should be crushed in a mortar and pestle or coffee grinder before being melted[2] in the hot strained decoction, or mixed into pill or powder form. Can also be melted in warm yellow wine and taken alone. Combining e jiao and wine enhances its ability to nourish and gently invigorate blood, and reduces its meaty richness. Unprocessed e jiao is used to nourish yin and moisten dryness; processing e jiao with pu huang (p.8) (*pu huang chao e jiao* 蒲黄炒阿胶) enhances its ability to stop bleeding; processing e jiao with powdered hai ge qiao (p.58) (*ge fen chao e jiao* 蛤粉炒阿胶, a combination also known as donkey skin gelatin pearls, *e jiao zhu* 阿胶珠) enhances its ability to moisten the Lungs and alleviate chronic dry cough and wheezing.

**Contraindications** Unprocessed e jiao can be difficult to digest, so should be used with care in patients with weak Spleen and Stomach qi, nausea, diarrhea and abdominal bloating, phlegm damp patterns and exterior disorders.

**Formulae** *Jiao Ai Tang* (chronic uterine bleeding from cold and deficiency); *Huang Lian E Jiao Tang* (post febrile yin damage with insomnia); *E Jiao Ji Zi Huang Tang* (spasms and tremors from yin and blood deficiency); *Bu Fei E Jiao Tang†* (hemoptysis from Lung yin deficiency with heat); *Bai Tou Weng Jia Gan Cao E Jiao Tang* (postpartum blood deficient type dysenteric disorder); *Huang Tu Tang* (rectal bleeding from Spleen yang deficiency); *Da Ding Feng Zhu* (spasms and tremors from yin and blood deficiency); *Yue Hua Wan†* (chronic cough and hemoptysis from Lung and Kidney yin deficiency); *Qing Zao Jiu Fei Tang* (cough from heat and dryness); *Zhu Ling Tang* (chronic urinary discomfort from Kidney yin deficiency with lingering damp heat); *Zhi Gan Cao Tang* (arrhythmia from qi and blood deficiency); *Shou Tai Wan* (habitual miscarriage from Kidney deficiency); & 10+ more in Appendix 7.

### Lóng Yǎn Ròu (Longan Arillus) longan fruit

**Preparation and use** Can be used alone as tea, or cooked with various foods in a similar fashion to lychees or raisins.

**Contraindications** Phlegm and damp, heat from qi constraint, or blockage of the qi dynamic.

**Formulae** *Gui Pi Tang* (shen disturbance and bleeding from Heart blood and Spleen qi deficiency)

---

1 Appendix 2, p.100
2 Appendix 6, p.108

| △ Indication / ▲ Strong Indication / E External Use / E Strong External Indication — INDICATIONS | Shu Di Huang 熟地黄 | Dang Gui 当归 | Bai Shao 白芍 | E Jiao 阿胶 | Long Yan Rou 龙眼肉 | Sang Shen 桑椹 | Gou Qi Zi 枸杞子 | Zhi He Shou Wu 制何首乌 | Sheng He Shou Wu 生何首乌 | | | ○ Function / ● Strong Function — FUNCTIONS |
|---|---|---|---|---|---|---|---|---|---|---|---|---|
| abscesses & sores – skin | | △ | | | | | | | ▲○ | | | alleviates malaria |
| amenorrhea – bld. def.; bld. stasis | ○ | ▲ | | | | | ○ | ○ | | | | augments essence |
| bleeding – deficiency type | | | | ▲ | | | ○ | | | | | brightens the eyes |
| bleeding – hemoptysis, yin def. | | | ○ | ▲ | | | | | | | | calms the Liver |
| bleeding – uterine; postpartum | △ | △ | △ | ▲ | ○ | | | | | | | calms the shen |
| cervical lymphadenitis (luo li) | | | | | | | | △○ | | | | clears toxic heat |
| constipation – blood def., dry | | ▲○ | | | | △ | | ▲ | | | | invigorates blood |
| cough – yin def., dry | | △○ | | △ | | ○ | △ | | ○ | | | moistens the Intestines |
| development – delayed | ▲ | | | ○ | | | △○ | △ | | | | moistens the Lungs |
| diabetes (xiao ke) | ▲ | | ○ | ○ | | △○ | △○ | | | | | nourishes yin |
| diarrhea – colicky pain during | ○ | ● | ▲○ | | | | | | | | | regulates menstruation |
| dizziness – blood & yin def. | ▲ | △ | △● | △ | △ | △ | △ | △ | | | | softens the liver |
| dizziness – ascendant yang | | | △ | ● | | | | △ | | | | stops bleeding |
| dysenteric disorder – pain of | | ○ | ▲○ | | | | | | | | | stops pain |
| dysmenorrhoea | ● | ▲ | ▲ | | | | | ○ | | | | tonifies Kidney yin |
| dysuria – blood, yin def. | | | | △ | | | | | | | | |
| ears – tinnitus, ↓hearing; Kid. def. | ▲ | | | | | △ | △ | △ | | | | |
| eyes – blurred vision, sporadic | ▲ | ▲ | △ | | | △ | ▲ | △ | | | | |
| eyes – weakness & loss of vision | ▲ | △ | | | | △ | ▲ | △ | | | | |
| fever – bone steaming; yin def. | ▲ | | | △ | | | | | | | | |
| hair – early greying & loss of | △ | | | | | △ | △ | ▲ | | | | |
| headache, dizziness – yang ↑ | | | △ | | | | | △ | | | | |
| hypertension | △ | | △ | | | △ | | △ | | | | |
| impotence; infertility | ▲ | △ | | | | | ▲ | △ | | | | **Domain (❖)** |
| insomnia, palpitations, anxiety | △ | △ | △ | △❖ | ▲ | △ | △❖ | | | | | Lung |
| leukorrhea – yin & blood def. | | | ▲ | | | | | △ | ❖ | | | Large Intestine |
| Liver & Kidney yin deficiency | ▲❖ | | | ❖ | | △❖ | ▲❖ | △❖ | ❖ | | | Kidney |
| malarial disorder – chronic | ❖ | ❖ | ❖ | ❖ | | ❖ | ❖ | ▲❖ | | | | Liver |
| masses – abdominal | | △❖ | | | ❖ | ❖ | | | | | | Heart |
| memory – poor | ▲ | △❖ | ❖ | | △❖ | | △ | ▲ | | | | Spleen |
| menstruation – irregular | ▲ | ▲ | △ | | | | | △ | | | | |
| miscarriage – threatened | | △ | | ▲ | | | | | | | | |
| numbness – extremities | | ▲ | △ | | | | | △ | | | | **Flavour, nature (◆)** |
| pain – & injury, trauma | | ▲◆ | | | | | | | | | | acrid |
| pain – abd.; bld. stag.; Liv. → Sp. | | △ | ▲ | | | | | ◆ | ◆ | | | astringent |
| pain – chest & hypochondriac | | | △◆ | | | | | ◆ | ◆ | | | bitter |
| pain – lower back, leg, knee | △ | | ◆ | | | | △ | △ | | | | sour |
| painful obst. – wind cold damp | ◆ | ▲◆ | | ◆ | ◆ | ◆ | ◆ | ◆ | ◆ | | | sweet |
| skin – dry, scaly, itchy; eczema | | ▲ | | | | ◆ | | △E | △E | | | cold |
| sperm – ↓ liquifaction, ↓ count | △ | | ◆ | | | | ▲ | ▲ | | | | cool |
| sweating – spontaneous; qi def. | | | △ | ◆ | | | ◆ | | ◆ | | | neutral |
| sweating – night; yin, bld. def. | ▲ | ◆ | △ | | | | △ | | | | | warm |
| tremor; spasm & cramp | ◆ | △ | ▲ | △ | | | | ◆ | | | | slightly warm |
| **Standard dosage range (g)** | 9–30 | 6–15 | 6–12 | 6–12 | 9–15 | 9–15 | 6–15 | 9–30 | 9–30 | | | |

**Sāng Shèn (Mori Fructus) mulberry fruit**

Placed in the yin tonic group in some texts.

**Preparation and use** Commonly cooked into a thick syrup with honey for prolonged use, with a dose of up to 30 grams of syrup, once or twice daily.

**Contraindications** Contraindicated in middle burner yang deficiency with diarrhea.

**Formulae** *Shou Wu Yan Shou Dan* (greying hair, dizziness and constipation from Liver and Kidney deficiency); *An Shen Wan* (insomnia and dream disturbed sleep from blood deficiency)

**Gǒu Qǐ Zǐ (Lycii Fructus) lycium fruit; Chinese wolfberry**

Placed in the yin tonic group in some texts.

**Preparation and use** Commonly cooked with nourishing foods such as chicken for postpartum weakness and convalescence for illness. These berries are quite tasty and can be cooked in the same fashion as raisins or currants.

**Contraindications** While generally better tolerated than most blood tonics, gou qi zi berries may nonetheless aggravate damp and cause diarrhea if overused. Caution in patients with middle burner yang deficiency and internal damp stagnation.

**Formulae** *Qi Ju Di Huang Wan* (Liver and Kidney yin deficiency); *Yi Guan Jian* (Liver yin deficiency); *Qi Bao Mei Ran Dan* (alopecia from Liver and Kidney deficiency); *Gui Lu Er Xian Jiao* (debility from essence deficiency); *Er Jing Wan* (general debility, visual and reproductive weakness from Liver and Kidney yin deficiency); *Zhu Jing Wan* (weak vision from Liver and Kidney deficiency); *Wu Zi Yan Zong Wan* (sperm disorders from Kidney deficiency); *Zan Yu Dan* (infertility from Kidney yang deficiency); *Nuan Gan Jian* (hypochondriac and groin pain from cold in the Liver channel or Liver yang deficiency) *You Gui Wan* (Kidney yang deficiency)

**Zhì Hé Shǒu Wū (Polygoni multiflori Radix preparata) processed fleeceflower root**

**Preparation and use** Processed he shou wu is used to tonify blood, the Liver and Kidneys, and augment essence.

**Contraindications** Zhi he shou wu is better tolerated than other blood tonics, and often used instead of shu di when the latter causes digestive upset. It retains some moistening and laxative effect, however, and is therefore contraindicated in patients with loose stools and those with phlegm damp.

**Formulae** *Qi Bao Mei Ran Dan* (alopecia from Liver and Kidney deficiency); *Shou Wu Yan Shou Dan* (greying hair, dizziness and constipation from Liver and Kidney deficiency); *Shou Wu He Ji* (hypertension, dizziness and numb extremities from Liver blood deficiency with ascendant yang); *Dang Gui Yin Zi* (chronic itchy skin disorder from blood deficiency)

**Shēng Hé Shǒu Wū (Polygoni multiflori Radix) fleeceflower root**

**Preparation and use** Unprocessed he shou wu has minimal tonic action and is used primarily to open the bowels, treat suppurative lesions and chronic malaria. To treat wind rash, unprocessed he shou wu may be used externally.

**Contraindications** Loose stools and diarrhea.

**Formulae** *He Ren Yin* (chronic malaria with qi and blood deficiency); *He Shou Wu Tang* (itchy rash from toxic heat in the skin)

Substances from other groups

Herbs from other groups with some blood tonic action include dan shen (p.6), ji xue teng (p.6), ren shen (p.74), dang shen (p.74), huang qi (p.74), da zao (p.74), lu rong (p.82) and rou gui (p.88).

Endnotes

† These formulae traditionally contain items from endangered animal species and/or obsolete toxic substances, and are unavailable in their original form.

# 17.3 TONIFYING – YIN

**Nán Shā Shēn (Adenophorae Radix) adenophora root**

Nan sha shen and bei sha shen are similar and can be used interchangeably, however nan sha shen is considered better when there is sticky phlegm, while bei sha shen is thought best when heat has damaged fluids.

**Preparation and use** When the fresh herb is available, up to 60 grams may be used. The dried herb is used for loosening sticky phlegm.

**Contraindications** Middle burner yang deficiency, cough and wheezing due to cold phlegm accumulation or wind cold exterior invasion. Incompatible[1] with li lu (p.22).

**Formulae** *Sang Xing Tang* (wind heat dryness common cold); *Yue Hua Tang* (cough and hemoptysis from Lung yin deficiency); *Yi Wei Tang* (Stomach yin deficiency); *Qing Zao Jiu Fei Tang* (cough from heat and dryness)

**Běi Shā Shēn (Glehniae Radix) glehnia root**

**Preparation and use** When the fresh herb is available, up to 30 grams may be used. The fresh herb is preferred for generating fluids.

**Contraindications** Middle burner yang deficiency, cough and wheezing due to cold phlegm accumulation or wind cold exterior invasion. Incompatible[2] with li lu (p.22).

**Formulae** *Sha Shen Mai Dong Tang* (Lung and Stomach dryness and yin deficiency); *Yi Guan Jian* (Liver and Stomach yin deficiency); *Bai Bu Tang* (chronic cough from Lung qi and yin deficiency)

**Mài Dōng (Ophiopogonis Radix) ophiopogon root**

**Preparation and use** In some parts of China the central core of the tuber is removed. The herb with and without the central core has slightly different uses. The herb with the core removed is thought better for nourishing Lung and Stomach yin, while the herb with the core retained (*lian xin mai dong* 连心麦冬) is better for nourishing the Heart and calming the *shen*.

**Contraindications** Middle burner yang deficiency, phlegm damp blocking the middle burner and Lungs, and externally induced cough.

**Formulae** *Qing Zao Jiu Fei Tang* (cough from heat and dryness); *Sheng Mai San* (qi and yin deficiency); *Sha Shen Mai Dong Tang* (dry cough from Lung and Stomach dryness); *Mai Men Dong Tang* (dry retching from Stomach yin deficiency); *Mai Wei Di Huang Wan* (chronic cough from Lung yin deficiency); *Zeng Ye Tang* (constipation from dry Intestines); *Tian Wang Bu Xin Dan* (Heart and Kidney yin deficiency); *Qing Ying Tang*† (heat in the ying level); *Zhu Ye Shi Gao Tang* (post febrile lingering heat with qi and fluid damage); *Yang Yin Qing Fei Tang* (chronic throat disorders from Lung yin deficiency); & 25+ more in Appendix 7.

**Tiān Dōng (Asparagi Radix) asparagus root**

**Contraindications** Middle burner yang deficiency with diarrhea, phlegm damp clogging the middle burner and Lungs or externally induced cough.

**Formulae** *Yue Hua Wan*† (chronic cough from Lung yin deficiency); *Er Dong Tang* (diabetes from heat in the upper burner); *San Cai Feng Sui Dan* (chronic cough from exhaustion of Lung and Kidney yin)

**Shí Hú (Dendrobi Herba) dendrobium orchid**

☸ Listed in Appendix 2 of CITES[3] which permits limited trade with appropriate documentation.

**Preparation and use** When the fresh herb is available, up to 30 grams can be used. The fresh herb is better for clearing heat, generating fluids and post febrile dryness. The dried herb is better for nourishing yin and moistening dryness from yin deficiency. The dried herb requires long cooking to extract its active components.

**Contraindications** Middle burner yang deficiency, internal damp, excess heat patterns, or in the early stages of a warm disease.

**Formulae** *Shi Hu Ye Guang Wan*† (visual weakness from Liver and Kidney yin deficiency); *Shi Hu Qing Wei San* (vomiting from Stomach heat and yin deficiency); *Qing Shu Yi Qi Tang* (qi and yin damage in the aftermath of a summerheat common cold)

---

1 Appendix 2, p.100
2 Ibid.

3 Appendix 4, p.105

| △ Indication / ▲ Strong Indication / E External Use / E Strong External Indication | Nan Sha Shen 南沙参 | Bei Sha Shen 北沙参 | Mai Dong 麦冬 | Tian Dong 天冬 | Shi Hu 石斛 | Yu Zhu 玉竹 | Bai He 百合 | Nü Zhen Zi 女贞子 | Mo Han Lian 墨旱莲 | Hei Zhi Ma 黑芝麻 | Gui Ban 龟板 | Bie Jia 鳖甲 | ○ Function / ● Strong Function — FUNCTIONS |
|---|---|---|---|---|---|---|---|---|---|---|---|---|---|
| amenorrhea | | | | | ○ | | | ○ | | | | △ | brightens the eyes |
| bleeding – heat in the blood | | | | | | | ○ | | ▲ | | | | calms the shen |
| bleeding – hematuria | | | ○ | | ○ | | | ○ | ▲ | | ● | ○ | clears heat from deficiency |
| bleeding – hemoptysis | △ | △ | △ | ▲ | | | △ | | △○ | | | | cools the blood |
| bleeding – uterine, menorrhagia | | | ○ | | | | | ○ | △ | | ▲ | | cools the Heart |
| bleeding – yin def. with heat | ○ | ○ | | ○ | | | | | ▲ | | | | cools the Lungs |
| constipation – dry, after fever | △ | △ | ▲ | △ | △ | △ | | | | △ | | ● | dissipates masses |
| cough – chronic dry | △○ | △ | △ | | | △ | | | | | | | expels phlegm |
| cough – Lung heat | △○ | △○ | △● | ▲○ | ● | △● | △ | | | | | | generates fluids |
| cough – dry sticky phlegm | ▲ | △ | △○ | | | | △ | | | ○ | | | moistens the Intestines |
| cough – yin deficiency | ▲ | △ | △ | △ | | △ | ▲ | | | | ● | ○ | pacifies ascendant yang |
| depression (*bai he* disease) | | | | | | | ▲ | | ● | | | | stops bleeding |
| development – delayed | | | ○ | | | | | ○ | ○ | ○ | ▲● | ○ | tonifies Kidney yin |
| diabetes (*xiao ke*) | | | ▲ | ▲ | △ | △ | | ○ | ○ | | ○ | ○ | tonifies Liver yin |
| dizziness, vertigo – yin def. | ● | ○ | ● | ○ | △ | △○ | ● | △ | △ | △ | ▲ | △ | tonifies Lung yin |
| ears – tinnitus, ↓hearing; Kid. def. | ○ | ○ | ● | | ● | ● | | △ | △ | △ | ▲ | | tonifies Stomach yin |
| eyes – weak vision from yin def. | | | | | ▲ | | | ▲ | △ | △ | | | |
| fever – bone steaming; yin def. | | | △ | △ | △ | | | △ | △ | △ | △ | ▲ | |
| fluids – damaged by febrile dis. | △ | △ | ▲ | △ | ▲ | ▲ | △ | | | | △ | △ | |
| hair – early greying & loss of | | | | | | | | ▲ | △ | △ | | | |
| hepatosplenomegaly | | | | | | | | | | | | ▲ | |
| insomnia | | | △ | | | | ▲ | | | | △ | | |
| lactation – insufficient | | | | | | | | | △ | | | | |
| malarial disorder – chronic | | | | | | | | | | | | ▲ | |
| masses – abdominal, bld. stasis | | | | | | | | | | | | ▲ | |
| muscle weakness & atrophy | | | | | | | | | | | ▲ | | **Domain (❖)** |
| nausea, vomiting (dry retching) | △❖ | △❖ | ▲❖ | ❖ | △ | ❖ | ❖ | | | | | | Lung |
| pain – lower back, leg, knee | | | | ❖ | △❖ | | | △❖ | △❖ | ❖ | △❖ | | Kidney |
| palpitations | | | △ | | | | △ | ❖ | ❖ | ❖ | △❖ | ❖ | Liver |
| skin – dry & itchy | ▲ | △ | ▲❖ | | | | ❖ | | | | ❖ | | Heart |
| spasm & tremor – internal wind | | | | | | △ | | | | | ▲ | △❖ | Spleen |
| sperm – poor liquefaction of | ❖ | ❖ | ❖ | | ❖ | ❖ | | | | | ▲ | | Stomach |
| sweating – night sweats | | | | | | | | △ | △ | △ | △ | ▲ | |
| throat – chronic sore & dry | △ | ▲ | △ | △ | △ | △ | △ | | | | | | |
| ulcers – mouth | | | △ | ▲ | | | | | | | | | **Flavour, nature (♦)** |
| voice – hoarse & dry; loss of | ▲ | △ | △ | △♦ | | | △ | ♦ | | | | | bitter |
| wheezing – yin & qi deficiency | △♦ | △♦ | △♦ | △ | | | ▲ | | | | | | slightly bitter |
| yin def. with ascendant yang | | | | | | | | | | | ▲♦ | △♦ | salty |
| yin deficiency – Heart | | | △ | | | | ▲ | | ♦ | | | | sour |
| yin deficiency – Kidney, Liver | ♦ | ♦ | ♦ | △♦ | △♦ | ♦ | ♦ | △♦ | △♦ | △♦ | △♦ | | sweet |
| yin deficiency – Lung | ▲ | △ | ▲ | △♦ | | △ | ▲ | | ♦ | | ♦ | ♦ | cold |
| yin deficiency – post febrile | △♦ | △♦ | ▲♦ | | ♦ | | ♦ | ♦ | | | | | cool |
| yin deficiency – Stomach | △ | △ | ▲ | △ | ▲ | ▲♦ | | | | | ♦ | | neutral |
| **Standard dosage range (g)** | 9–15 | 9–15 | 9–15 | 6–15 | 6–15 | 9–15 | 9–30 | 9–15 | 9–30 | 9–30 | 9–30 | 9–30 | |

**Yù Zhú** (Polygonati odorati Rhizoma) Solomon's Seal rhizome

**Preparation and use** In severe cases up to 30 grams can be used. Unprocessed yu zhu is used for yin deficiency with obvious heat; when steamed (*zheng yu zhu* 蒸玉竹), its ability to nourish yin is enhanced and it is better for yin deficiency with damaged fluids.

**Contraindications** Middle burner yang deficiency and phlegm damp blocking the middle burner.

**Formulae** *Jia Jian Wei Rui Tang* (wind heat common cold with underlying yin deficiency); *Sha Shen Mai Dong Tang* (Lung and Stomach dryness and yin deficiency); *Yi Wei Tang* (Stomach yin deficiency)

**Bǎi Hé** (Lilii Bulbus) lily bulb

**Preparation and use** Unprocessed bai he is used to cool the Heart and calm the *shen*; stir frying with honey (*zhi bai he* 炙百合) enhances its ability to moisten the Lungs and stop cough. Bai he is a popular food item and commonly cooked with rice porridge (*zhou* 粥) for patients with chronic insomnia and anxiety from yin deficiency.

**Contraindications** Contraindicated in middle burner yang deficiency and externally induced coughs.

**Formulae** *Bai He Gu Jin Tang* (cough and hemoptysis from Lung yin deficiency); *Bai He Di Huang Tang* (post febrile irritability and insomnia); *Bai He Hua Shi San* (chronic fever from lingering heat in the qi level)

**Nǚ Zhēn Zǐ** (Ligustri Fructus) privet fruit

**Preparation and use** The fruits should be crushed before decoction.

**Contraindications** Middle burner yang deficiency.

**Formulae** *Er Zhi Wan* (fever and bone steaming from Kidney yin deficiency); *Shou Wu Yan Shou Dan* (greying hair, dizziness and constipation from Liver and Kidney deficiency); *An Shen Bu Xin Wan* (*shen* disturbances from Heart yin and blood deficiency)

**Mò Hàn Lián** (Ecliptae Herba) eclipta

Also known as hàn lián cǎo 旱莲草.

**Contraindications** Middle burner yang deficiency and Kidney yang deficiency.

**Formulae** *Er Zhi Wan* (fever and bone steaming from Kidney yin deficiency); *Shou Wu Yan Shou Dan* (greying hair, dizziness and constipation from Liver and Kidney deficiency)

**Hēi Zhī Ma** (Sesami Semen nigrum) black sesame seed

**Preparation and use** Stir frying the seeds (*chao zhi ma* 炒芝麻) before decoction or crushing to paste enhances their ability to tonify the Liver and Kidneys.

**Contraindications** Diarrhea and loose stools from Spleen deficiency.

**Formulae** *Shou Wu Yan Shou Dan* (greying hair, dizziness and constipation from Liver and Kidney deficiency); *Xiao Feng San* (itchy wind rash); *Qing Zao Jiu Fei Tang* (cough from heat and dryness)

**Guī Bǎn** (Testudinis Plastrum) Chinese pond turtle plastron

🐢 Listed in Appendix 3 of CITES[1].

**Preparation and use** When decocted the shell is crushed and cooked for 30 minutes[2] prior to the other herbs. Unprocessed gui ban is preferred for nourishing yin; processing with vinegar (*cu gui ban* 醋龟板) enhances its ability to target the Liver, pacify ascendant yang and stop bleeding; processing with wine (*jiu gui ban* 酒龟板) enhances its ability to invigorate qi and blood, and is used for weakness and atrophy patterns. A cheaper processed variant (*gui ban jiao* 龟板胶; turtle plastron glue) is available in hard resinous blocks. This can be pulverized in a coffee grinder, taken separately as powder or dissolved in the strained decoction.

**Contraindications** Pregnancy[3], middle burner yang deficiency, cold damp blocking the middle burner or exterior conditions.

**Formulae** *Da Bu Yin Wan* (bone steaming fever from Kidney yin deficiency); *Zhen Gan Xi Feng Tang* (yin deficiency with ascendant yang); *San Jia Fu Mai Tang†* (post febrile yin deficiency with tremor and spasm); *Hu Qian Wan†* (weakness and atrophy of the legs from Liver and Kidney deficiency); *Gu Jing Wan* (uterine bleeding from yin deficiency with heat)

**Biē Jiǎ** (Trionycis Carapax) Chinese softshell turtle shell

🐢 Listed in Appendix 3 of CITES[4].

**Preparation and use** Used in decoction, this substance should be cooked for 30 minutes[5] prior to the other herbs. Unprocessed bie jia has the greatest ability to nourish yin and pacify ascendant yang; processing with vinegar (*cu bie jia* 醋鳖甲) enhances its ability to soften hardness and dissipate masses.

**Contraindications** Pregnancy, middle burner yang deficiency, cold damp blocking the middle burner or in patients with exterior conditions.

**Formulae** *Qing Hao Bie Jia Tang* (post febrile lingering fever, night sweats and heat); *Qing Gu San* (bone steaming fever); *Qin Jiao Bie Jia Tang* (bone steaming fever and night sweats from yin deficiency); *Bie Jia Wan* (abdominal masses); *San Jia Fu Mai Tang* (post febrile yin deficiency with tremor and spasm); *Da Ding Feng Zhu* (spasms and tremors from yin and blood deficiency)

## Substances from other groups

Herbs from other groups with some ability to nourish and tonify yin include zhi mu (p.32), sheng di huang (p.40), xuan shen (p.40), lu dou yi (p.48), huang jing (p.74), xi yang shen (p.74), shan yao (p.74), zhi he shou wu (p.78), gou qi zi (p.78), sang shen (p.78), shu di huang (p.78), bai shao (p.78) and tu si zi (p.84).

## Endnotes

† These formulae traditionally contain items from endangered animal species and/or obsolete toxic substances, and are unavailable in their original form.

---

1 Appendix 4, p.105
2 Appendix 6, p.108
3 Gui ban jiao is not contraindicated.
4 Appendix 4, p.105
5 Appendix 6, p.108

| Indications | Lu Rong 鹿茸 | Ge Jie 蛤蚧 | Dong Chong Xia Cao 冬虫夏草 | Zi He Che 紫河车 | Ba Ji Tian 巴戟天 | Xian Ling Pi 仙灵脾 | Xian Mao 仙茅 | Rou Cong Rong 肉苁蓉 | Suo Yang 锁阳 | Bu Gu Zhi 补骨脂 | Yi Zhi Ren 益智仁 | Hu Tao Ren 胡桃仁 | Functions |
|---|---|---|---|---|---|---|---|---|---|---|---|---|---|
| appetite – loss of | | ○ | | | | | | | | | △ | ○ | aids Kidney grasping qi |
| bleeding – hemoptysis, yin def. | ● | ○ | ▲○ | △○ | | | | ○ | | | | | augments essence |
| bleeding – uterine | △ | | | | ○ | ○ | ● | △ | | | △ | | dispels wind damp |
| blood & qi deficiency | △ | | | △ | | | | ● | ○ | | | ○ | moistens the Intestines |
| bones – poor healing of broken | △ | | | | | | | | | ○ | ○ | | restrains urine |
| cold – intolerance, limbs | △ | ● | ○ | ○ | | ▲ | ▲ | | | | | ○ | stops cough & wheeze |
| constipation – atonic; dry | ○ | | | | | | | ▲ | ▲ | | | △ | strengthens sinew & bone |
| cough – chronic; Lu. & Kid def. | | ▲○ | ▲○ | △○ | | △ | | | | | | △○ | tonifies Lung qi |
| debility – generalized chronic | △● | ○ | ▲○ | △○ | ○ | ● | ● | ○ | ○ | ○ | ○ | ○ | tonifies Kidney yang |
| development – delayed | ▲ | | ○ | | | | | | | | | | tonifies Lung yin |
| diarrhea – chronic, cockcrow | | △ | | | | | | | | ▲○ | △○ | | tonifies Spleen yang |
| dizziness | △ | | △○ | △ | | △ | △ | | | | | | transforms phlegm |
| ears – tinnitus, hearing loss | △ | | △ | △ | | | | | | | | | |
| fever – bone steaming; yin def. | | △ | △ | ▲ | | | | | | | | | |
| hemiplegia | | | | | | △ | ▲ | | △ | | | | |
| hypertension – menopausal | | | | | | ▲ | ▲ | | | | | | |
| impotence – Kidney yang def. | ▲ | △ | △ | △ | △ | ▲ | ▲ | △ | △ | △ | | | |
| infertility – Kidney yang def. | ▲ | | | ▲ | ▲ | △ | △ | △ | △ | | | | |
| lactation – insufficient | | | | △ | | | | | | | | | |
| leukorrhea – Sp. & Kid. def. | △ | | | | △ | | | △ | | | | | |
| libido – low, loss of | △ | △ | △ | △ | △ | ▲ | △ | △ | △ | △ | | | |
| memory – poor | ▲ | | | | | △ | | △ | | | △ | △ | |
| menstruation – irregular | | | | | △ | △ | | | | | | | |
| muscle weakness & atrophy | △ | | | | △ | △ | | | ▲ | | | | |
| numbness – extremities | | | | | | △ | △ | | | | | | |
| pain – abdominal; def., cold | | | | | △ | | ▲ | | | △ | △ | | **Domain (❖)** |
| pain – back, from kidney stones | | ❖ | ❖ | ❖ | | | | | | | | △❖ | Lung |
| pain – joint, with stiffness | | | | | △ | △ | ▲ | ❖ | ❖ | | | ❖ | Large Intestine |
| pain – lower back, leg, knee | △❖ | ❖ | △❖ | △❖ | △❖ | △❖ | ▲❖ | △❖ | ❖ | △❖ | ❖ | △❖ | Kidney |
| painful obst. – wind cold damp | ❖ | | | ❖ | △ | △❖ | ▲❖ | | ❖ | | | | Liver |
| postpartum convalescence | | | △ | △ | | | | | | ❖ | ❖ | | Spleen |
| salivation – excessive, drooling | | | | | | | | | | | ▲ | | |
| skin – vitiligo | | | | | | | | | | △ E | | | |
| sperm – poor motility, ↓count | ▲ | | △ | | | ▲ | | | | △ | | | **Flavour, nature (◆)** |
| sperm – involuntary loss of | | | △ | | △ | | | ◆ | | △ | ▲ | | slightly toxic |
| sweating – night; yin def. | | △ | △ | ▲ | ◆ | ◆ | | ◆ | | ◆ | ◆ | | acrid |
| sweating – spontaneous; qi def. | | | ▲ | | | | | | | ◆ | | | bitter |
| ulcers – skin, chronic | ▲◆ | ◆ | | ◆ | | | | ◆ | | | | | salty |
| urination – enuresis, nocturia | △◆ | △ | | ◆ | △◆ | △◆ | △ | ◆ | | △◆ | ▲ | ◆ | sweet |
| urine – frequent, incontinence | △ | △ | | | △ | △ | △◆ | △ | △ | ▲◆ | ▲ | | hot |
| vomiting, nausea – Spleen def. | ◆ | | ◆ | ◆ | | ◆ | | ◆ | ◆ | | △◆ | ◆ | warm |
| wheezing – Lung & Kidney def. | | ▲ | △ | △ | ◆ | △ | | | | △ | | △ | slightly warm |
| | | ◆ | | | | | | | | | | | neutral |
| **Standard dosage range (g)** | 1–3 | 1–2 | 6–9 | 1.5–3 | 9–15 | 9–15 | 3–9 | 9–21 | 9–15 | 6–15 | 3–9 | 9–30 | |

Legend:
△ Indication
▲ Strong Indication
E External Use
E Strong External Indication
○ Function
● Strong Function

**Lù Róng** (Cervi Cornu pantotrichum) deer velvet; the immature horn removed before maturation

**Preparation and use** Not suitable for decoction. Taken directly[1] in capsules or alcohol tincture. Lu rong is quite heating and can lead to ascendant yang and the generation of internal wind in some patients. Best to start with a small dose and gradually increase it, over a week or two, to test its effect. Other products derived from deer antlers include:

The mature horn (*lu jiao* (鹿角)) shed by the deer each season. Similar to lu rong, but weaker in tonifying yang. It invigorates blood and is preferred for yin sores, the early stages of breast abscess, lower back pain and blood stasis type pain. The dose is 6–15 grams, powdered and taken separately.

The resinous extract of boiled down antlers (*lu jiao jiao* (鹿角胶)). This inexpensive product is a common substitute for lu rong. It is weaker than lu rong in tonifying yang, but can stop bleeding, and is preferred for yin sores and bleeding disorders from yang deficiency. It comes in hard resinous blocks which are pulverized in a coffee grinder before use. The dose is 6–12 grams melted in the strained decoction, or taken separately in alcohol tincture or as powder.

**Contraindications** All varieties are contraindicated in yin deficiency with heat and ascendant yang, heat in the blood, warm diseases, phlegm heat in the Lungs or other heat patterns.

**Formulae** *Jia Wei Di Huang Wan*† (failure to thrive); *Yang He Tang* (yin sores); *Shen Rong Gu Ben Wan* (infertility and urinary frequency from Kidney yang deficiency); *Ren Shen Lu Rong Wan* (impotence from Kidney yang deficiency); *Gui Lu Er Xian Jiao* (debility from essence deficiency); *Si Jing Wan* (premature ejaculation and weakness from Kidney deficiency); *You Gui Wan* (Kidney yang deficiency)

**Gé Jiè** (Gecko) gecko

**Preparation and use** Mostly used alcohol extract, pills or powder. When used as powder, the dose is 1–2 grams daily. Rarely decocted, but if so up to 6 grams can be used per bag.

**Contraindications** Wind cold and excess heat patterns with cough and wheezing.

**Formulae** *Ren Shen Ge Jie San* (cough and wheeze from Lung and Kidney deficiency)

**Dōng Chóng Xià Cǎo** (Cordyceps) cordyceps fungus

**Preparation and use** An expensive substance, best powdered and taken directly in doses of 1.5–3 grams. Can be decocted in doses of 6–9 grams, and used in cooking, particularly with chicken, duck or pork, for general weakness, postpartum recovery or the convalescent stage of any severe illness. It needs to be taken for a long time for optimum effect.

**Contraindications** Exterior patterns and cough due to Lung heat.

**Formulae** *Dong Chong Ji Jing* (convalescence from illness or debility)

**Zǐ Hé Chē** (Hominis Placenta) human placenta

**Preparation and use** Powdered, placed in capsules and taken 2–3 times daily. In severe case the dose may be doubled. Not suitable for decoction.

**Contraindications** Not used alone in yin deficiency with heat.

**Formulae** *He Che Da Zao Wan* (chronic wheezing, cough and sweats from Lung and Kidney yin deficiency)

**Bā Jǐ Tiān** (Morindae officinalis Radix) morinda root

**Contraindications** Yin deficiency with heat, excess heat patterns, difficult urination or dry type constipation.

**Formulae** *Ba Ji Wan*[2] (irregular menstruation and dysmenorrhea from lower burner yang deficiency); *Ba Ji Wan*[3] (chronic pain in the low back and legs from Liver and Kidney deficiency); *Er Xian Tang* (hypertension and menopausal symptoms from Kidney yin and yang deficiency); *Zan Yu Dan* (impotence and infertility from Kidney yang deficiency); *Jin Gang Wan* (weakness and atrophy from Kidney deficiency)

**Xiān Líng Pí** (Epimedii Herba) epimedium leaf

Also known as yín yáng huò 淫羊藿.

**Preparation and use** This herb is quite drying and is not suitable for prolonged use when unprocessed (more than 6-8 weeks) as it can deplete yin. Processing with wine (*jiu ling pi* 酒灵脾) enhances its ability to dispel wind damp; processing with rendered sheep fat (*zhi ling pi* 炙灵脾) enhances its ability to warm yang, stimulate the libido and treat impotence. Both these treatments moderate its acrid warmth and reduces its tendency to damage yin. Commonly used in alcohol extract.

**Contraindications** Yin deficiency with heat.

**Formulae** *Er Xian Tang* (hypertension and menopausal symptoms from Kidney yin and yang deficiency); *Xian Ling Pi San* (wind cold damp painful obstruction and numbness); *Zan Yu Dan* (infertility from Kidney yang deficiency); *Gu Zhi Zeng Sheng Wan* (bony proliferation, osteophytes)

**Xiān Máo** (Curculiginis Rhizoma) golden eye-grass rhizome

**Preparation and use** Commonly used in alcohol extract. Not suitable for prolonged use, no more than 4–6 weeks at a time without a break, as symptoms of toxicity[4] may occur. The maximum recommended dose should not be exceeded.

**Contraindications** Yin deficiency with heat.

**Formulae** *Er Xian Tang* (hypertension and menopausal symptoms from Kidney yin and yang deficiency); *Zan Yu Dan* (infertility from Kidney yang deficiency)

**Ròu Cōng Róng** (Cistanches Herba) broomrape stem

⚙ Listed in Appendix 2 of CITES[5] which permits limited trade with appropriate documentation.

**Preparation and use** In severe cases, or when used alone, up to 30 grams may be prescribed.

**Contraindications** Yin deficiency with heat and ascendant yang, Spleen deficiency diarrhea or excess heat type constipation.

**Formulae** *Ma Ren Cong Rong Tang* (constipation in postpartum women with blood deficiency); *Ji Chuan Jian* (constipation from yang deficiency); *Rou Cong Rong Wan* (impotence from Kidney yang deficiency); *Si Jing Wan* (premature ejaculation and weakness from Kidney deficiency); *Jin Gang Wan* (weakness and atrophy from Kidney deficiency); *Gu Zhi Zeng Sheng Wan* (bony proliferation, osteophytes); *Yang Qi Shi Wan*[6] (infertility and sperm disorders from yang deficiency)

**Suǒ Yáng** (Cynomorii Herba) cynomorium stem

**Contraindications** Yin deficiency with heat and ascendant yang, Spleen deficiency diarrhea or excess heat type constipation.

**Formulae** *Hu Qian Wan*† (weakness and atrophy from Kidney deficiency); *Suo Yang Gu Jing Wan* (frequent urination and premature ejaculation from Kidney deficiency); *Gu Ben Suo Jing Wan* (nocturia and night sweats from yang deficiency)

**Bǔ Gǔ Zhī** (Psoraleae Fructus) psoralea fruit

Also known as pò gù zhǐ 破故纸.

**Preparation and use** Used topically to treat vitiligo, bu gu zhi is crushed and steeped in yellow wine, with the resulting extract applied to the affected area which is then exposed to sunlight for 5–10 minutes, or ultraviolet light for 2–5 minutes once daily, after which the area is washed. If blistering or rash appears, administration should cease.

**Contraindications** Yin deficiency with heat, internal excess heat patterns, wet dreams, dysuria and hematuria, constipation or indefinable epigastric discomfort.

**Formulae** *Si Shen Wan* (chronic diarrhea from Spleen and Kidney yang deficiency); *Po Gu Zhi Wan* (nocturia, enuresis and frequent urination from Kidney deficiency); *Qing E Wan* (backache from Kidney deficiency); *Bu Gu Zhi Wan* (impotence and night sweats from Kidney yang deficiency); *Qi Bao Mei Ran Dan* (alopecia from Liver and Kidney deficiency)

---

1 Appendix 6, p.108
2 *He Ji Ju Fang* (Imperial Grace Formulary of the Tai Ping Era)
3 *Tai Ping Sheng Hui Fang* (Formulas from Benevolent Sages Compiled during the Taiping Era)

4 Appendix 3.2, p.104
5 Appendix 4, p.105
6 *Fu Ke Yu Chi* (Jade Rule Gynecology)

| Indications | Xu Duan 续断 | Du Zhong 杜仲 | Gou Ji 狗脊 | Gu Sui Bu 骨碎补 | Tu Si Zi 菟丝子 | Jiu Cai Zi 韭菜子 | Sha Yuan Zi 沙苑子 | Hu Lu Ba 葫芦巴 | Yang Qi Shi 阳起石 | Functions |
|---|---|---|---|---|---|---|---|---|---|---|
| abscesses & sores – skin | △○ | ○ | | | ○ | | | | | calms fetal restlessness |
| abscess – breast, mastitis | △ | | | | ● | | ○ | | | brightens the eyes |
| alopecia | | | ○ | E | | | | | | dispels wind damp |
| bleeding – uterine | ▲○ | ▲ | | | △ | | | △ | | invigorates blood |
| bones – poor healing of broken | ▲ | | | ▲ | ○ | | | | | nourishes yin |
| diabetes (*xiao ke*) | ● | | | ○ | △ | | | | | promotes healing |
| diarrhea – Spleen & Kidney def. | | | | △ | ▲○ | | | | | restrains urine |
| dizziness | | △ | | | △○ | ○ | ● | | | secures essence |
| dysmenorrhea – def., cold | | | | | ○ | | | △ | | stops diarrhea |
| ears – tinnitus, hearing loss | ● | ○ | ○ | ▲● | △ | | △ | | | strengthens sinew & bone |
| eyes – corneal opacity, cataract | ○ | ● | ○ | ○ | ● | ○ | ▲○ | | | tonifies Liver & Kidneys |
| eyes – weak, blurring vision | | | | | △ | | ▲ | ○ | ○ | warms the Kidneys |
| gingivitis, oral inflammation | | | | ▲ E | | | | | | |
| hypertension – Kidney def. | | ▲ | | | | | | | | |
| impotence – Kidney yang def. | △ | △ | △ | | △ | △ | △ | ▲ | △ | |
| infertility – Kidney yang def. | | | | | △ | △ | | ▲ | | |
| leg qi – cold damp | | | △ | | | | | △ | | |
| leukorrhea – Sp. & Kid. def. | △ | | △ | | △ | △ | △ | | | |
| libido – low, loss of | | | | | △ | △ | △ | △ | | |
| lower back, legs – weak, cold | ▲ | ▲ | △ | △ | △ | △ | △ | △ | △ | |
| miscarriage – threat of; recurrent | ▲ | ▲ | | | ▲ | | | | | |
| pain – abdominal; def., cold | | | | | | | | △ | | |
| pain – back, during menses | △ | ▲ | | | | | | | | |
| pain – joint, with stiffness | △ | △ | ▲ | △ | | | | | | |
| pain – lower back, leg, knee | ▲ | ▲ | △ | ▲ | △ | △ | △ | △ | △ | |
| pain – lower back; acute trauma | △ E | | | △ | | | | | | |
| pain – spine, with stiffness | | | ▲ | | | | | | | |
| pain – testicular, from cold | | | | | | | | ▲ | | |
| painful obst. – wind cold damp | △ | △ | ▲ | △ | | | | | | |
| pregnancy – bleeding during | ▲ | ▲ | | | | | | | | **Domain (❖)** |
| sinew & bones – damage to | △ ❖ | ❖ | ❖ | ▲ ❖ | ❖ | ❖ | ❖ | ❖ | ❖ | Kidney |
| sperm – poor motility, ↓count | ❖ | ❖ | ❖ | ❖ | ▲ ❖ | ❖ | ❖ | ❖ | | Liver |
| sperm – involuntary loss of | | | | | △ ❖ | △ | ▲ | △ | | Spleen |
| sprains & strains | △ | | | ▲ | | | | | | |
| teeth – loose or loss of | | | | ▲ E | | | | | | |
| toothache – Kidney deficiency | | | | ▲ | | | | | | **Flavour, nature (♦)** |
| traumatic injury | △ E ♦ | | | ▲ | ♦ | ♦ | | | | acrid |
| urination – frequent, nocturia | ♦ | △ | △ ♦ | △ ♦ | ▲ | | △ | ♦ | | bitter |
| urination – incontinence of | | | △ | | ▲ | △ | △ | | ♦ | salty |
| | ♦ | | ♦ | | ♦ | | | | | sweet |
| | | ♦ | ♦ | ♦ | | ♦ | ♦ | ♦ | | warm |
| | ♦ | | | | | | | | ♦ | slightly warm |
| | | | | | ♦ | | | | | neutral |
| **Standard dosage range (g)** | 9–18 | 9–15 | 9–15 | 9–18 | 9–15 | 6–15 | 9–18 | 3–9 | 3–6 | |

Legend:
△ Indication
▲ Strong Indication
E External Use
E Strong External Indication
○ Function
● Strong Function

**Yì Zhì Rén (Alpiniae oxyphyllae Fructus) black cardamon**

**Preparation and use** Usually stir fried (*chao yi zhi ren* 炒益智仁) to remove the outer shell and release the seeds. Can be processed with salt (*yan yi zhi ren* 盐益智仁) to focus its action on the Kidneys and alleviate frequent urination. The seeds are crushed before decoction.

**Contraindications** Yin deficiency with heat; urinary frequency from damp heat in the lower burner.

**Formulae** *Suo Quan Wan* (frequent urination from Kidney deficiency); *Yi Zhi San* (diarrhea and excessive salivation from Spleen yang deficiency); *Bi Xie Fen Qing Yin* (turbid urine from Kidney deficiency)

**Hú Táo Rén (Juglandis Semen) walnut kernel**

Also known as hé táo rén 核桃仁.

**Preparation and use** Used for wheezing and cough, the skin should be left on; when used for constipation the skin should be removed. Should not be taken with strong tea. Hu tao ren is often ground into a paste with black sesame seeds (hei zhi ma p.80) and honey to treat constipation in the elderly.

**Contraindications** Diarrhea and loose stools, phlegm heat type wheezing and cough, yin deficiency with heat, and internal excess heat patterns with epistaxis and hematemesis.

**Formulae** *Ren Shen Hu Tao Tang* (chronic wheezing from Lung and Kidney deficiency); *San Jin Hu Tao Tang* (Kidney stones); *Qing E Wan* (backache from Kidney deficiency)

**Xù Duàn (Dipsaci Radix) Japanese teasel root**

Also known as jiē gǔ cǎo 接骨草 (set bone grass).

**Preparation and use** Unprocessed to tonify the Liver and Kidneys and strengthen sinews and bones; stir frying (*chao xu duan* 炒续断) enhances its ability to calm fetal restlessness and support women prone to miscarriage; charring (*xu duan tan* 续断炭) enhances its ability to stop uterine bleeding and bleeding during pregnancy; processing with wine (*jiu xu duan* 酒续断) enhances its ability to promote knitting of bones and alleviate wind damp pain.

**Contraindications** Pain from wind damp heat.

**Formulae** *Shou Tai Wan* (threatened or habitual miscarriage from Kidney deficiency); *Jie Gu Dan* (slow healing broken bones); *Xu Duan Wan* (chronic back pain from Kidney deficiency); *Ai Fu Nuan Gong Wan* (infertility from Kidney deficiency); *Jia Wei Si Wu Tang* (menorrhagia from Liver and Kidney deficiency); *San Bi Tang* (qi and blood deficiency type painful obstruction)

**Dù Zhòng (Eucommiae Cortex) eucommia bark**

**Preparation and use** In severe cases, up to 60 grams may be used. Charred du zhong (*du zhong tan* 杜仲炭) is best for uterine bleeding and bleeding during pregnancy; processing with salt (*yan du zhong* 盐杜仲) enhances its ability to target the Kidneys, stabilize pregnancy and relieve lower back pain.

**Contraindications** Yin deficiency with heat.

**Formulae** *Du Zhong Wan* (weakness, backache and bleeding during pregnancy); *Qing E Wan* (backache from Kidney deficiency); *Du Huo Ji Sheng Tang* (wind damp painful obstruction with Liver and Kidney deficiency); *Jin Gang Wan* (weakness and atrophy from Kidney deficiency); *Tian Ma Gou Teng Yin* (dizziness and headache from ascendant Liver yang)

**Gǒu Jǐ (Cibotii Rhizoma) chain fern rhizome**

⬛ Listed in Appendix 2 of CITES[1] which permits limited trade with appropriate documentation.

**Preparation and use** Unprocessed gou ji is best for wind damp painful obstruction; steamed gou ji (*shu gou ji* 熟狗脊) is less bitter and drying, more tonic to the Liver and Kidneys, and preferred for pain and weakness from Liver and Kidney deficiency.

**Contraindications** Yin deficiency with heat, or in patterns of difficult or painful urination.

**Formulae** *Gou Ji Yin* (lower back, spine and leg pain from wind damp)

**Gǔ Suì Bǔ (Drynariae Rhizoma) drynaria rhizome**

Placed in the blood invigorating group in some texts.

**Preparation and use** Processed in hot sand before decoction (*sha tang gu sui bu* 砂烫骨碎补) to soften and remove the outer fibres, and facilitate extraction. For topical use on alopecia an alcohol extract of the herb can be massaged into the affected area.

**Contraindications** Yin deficiency with heat, in excess fire type toothache, or in the absence of blood stasis.

**Formulae** *Gu Sui Bu San*† (acute pain and damage to sinews and bones from trauma); *Jie Gu Dan* (slow healing broken bones); *Gu Zhi Zeng Sheng Wan* (bony proliferation, osteophytes)

**Tù Sī Zǐ (Semen Cuscutae) cuscuta seed**

**Preparation and use** A mild herb suitable for yin and yang deficiency patterns, as long as there is no significant heat.

**Contraindications** Yin deficiency with heat, or in patients with constipation or painful or concentrated urination.

**Formulae** *Tu Si Zi Wan* (nocturia from Kidney deficiency); *Wu Zi Yan Zong Wan* (sperm disorders from Kidney deficiency); *Fu Tu Dan* (leukorrhea from Kidney deficiency); *Zhu Jing Wan* (weak vision from Liver and Kidney deficiency); *Shou Tai Wan* (habitual miscarriage from Kidney deficiency); *Pi Shen Shuang Bu Wan* (chronic diarrhea from Spleen and Kidney deficiency); & 10+ more in Appendix 7.

**Jiǔ Cài Zǐ (Semen Allii Tuberosi) chinese leek seed**

**Preparation and use** Usually stir fried (*chao jiu cai zi* 炒韭菜子) to enhance its ability to warm the Kidneys and secure jing.

**Contraindications** Yin deficiency with heat.

**Formulae** *Zan Yu Dan* (infertility from Kidney yang deficiency)

**Shā Yuàn Zǐ (Astragali complanati Semen) astragalus seed**

Also known as shā yuàn jí lí 沙苑蒺藜.

**Preparation and use** Unprocessed for visual problems; stir frying (*chao sha yuan zi* 炒沙苑子) enhances its ability to secure essence and is preferred for frequent urination and fluid leakage; processing with salt (*yan sha yian zi* 盐沙苑子) enhances its ability to tonify the Liver and Kidneys and is preferred for lower back pain and tinnitus.

**Contraindications** Yin deficiency with heat; difficult urination.

**Formulae** *Jin Suo Gu Jing Wan* (frequent urination and loss of essence from Kidney deficiency)

**Hú Lú Bā (Trigonellae Semen) fenugreek seed**

**Preparation and use** Unprocessed for leg and abdominal pain from cold; processing with salt (*yan hu lu ba* 盐葫芦巴) enhances its ability to target the Kidneys and is preferred for testicular pain, dysmenorrhea, impotence and lower back pain.

**Contraindications** Yin deficiency with heat or damp heat patterns. Caution during pregnancy[2].

**Formulae** *Hu Lu Ba Wan* (cold type testicular pain and swelling)

**Yáng Qǐ Shí (Actinolitum) actinolite; silicate mineral with the chemical composition $Ca_2Mg_5Si_8O2_2(OH)_2$**

**Preparation and use** Not suitable for prolonged use. Only used in pills and powder form, and calcined (*duan yang qi shi* 煅阳起石) before use to enable pulverization.

**Contraindications** Yin deficiency with heat.

**Formulae** *Yang Qi Shi Wan*[3] (infertility and sperm disorders from yang deficiency); *Yang Qi Shi Wan*[4] (infertility from cold in the Uterus)

**Substances from other groups**

Herbs from other groups with some yang warming effect include liu huang (p.24), she chuang zi (p.24), jiu xiang chong (p.66), zhong ru shi (p.68), zi shi ying (p.72), zhi fu zi (p.88), rou gui (p.88) and ding xiang (p.88).

**Endnotes**

† These formulae traditionally contain items from endangered animal species and/or obsolete toxic substances, and are unavailable in their original form.

1 Appendix 4, p.105

2 Chen (2004)
3 *Fu Ke Yu Chi* (Jade Rule Gynecology)
4 *He Ji Ju Fang* (Imperial Grace Formulary of the Tai Ping Era)

Legend:
- △ Indication
- ▲ Strong Indication
- E External Use
- **E** Strong External Indication
- ○ Function
- ● Strong Function

| INDICATIONS | Ban Zhi Lian 半枝莲 | Huang Yao Zi 黄药子 | Shan Ci Gu 山慈姑 | Teng Li Gen 藤梨根 | Shu Yang Quan 蜀羊泉 | Long Kui 龙葵 | She Mei 蛇莓 | Tian Kui Zi 天葵子 | Xi Shu 喜树 | Chang Chun Hua 长春花 | Nong Ji Li 农吉利 | Zhong Jie Feng 肿节风 | FUNCTIONS |
|---|---|---|---|---|---|---|---|---|---|---|---|---|---|
| abscess – breast | | | | △ | | ○ | | △ | | | | | alleviates dysuria |
| abscess – Intestinal | △ | | | | | | | | | ○ | | △ | breaks up blood stasis |
| abscess – Lung | △ | | | | | | | | | ○ | | | calms the Liver |
| abscesses & sores – skin | △○ | △○ | △○ | ○ | △○ | △E○ | △E○ | ▲○ | △E○ | ○ | ○ | △E○ | clears toxic heat |
| ascites – from cirrhosis | △ | ○ | | | | | | | | | | | cools the blood |
| bleeding – hemoptysis, nose | | △ | | ○ | ○ | | | △ | | | | | dispels wind & damp |
| bleeding – uterine | | △○ | ○ | | | | △ | ○ | | | ○ | | dissipates masses |
| burns & scalds | | | | ○ | | ○ | E | | | | | | invigorates blood |
| cancer – bladder | ○ | | | | △ | △○ | | △ | △ | | | | promotes urination |
| cancer – breast | | ○ | ▲ | | | △ | △○ | △ | △ | △ | | | stops bleeding |
| cancer – cervical | | E | △ | | △ | △E | △○ | | | | △E | | stops cough |
| cancer – esophagus | △ | △ | △ | △ | △ | | | | | | | △ | |
| cancer – intestine | △ | △ | | △ | | | | △ | | | | △ | |
| cancer – leukemia; blood | | | | | | | | ▲ | △ | | | △ | |
| cancer – liver | ▲ | △ | | | △ | △ | | △ | △ | | | | |
| cancer – lung | △ | | △ | | | | | △ | | | | | |
| cancer – lymphoma | | | | | | | | △ | | △ | | | |
| cancer – nasopharyngeal | △ | | △ | | △ | | △ | △ | | | | | |
| cancer – pancreas | | | | | | | | | | | △ | | |
| cancer – rectum | | △ | | △ | | | | △ | | | | | |
| cancer – skin (SCC, BCC) | | | △ | | | | | | | | △E | | |
| cancer – stomach | △ | △ | | △ | | △ | △ | △ | | | △ | △ | **Domain (❖)** |
| cancer – testicular | ❖ | ❖ | | | | ❖ | ❖ | | | △ | ❖ | | Lung |
| cancer – thyroid | | ▲ | △ | | | | △ | | ❖ | | | ❖ | Large Intestine |
| cancer – uterine, ovarian | | △ | | ❖ | | ❖ | | ❖ | ❖ | △ | | ❖ | Bladder |
| cervical lymphadenitis (luo li) | ❖ | ❖ | △❖ | | ❖ | | ❖ | △❖ | ❖ | | | ❖ | Liver |
| cirrhosis of the liver – early | | △ | | | ❖ | | | | | | | | Gallbladder |
| cough – Lung heat | | △ | ❖ | | | | △ | ❖ | | ❖ | ❖ | | Spleen |
| cough – whooping | ❖ | △ | | | ❖ | | △❖ | | ❖ | | ❖ | | Stomach |
| dysuria – damp heat; blood | △ | | | | | △ | | | | | | | |
| edema | △ | | | | | △ | | | | | | | |
| hepatitis – chronic | △ | | | | | | | | | | | | |
| hepatosplenomegaly | △ | ◆ | △ | | | | | | ◆ | ◆ | ◆ | | **Flavour, nature (◆)** |
| hypertension | | | ◆ | | | ◆ | | | | △ | | | toxic |
| jaundice – damp heat | ◆ | | ◆ | △ | △ | | | | | | | ◆ | slightly toxic |
| leukorrhea – damp heat | | | | ◆ | △ | | | | | | | | acrid |
| nodules & masses – phlegm | | △◆ | △ | | ◆ | | | ◆ | ◆ | ◆ | ◆ | ◆ | astringent |
| painful obst. – wind damp | ◆ | | | △ | △ | | ◆ | | | | | △ | bitter |
| skin – itchy wind/damp rash | | E | | | ◆ | △E | △E | △E | | | | | slightly bitter |
| snakebite | △ | △ | | | | | △E | △◆ | | | | | sour |
| throat – sore; acute | △◆ | △ | | ◆ | ◆ | △ | △ | | | | | | sweet |
| thyroid – nodules, goitre | | ▲◆ | △◆ | | | ◆ | ◆ | ◆ | ◆ | ◆ | | | cool |
| | | | | | | | | | | | ◆ | ◆ | cold |
| | | | | | | | | | | | ◆ | ◆ | neutral |
| **Standard dosage range (g)** | 9–30 | 9–15 | 3–6 | 15–30 | 9–24 | 15–30 | 9–30 | 3–9 | *see* p.87 | 9–15 | 6–12 | 6–15 | |

### Bàn Zhī Lián (Scutellariae barbate Herba) bearded scullcap

**Preparation and use** If the fresh herb is available, 30–60 grams may be used.

**Contraindications** Caution during pregnancy.

### Huáng Yào Zǐ (Dioscoreae bulbiferae Rhizoma) aerial yam

**Preparation and use** Taken directly in pill or powder form the dose is 1–2 grams, two or three times daily. The crushed fresh tubers can be applied topically.

**Contraindications** Patients with pre–existing organic liver disease. Caution in patients with middle burner deficiency or Liver and Kidney deficiency. Not suitable for prolonged or excessive use as toxic effects[1] can occur. The maximum dose should not be exceeded and liver function should be monitored periodically while taking this herb.

**Formulae** *Xiao Ying Tang* (goitre and thyroid nodules)

### Shān Cí Gū (Cremastrae/Pleiones Pseudobulbus) cremastra or pleione orchid bulbs

🔸 Listed in Appendix 2 of CITES[2] which permits limited trade with appropriate documentation.

**Contraindications** Caution in weak and deficient patients.

**Formulae** *Zi Jin Ding*† (toxic lesions and summerheat stroke)

### Téng Lí Gēn (Actinidia arguta Radix) hardy kiwifruit root

**Preparation and use** For cancer, the dosage range is 60–120 grams per day for fifteen days. The decoction should be cooked on a low heat for around 3 hours and taken in several doses throughout the day. Avoid shallots (scallions), ginger and fermented fish products during this time.

**Contraindications** None noted.

### Shǔ Yáng Quán (Solani lyratum Herba) climbing nightshade

Also known as bái yīng 白英.

**Preparation and use** The crushed fresh herb can be applied topically.

**Contraindications** Caution in patients with middle burner yang deficiency.

### Lóng Kuí (Solani nigri Herba) black nightshade aerial parts

**Preparation and use** The crushed fresh herb can be applied topically.

**Contraindications** Pregnancy. Not suitable for prolonged or excessive use as toxic effects[3] may occur.

### Shé Méi (Potentilla indica Herba) mock strawberry aerial parts (formerly Duchesnea indica)

**Contraindications** None noted.

### Tiān Kuí Zǐ (Semiaquilegiae Radix) semiaquilegia root

**Contraindications** Caution in patients with middle burner yang deficiency.

**Formulae** *Wu Wei Xiao Du Yin* (abscesses and sores from toxic heat)

### Xǐ Shù (Camptotheca acuminata Fructus et Radix) cancer tree fruit and root

**Preparation and use** The dosage of the fruit is 3–9 grams, and the root 9–15 grams. This plant is the source of the chemotherapeutic alkaloid camptothecine.

**Contraindications** Not suitable for prolonged or excessive use as toxic effects[4] may occur.

### Cháng Chūn Huā (Catharanthus roseus Flos) madagascar periwinkle

**Preparation and use** This plant is the source of the chemotherapeutic agents vincristine and vinblastine, used in the treatment of leukemia.

**Contraindications** Not suitable for prolonged or excessive use as toxic effects[5] may occur.

### Nóng Jí Lì (Crotalariae Herba) purpleflower crotalaria; rattlebush

Also known as yě bǎi hé 野百合.

**Contraindications** Not suitable for prolonged or excessive use as toxic effects[6] may occur.

### Zhǒng Jié Fēng (Sarcandrae Herba) glabrous sarcandra

**Preparation and use** Mostly used unprocessed, but can be processed with alcohol (*jiu zhong jie feng* 酒肿节风) to enhance its ability to dispel wind damp and stop pain.

**Contraindications** None noted.

### Substances from other groups

Herbs from other groups with some tumour resolving activity include e zhu (p.10), san leng (p.10), shui hong hua zi (p.10), shui zhi (p.10), di bie chong (p.10), meng chong (p.10), wa leng zi (p.10), ban bian lian (p.20), bai hua she she cao (p.36), shan dou gen (p.36), gui zhen cao (p.36), qing dai (p.36), feng wei cao (p.38), chan su (p.50), mao zhua cao (p.54) and ba yue zha (p.66).

### Endnotes

† These formulae traditionally contain items from endangered animal species and/or obsolete toxic substances, and are unavailable in their original form.

---

1 Appendix 3.1, p.101
2 Appendix 4, p.105
3 Appendix 3.2, p.103

4 Appendix 3.1, p.101
5 Ibid.
6 Ibid.

| | Zhi Fu Zi 制附子 | Gan Jiang 干姜 | Rou Gui 肉桂 | Wu Zhu Yu 吴茱萸 | Hua Jiao 花椒 | Hu Jiao 胡椒 | Bi Ba 荜茇 | Gao Liang Jiang 高良姜 | Xiao Hui Xiang 小茴香 | Ding Xiang 丁香 | Ba Jiao Hui Xiang 八角茴香 | | FUNCTIONS |
|---|---|---|---|---|---|---|---|---|---|---|---|---|---|
| **INDICATIONS** — △ Indication, ▲ Strong Indication, E External Use, **E** Strong External Indication | | | | | | | | | | | | | ○ Function, ● Strong Function |
| abscess & sores – yin, cold | △ | | ▲ | ○ | | | | | | ○ | | | directs qi downward |
| acid reflux, heartburn – St. cold | ● | ● | ○ | ▲○ | ○ | ○ | ○ | ○ | ○ | ○ | ○ | | disperses cold |
| appetite – loss of | | △ | | | ○ | △ | | | △ | | △ | | kills parasites |
| bleeding – GIT; def., cold | ● | ▲ | | | | | | | | | | | promotes fluid metabolism |
| bleeding – uterine; def., cold | | △ | | | | | | | ● | ○ | | | regulates qi |
| cold intolerance, cold limbs | ▲● | △○ | △ | | | | | | | | | | restores collapsing yang |
| collapsing yang (shock) | ▲● | △● | ○ | ● | ○ | ○ | ○ | ● | ● | ○ | ○ | | stops pain |
| cough – phlegm damp; thin | | ▲ | | ● | | | | ○ | | | | | stops vomiting |
| diarrhea – cockcrow | △ | △○ | △ | ▲ | △ | | | | | | | | transforms thin phlegm |
| diarrhea – cold; yang def. | ▲○ | ▲ | △○ | △ | △ | △ | △ | △ | | △○ | | | warms Kidney yang |
| dysmenorrhea – def., cold | △ | ○ | ▲ | △ | | | | | | | | | warms the Lungs |
| edema – yang deficiency | ▲○ | ● | ○ | ○ | ○ | ○ | ○ | ● | ○ | ○ | ○ | | warms the middle burner |
| headache – vertex, migraine | | | | ▲ | | | | | | | | | |
| Heart yang deficiency | ▲ | | | | | | | | | | | | |
| hiccup – cold, yang deficiency | | | | | | | | △ | | ▲ | | | |
| impotence – Kidney yang def. | △ | | △ | | | | | | | △ | | | |
| infertility – Kidney yang def. | △ | | △ | | | | | | | | | | |
| Kidney yang deficiency | ▲ | | △ | | | | | | | | | | |
| leukorrhea – cold damp | | | | | | | | | | △ | | | |
| Liver qi invading the stomach | | | | △ | | | | | | | | | |
| menses – irregular; def., cold | | | △ | | | | | | | | | | |
| morning sickness | | | | | | | | | | △ | | | |
| nipples – cracking & pain of | | | | | | | | | | E | | | |
| pain – abdominal, epigastric | ▲ | ▲ | △ | △ | △ | △ | △ | ▲ | △ | △ | △ | | |
| pain – abdominal, from worms | | | | | △ | | | | | | | | **Domain (❖)** |
| pain – chest, angina; cold | ▲ | ❖ | | | | | | | | | | | Lung |
| pain – facial, neuralgia | △ | | | ▲ | | ❖ | ❖ | | | | | | Large Intestine |
| pain – joint, cold damp | ▲❖ | | △❖ | | ❖ | | | | ❖ | ❖ | ❖ | | Kidney |
| pain – lower back, leg, knee | ▲ | | ❖ | ❖ | | | | | △❖ | △ | △❖ | | Liver |
| pain – testicular; cold, yang def. | ❖ | ❖ | △❖ | △ | △ | | | △ | ▲ | △ | △ | | Heart |
| painful obst. – wind cold damp | ▲❖ | ❖ | △❖ | ❖ | ❖ | | | ❖ | ❖ | ❖ | ❖ | | Spleen |
| parasites – roundworms | | ❖ | | ❖ | △❖ | ❖ | ❖ | ❖ | ❖ | ❖ | | | Stomach |
| shock – hemorrhagic | ▲ | △ | | | | | | | | | | | |
| skin – eczema, genital itch | | | | | E | | | | | | | | |
| Spleen yang deficiency | △ | ▲ | △ | | | | | | | | | | **Flavour, nature (♦)** |
| sweating – profuse, in shock | ▲♦ | △ | | | | | | | | | | | toxic |
| toothache – cold | | | | ♦ | E♦ | E | E | | | E | | | slightly toxic |
| ulcers – mouth | ♦ | ♦ | ♦ | E♦ | ♦ | ♦ | ♦ | ♦ | ♦ | ♦ | ♦ | | acrid |
| urination – frequent, nocturia | △ | | △ | ♦ | | | | | | | | | bitter |
| urination – scanty, with edema | ▲ | | ♦ | | | | | | | | ♦ | | sweet |
| vomiting, nausea – def., cold | △ | ▲ | | ▲ | △ | △ | △ | ▲ | △♦ | △♦ | △♦ | | warm |
| wheezing – Kidney deficiency | △ | | △ | ♦ | ♦ | ♦ | ♦ | ♦ | | | | | hot |
| wheezing – phlegm damp, thin | ♦ | △♦ | ♦ | | | | | | | | | | very hot |
| **Standard dosage range (g)** | 3–15 | 3–9 | 1–2 | 1–5 | 3–6 | 2–3 | 2–5 | 3–9 | 6–9 | 1–3 | 3–9 | | |

**Zhì Fù Zǐ** (Aconiti Radix lateralis preparata) processed aconite accessory root

**Preparation and use** Unprocessed fu zi is toxic[1]. Only the processed root is used internally. When used in decoction, zhi fu zi should be boiled for 30–60 minutes[2] prior to the other herbs, especially when used in doses of 9 grams or more to ensure decomposition of remaining toxic alkaloids. The larger the dose, the longer the cooking time required for safety. When used in pill or powder form the ingested daily dose is smaller, usually between 1–3 grams. Do not take with alcohol as it facilitates absorption of the toxic alkaloids and increases the potential for side effects.

**Contraindications** Pregnancy, 'true heat, false cold', excess heat patterns, and yin deficiency with internal heat or ascendant yang. Traditionally incompatible[3] with bai ji (p.14), bai lian (p.38), zhi ban xia (p.54), gua lou (p.56), chuan bei mu (p.56) and zhe bei mu (p.56).

**Formulae** *Si Ni Tang* (yang collapse; shock); *Jin Gui Shen Qi Wan* (Kidney yang deficiency); *You Gui Wan* (Kidney yang deficiency); *Fu Zi Li Zhong Wan* (Spleen yang deficiency); *Zhen Wu Tang* (edema from Heart and Kidney yang deficiency); *Fu Zi Tang* (cold damp painful obstruction); *Yin Chen Zhu Fu Tang* (yin jaundice from Spleen yang deficiency and cold damp); *Gui Zhi Jia Fu Zi Tang* (incessant sweating from yang deficiency); *Ma Huang Fu Zi Xi Xin Tang* (wind cold common cold in a patient with yang deficiency); *Yi Yi Fu Zi Bai Jiang Tang* (chronic Intestinal abscess); *Gui Zhi Shao Yao Zhi Mu Tang* (painful obstruction; heat concentrated in a joint); & 15+ more in Appendix 7.

**Gān Jiāng** (Zingiberis Rhizoma) dried ginger

**Preparation and use** For bleeding from cold and deficiency, quick fried gan jiang (*pao jiang* 炮姜, p.14) is preferred.

**Contraindications** Pregnancy, excess heat patterns, yin deficiency with heat or bleeding from heat in the blood.

**Formulae** *Si Ni Tang* (yang collapse; shock); *Li Zhong Wan* (Spleen yang deficiency); *Da Jian Zhong Tang* (acute abdominal pain from cold); *Xiao Qing Long Tang* (wind cold with thin phlegm congestion); *Wu Mei Wan* (*jue yin* syndrome; chronic diarrhea; roundworms); *Wen Pi Yin* (chronic constipation from Spleen yang deficiency); *Shi Pi Yin* (edema and watery diarrhea from Spleen yang deficiency); *Ban Xia Xie Xin Tang* (qi dynamic blockage from heat and cold in the middle burner); *Chai Hu Gui Zhi Gan Jiang Tang* (*shao yang* syndrome with phlegm damp [thin mucus] interiorly); & 20+ more in Appendix 7.

**Ròu Guì** (Cinnamomi Cortex) cinnamon bark

**Preparation and use** Usually taken separately or added as powder to the strained decoction. When decocted, the dose is increased to 2–5 grams, added at the end.

**Contraindications** Pregnancy, excess heat, yin deficiency with heat or ascendant yang, or bleeding from heat. Antagonistic[4] to chi shi zhi (p.4).

**Formulae** *Jin Gui Shen Qi Wan* (Kidney yang deficiency); *Shi Quan Da Bu Tang* (qi and blood deficiency with cold; chronic ulcers); *Yang He Tang* (yin sores); *Du Huo Ji Sheng Tang* (wind damp painful obstruction with Liver and Kidney deficiency); *Shao Fu Zhu Yu Tang* (dysmenorrhea from cold and blood stasis in the lower burner); *Ai Fu Nuan Gong Wan* (infertility, dysmenorrhea and irregular menses from Kidney deficiency); *Hei Shen San* (postpartum blood stasis); & 30+ more in Appendix 7.

**Wú Zhū Yú** (Evodiae Fructus) evodia fruit

**Preparation and use** Processed for internal use by soaking in several changes of water or a decoction of gan cao (p.74) before drying in the sun. This ameliorates its harsh acrid dryness. The unprocessed herb is peppery, slightly toxic[5], and used externally. For mouth and tongue ulcers, unprocessed wu zhu yu is mixed with vinegar and applied to the KI-1 (*yǒng quán*) acupoint. Processing with salt (*yan wu zhu yu* 盐吴茱萸) enhances its ability to treat genital pain; stir frying with huang lian (p.42) (*huang lian chao zhu yu* 黄连炒茱萸), enhances its ability to treat heartburn; stir frying with ginger (*jiang chao zhu yu* 姜炒茱萸), enhances its ability to treat nausea and dry retching; processing with vinegar (*cu zhu yu* 醋茱萸) enhances its ability treat the Liver and stop pain. Not suited to prolonged use.

**Contraindications** Excess heat patterns; yin deficiency with heat.

**Formulae** *Wu Zhu Yu Tang* (headache and vomiting from yang deficiency with Liver and Spleen disharmony); *Si Shen Wan* (chronic diarrhea from Spleen and Kidney yang deficiency); *Dao Qi Tang* (cold type testicular pain); *Wen Jing Tang* (infertility and dysmenorrhea from *chōng mài / rèn mài* deficiency); *Zuo Jin Wan* (heartburn and acid reflux from Liver and Stomach disharmony); *Can Shi Tang* (sudden turmoil from damp heat)

**Huā Jiāo** (Zanthoxyli Pericarpium) Sichuan pepper

Also known as chuān jiāo 川椒. The tiny black seeds extracted from within the outer shell are known as jiāo mù 椒目 (Zanthoxyli Semen). They promote fluid metabolism and are used for relatively severe edema, ascites and wheezing with profuse phlegm damp.

**Preparation and use** For toothache, a strong decoction can be held in the mouth and used as a mouthwash, or applied directly as a powder.

**Contraindications** Yin deficiency patterns with heat. Caution during pregnancy. Overdosage can cause toxic[6] symptoms.

**Formulae** *Da Jian Zhong Tang* (acute abdominal pain from cold); *Wu Mei Wan* (roundworms; *jue yin* syndrome; chronic diarrhea); *She Chuang Zi San* (a wash for itching from numerous causes)

**Hú Jiāo** (Piperis Fructus) black and white pepper

**Preparation and use** Taken directly as powder the dose is 0.5–1 gram.

**Contraindications** Not to be used in therapeutic doses during pregnancy[7]; yin deficiency with heat.

**Bì Bá** (Piperis longi Fructus) long pepper fruit

**Contraindications** Yin deficiency with heat.

**Formulae** *Da Yi Han Wan* (abdominal pain and diarrhea from Spleen yang deficiency)

**Gāo Liáng Jiāng** (Alpiniae officinarum Rhizoma) galangal root

**Contraindications** Yin deficiency with heat, vomiting from Stomach fire, epigastric pain from Stomach qi deficiency, or diarrhea from heat.

**Formulae** *Liang Fu Wan* (cold type genital pain); *An Zhong San* (epigastric pain from cold); *Cao Guo Yin* (cold damp malarial disorder)

**Xiǎo Huí Xiāng** (Foeniculi Fructus) fennel seed

**Preparation and use** The acrid nature and qi regulating action of unprocessed seeds is quite strong; stir frying (*chao hui xiang* 炒茴香) moderates its strong mobilizing nature and enhances its ability to warm the middle burner and stop nausea and vomiting from cold in the Stomach; processing with salt (*yan hui xiang* 盐茴香) enhances its ability to influence the lower burner, dispel cold and alleviate genital pain.

**Contraindications** Caution (unprocessed) during pregnancy or in yin deficiency patterns with heat.

**Formulae** *Tian Tai Wu Yao San* (cold type abdominal and genital pain); *Nuan Gan Jian* (testicular pain from cold in the Liver channel); *An Zhong San* (epigastric pain from cold)

**Dīng Xiāng** (Caryophylli Flos) clove flower bud

**Contraindications** Excess heat and yin deficiency patterns with heat. Antagonistic[8] to yu jin (p.8).

**Formulae** *Ding Xiang Shi Di Tang* (incessant hiccups from Spleen yang deficiency); *Ding Kou Li Zhong Wan* (acid reflux, abdominal pain and vomiting from yang deficiency); & 10 more in Appendix 7.

**Bā Jiǎo Huí Xiāng** (Illicium verum Fructus) star anise fruit

Also known as dà huí xiāng 大茴香.

**Contraindications** Caution in yin deficiency with heat.

Substances from other groups

Herbs from other groups with some interior warming action include rou dou kou (p.4), pao jiang (p.14), zao xin tu (p.14), sha ren (p.16), bai dou kou (p.16), cao dou kou (p.16), cao guo (p.16), gui zhi (p.28), sheng jiang (p.28), bai jie zi (p.54), ba dou shuang (p.62), wu yao (p.64), chen xiang (p.64), tan xiang (p.64), zhong ru shi (p.68) and zi shi ying (p.72).

---

1 Appendix 3.1, p.102
2 Appendix 6, p.108
3 Appendix 2, p.100
4 Appendix 2, p.100
5 Appendix 3.2, p.104

---

6 Appendix 3.2, p.103
7 The quantity used to season food is safe.
8 Appendix 2, p.100

Legend:
△ Indication
▲ Strong Indication
E External Use
E Strong External Indication
○ Function
● Strong Function

| INDICATIONS | Du Huo 独活 | Qiang Huo 羌活 | Wei Ling Xian 威灵仙 | Mu Gua 木瓜 | Cang Er Zi 苍耳子 | Can Sha 蚕沙 | Shen Jin Cao 伸筋草 | Xia Tian Wu 夏天无 | Song Jie 松节 | Tou Gu Cao 透骨草 | Hai Feng Teng 海风藤 | Qing Feng Teng 青风藤 | FUNCTIONS |
|---|---|---|---|---|---|---|---|---|---|---|---|---|---|
| common cold – wind cold | △ | ▲ | | ○ | | | ○ | | | | | | alleviates spasm |
| common cold – wind damp | ● | ▲● | ● | | ○ | ○ | ○ | ○ | ○ | ○ | ○ | ○ | dispels wind damp |
| food stagnation | | | ○ | △ | | | | | | | | | disperses phlegm |
| headache – frontal, wind cold | | | | ○ | △ | ○ | | | | | | | harmonizes the Stomach |
| headache – occipital | △ | ▲ | | | | | | ○ | | ○ | | | invigorates blood |
| headache – sinus | | | | | ▲● | | | | | | | | opens nose & sinuses |
| headache – wind cold, damp | △○ | ▲○ | | | | | | | | | | | releases the exterior |
| leg qi – cold damp | | | ○ | △ | | | | | | ○ | | △ | softens hardness |
| masses – abdominal, bld. stasis | | | △● | | | | ○ | | | △○ | ○ | ○ | unblocks channels |
| masses – phlegm | | | △ | | | | | | | | | | |
| nasosinusitis (bi yuan) | | | | | ▲ | | | | | | | | |
| nodules & masses – phlegm | | | △ | | | | | | | | | | |
| numbness – extremities | | | ▲ | | △ | | △ | △ | | | | | |
| osteophytes, bony deformity | | | ▲ | | | | | | | ▲ | | | |
| pain – & injury, trauma | | | | | | | △ | △ | △ | ▲ | △ | | |
| pain – abdominal, cold damp | | | | △ | | | | | | | | | |
| pain – abdominal, blood stasis | | | | | | | | △ | | | | | |
| pain – arm, shoulder, neck | | ▲ | △ | | △ | | | | △ | ▲ | | △ | |
| pain – extremities, fingers/toes | △ | △ | ▲ | △ | | | △ | △ | | ▲ | △ | | |
| pain – lower back, leg, knee | ▲ | | △ | △ | | △ | △ | | | | △ | | |
| pain – muscle; wind cold, damp | △ | ▲ | △ | ▲ | | | | | | | △ | △ | |
| painful obst. – wind cold damp | ▲ | ▲ | △ | | | △ | | | △ | | △ | | |
| painful obst. – wind damp | △ | △ | ▲ | △ | △ | △ | △ | △ | △ | △ | △ | △ | |
| shingles | | | | | | | E | | | | | | |
| skin – eczema, dermatitis | △ | | | | ▲ | △ E | | | | E | | | |
| skin – itchy wind rash; urticaria | △ | | | | △ | △ E | | | | E | | △ | **Domain** (❖) |
| skin – numbness of | | | ▲ | | △ ❖ | | △ | △ | | | | | Lung |
| skin – psoriasis | ❖ | ❖ | | | △ | | | | | ❖ | | | Kidney |
| spasm & cramp – calf | ❖ | ❖ | ❖ | ▲ | | △ | | | | | | | Bladder |
| spasm & cramp – bld., yin def. | ❖ | | | △ ❖ | ❖ | ❖ | ❖ | ❖ | ❖ | ❖ | ❖ | ❖ | Liver |
| spasm & cramp – Liv. → Sp. | | | | △ ❖ | | ❖ | | | | | | | Spleen |
| sudden turmoil disorder | | | | △ | | △ ❖ | | | | | | | Stomach |
| throat – fish bone stuck in | | | △ | | | | | | | | | | |
| toothache; jaw pain – cold | △ | | | | | | | | | | | | |
| vomiting, diarrhea – acute | | | | | △ | | △ | | | | | | **Flavour, nature** (♦) |
| | | | | | ♦ | | | | | | | ♦ | slightly toxic |
| | ♦ | ♦ | ♦ | | ♦ | ♦ | ♦ | ♦ | | ♦ | ♦ | | acrid |
| | ♦ | ♦ | | | ♦ | | | | ♦ | | | ♦ | bitter |
| | | | ♦ | | | | | | | | | | salty |
| | | | | ♦ | | | | | | | | | sour |
| | | | | | | ♦ | | | | | | | sweet |
| | | | | | | | | | | | | ♦ | neutral |
| | ♦ | ♦ | ♦ | ♦ | ♦ | | ♦ | ♦ | ♦ | ♦ | ♦ | ♦ | warm |
| **Standard dosage range (g)** | 3–9 | 3–9 | 6–9 | 6–12 | 3–9 | 6–9 | 6–15 | 6–15 | 9–15 | 9–15 | 9–15 | 9–15 | |

**Dú Huó (Angelicae pubescentis Radix) pubescent angelica root**

**Contraindications** Internal wind. Caution in patients with yin or blood deficiency.

**Formulae** *Du Huo Ji Sheng Tang* (wind damp painful obstruction with Kidney deficiency); *Du Huo Xi Xin Tang* (toothache and jaw pain from wind cold); *Juan Bi Tang* (wind damp painful obstruction); *Qin Jiao Ji Sheng Tang* (postpartum joint pain from blood deficiency with wind); *Qiang Huo Sheng Shi Tang* (headache from wind damp); *Da Qin Jiao Tang* (hemiplegia with blood deficiency); *Shu Jin Huo Xue Tang* (hemiplegia and wind damp painful obstruction with blood stasis); *Jing Fang Bai Du San* (wind cold common cold); *Si Wu Xiao Feng Yin* (itchy wind rash)

**Qiāng Huó (Notopterygii Rhizoma seu Radix) notopterygium root**

Placed in the exterior releasing group in some texts.

**Contraindications** Pain associated with blood deficiency.

**Formulae** *Qiang Huo Sheng Shi Tang* (wind damp headache); *Chuan Xiong Cha Tiao San* (wind headache); *Juan Bi Tang* (wind damp painful obstruction); *Dang Gui Nian Tong Tang* (leg pain and swelling from damp heat); *Jiu Wei Qiang Huo Tang* (wind cold common cold); *Zai Zao San* (wind cold in a patient with yang deficiency); *Lian Qiao Bai Su San* (mumps and suppurative sores from toxic heat); *Shen Tong Zhu Yu Tang* (chronic musculoskeletal pain from blood stasis); *Yu Zhen San* (tetanic spasms); *Xin Yi San* (wind cold headache and nasal congestion); *Zi Ran Tong San* (slow healing broken bones); & 15+ more in Appendix 7.

**Wēi Líng Xiān (Clematidis Radix) Chinese clematis root**

**Preparation and use** Mostly used unprocessed, but processing with wine (*jiu wei ling xian* 酒威灵仙) enhances its warmth and ability to dispel cold from the joints. To dissolve clumped fish bones[1], 30 grams may be boiled with vinegar and used as a gargle.

**Contraindications** Caution during pregnancy[2] and in patients with qi and blood deficiency. Not suitable for prolonged or excessive use as it can easily deplete qi.

**Formulae** *Shen Ying Wan* (wind damp painful obstruction); *Shu Jin Huo Xue Tang* (hemiplegia and wind damp painful obstruction with blood stasis); *Hai Tong Pi Jiu* (alcohol extract for wind damp painful obstruction); *Sang Zhi Tang* (shoulder pain and stiffness from wind damp); *Xian Ling Pi San* (wind cold damp painful obstruction)

**Mù Guā (Chaenomelis Fructus) Chinese quince**

**Preparation and use** Mostly used unprocessed, but can be stir fried (*chao mu gua* 炒木瓜) to enhance its ability to harmonize the Stomach.

**Contraindications** Heat from qi constraint; pain and swelling of the legs in patients with scanty concentrated urine.

**Formulae** *Mu Gua Tang* (smooth and skeletal muscle cramps accompanying severe vomiting and diarrhea; sudden turmoil from cold); *Mu Gua Jian* (wind damp leg pain); *Ji Ming San* (weakness, pain and swelling of the legs from cold damp); *Can Shi Tang* (sudden turmoil from damp heat); *Jing Wan Hong* (ointment for burns and non healing sores); *Wu Jia Pi San*[3] (wind damp painful obstruction and spasm)

**Cāng Ěr Zǐ (Xanthii Fructus) cockleburr fruit**

**Preparation and use** For internal use, the stir fried form (*chao cang er zi* 炒苍耳子) is preferred as this reduces its toxicity while preserving its acrid dispersing nature. Can be used unprocessed topically as a wash for itchy skin conditions.

**Contraindications** Headache and musculoskeletal pain from blood deficiency. Not suitable for prolonged or excessive use as symptoms of toxicity[4] may occur.

**Formulae** *Cang Er Zi San* (acute and chronic sinus congestion with frontal headache); *Xian Ling Pi San* (wind cold damp painful obstruction); *Xi Xian Jiu* (alcohol extract for wind damp painful obstruction and hemiplegia)

**Cán Shā (Bombycis Faeces) silkworm droppings**

**Preparation and use** Cooked in a cloth bag[5].

**Contraindications** None noted.

**Formulae** *Xuan Bi Tang* (wind damp heat painful obstruction); *Can She Tang* (stubborn wind damp painful obstruction); *Can Shi Tang* (sudden turmoil from damp heat)

**Shēn Jīn Cǎo (Lycopodii Herba) common clubmoss**

**Preparation and use** Can be cooked into a concentrate and mixed with a suitable carrier, such as sorbolene or sterile honey, to form an ointment for topical application.

**Contraindications** Pregnancy.

**Formulae** *Shu Jin Huo Xue Fang* (an external poultice for post traumatic spasm and pain); *Can She Tang* (stubborn wind damp painful obstruction)

**Xià Tiān Wú (Corydalis decumbens Rhizoma) rhizome of decumbent corydalis**

**Contraindications** Pregnancy.

**Sōng Jié (Pini Lignum nodi) knotty pine wood**

**Contraindications** Caution in patients with yin or blood deficiency.

**Formulae** *Wu Jia Pi San*[6] (developmental delay in children); *Gou Ji Yin* (lower back, spine and leg pain from wind damp)

**Tòu Gǔ Cǎo (Speranskia Herba) garden balsam**

**Preparation and use** For acute and slow healing trauma, tou gu cao can be used internally and applied topically as a poultice.

**Contraindications** Pregnancy.

**Formulae** *Tou Gu Cao Wan*† (acute and chronic wind damp painful obstruction); *Zheng Gu Tang Yao* (poultice for persistent pain and slow healing following trauma); *Can She Tang* (stubborn wind damp painful obstruction)

**Hǎi Fēng Téng (Piperis kadsurae Caulis) kadsura pepper stem**

**Contraindications** None noted.

**Formulae** *Tou Gu Cao Wan*† (acute and chronic wind damp painful obstruction); *Juan Bi Tang* (wind damp painful obstruction); *Xi Xian Jiu* (alcohol extract for wind damp painful obstruction and hemiplegia); *Gou Ji Yin* (lower back, spine and leg pain from wind damp)

**Qīng Fēng Téng (Sinomenii Caulis) orient vine**

**Contraindications** Do not exceed the recommended dosage range or symptoms of toxicity[7] may occur.

**Endnotes**

† These formulae traditionally contain items from endangered animal species and/or obsolete toxic substances, and are unavailable in their original form.

---

1 These are the fine bones typical of fresh water fish such as carp. Not suitable for large bones.
2 Chen (2004)
3 *Bao Ying Cuo Yao* (Outline of Infant Care)

4 Appendix 3.2, p.103
5 Appendix 6, p.109
6 *Shen Shi Zun Sheng Shu* (Master Shen's Book for Revering Life)
7 Appendix 3.2, p.104

△ Indication
▲ Strong Indication
E External Use
E Strong External Indication

○ Function
● Strong Function

| INDICATIONS | Bai Hua She 白花蛇 | Xu Chang Qing 徐长卿 | Qin Jiao 秦艽 | Ren Dong Teng 忍冬藤 | Sang Zhi 桑枝 | Xi Xian Cao 豨莶草 | Chou Wu Tong 臭梧桐 | Hai Tong Pi 海桐皮 | Luo Shi Teng 络石藤 | Lao Guan Cao 老鹳草 | Chuan Shan Long 穿山龙 | Si Gua Luo 丝瓜络 | FUNCTIONS |
|---|---|---|---|---|---|---|---|---|---|---|---|---|---|
| abscess – breast; mastitis | ● | | | △ | | | | | | | | △ | alleviates spasm |
| abscesses & sores – skin | | △E | | △E | | △E○ | ○ | | △ | △E | △ | | calms the Liver |
| constipation | | | △● | | | | | | | | ○ | | clears heat, damp heat |
| convulsions – chronic childhood | △ | | | ○ | | ○ | | | ○ | ○ | | | clears toxic heat |
| cough – Lung heat | ○ | | | | | | | | | | △ | △ | dispels wind |
| dysenteric dis. – damp heat | | ○ | ○ | ○ | ○ | ○ | ○ | △○ | ○ | △○ | ○ | ○ | dispels wind damp |
| dysmenorrhea | ○ | △ | | | | | | | | | | | extinguishes wind |
| dysuria – damp heat | | △○ | | | | | | | | | ○ | ○ | invigorates blood |
| edema | | △ | | | △ | | | | △○ | | | | kills parasites |
| fever – bone steaming; yin def. | | ▲ | | | | | | | | | ○ | | stops cough |
| hemiplegia | △○ | ○ | △ | | △ | ▲○ | △ | ○ | | | | | stops itch |
| hypertension – yang ↑ | | | | | | △ | △ | | | | | | |
| jaundice – damp heat | | | △ | | | △ | | | | | | | |
| lactation – insufficient | | | | | | | | | | | | △ | |
| leprosy – numbness of | △ | | | | | | | | | | | | |
| malarial disorder | | | | | | △ | △ | | | | | | |
| numbness – extremities | ▲ | | | △ | | △ | △ | | | △ | △ | △ | |
| pain – & injury, trauma | | △ | | | | | | | | △ | △ | △ | |
| pain – abdominal, cold | | △ | | | | | | | | | | | |
| pain – abdominal, heat | | | | △ | | | | | | | | | |
| pain – chest, angina; bld stasis | | | | | | | | | | | △ | △ | |
| pain – extremities, fingers/toes | | | | △ | △ | | | | △ | △ | | | |
| pain – hypochondriac | | | | | | | | | | | | △ | **Domain (❖)** |
| pain – lower body, leg, knee | | △ | | ❖ | | △ | | △ | | | △❖ | ❖ | Lung |
| pain – shoulder & arm | | | △ | ❖ | ▲ | | | | | ❖ | | ❖ | Large Intestine |
| pain – tumours, post surgical | | △ | | | | ❖ | | | | | | | Kidney |
| painful obst. – wind damp | △❖ | △❖ | △❖ | | △❖ | ▲❖ | △❖ | △❖ | △❖ | △❖ | △❖ | △❖ | Liver |
| painful obst. – wind damp heat | | ▲❖ | ▲ | △ | △ | | | ▲ | ▲ | △ | ▲ | | Gallbladder |
| paralysisw – facial | △ | | △ | | △ | △ | △ | | ❖ | | | | Heart |
| seizures, epilepsy | △ | ❖ | ❖ | ❖ | | | | | | | | ❖ | Stomach |
| skin – eczema, dermatitis | ▲ | ▲E | | | | ▲E | △E | E | | △E | | | |
| skin – itchy wind rash; urticaria | ▲ | ▲E | | △ | | ▲E | △E | E | | △E | | | |
| skin – scabies | | | | | | | | E | | | | | **Flavour, nature (◆)** |
| skin – vitiligo | ◆ | | | | △ | | | | | | | | toxic |
| spasm & cramp – skeletal mm. | △ | | △ | △ | △ | | | △ | △ | △ | ◆ | △ | slightly toxic |
| spasm – tetanic | △ | ◆ | ◆ | | | | ◆ | ◆ | | ◆ | | | acrid |
| throat – sore; acute | | ◆ | △ | ◆ | ◆ | ◆ | ◆ | ◆ | △◆ | ◆ | ◆ | | bitter |
| tremors | △◆ | | | | | | | | | | | | salty |
| toothache | ◆ | △ | | ◆ | | | ◆ | △ | | | | ◆ | sweet |
| | | | | | | | ◆ | | ◆ | | | | cool |
| | | | ◆ | | | ◆ | | | | | | | cold |
| | | | | | ◆ | | | | | ◆ | | ◆ | neutral |
| | ◆ | ◆ | | | | | | | | | | | warm |
| **Standard dosage range (g)** | 3–9 | 9–15 | 6–12 | 15–30 | 15–30 | 9–15 | 6–15 | 6–12 | 6–15 | 9–30 | 9–15 | 9–15 | |

## Bái Huā Shé (Agistrokodon/Bungarus) dried snake

Also known as qí shé 蘄蛇.

**Preparation and use** Mostly taken as pills, powder or alcohol extract. For internal use, the snake is processed with wine (*jiu zhi bai hua she* 酒制白花蛇) before being made into pills or powder. When taken directly as powder the dose is 1–1.5 grams, two or three times daily. The most popular delivery method is to soak a processed snake in grain alcohol, with a dose (10-15ml) taken in addition to any appropriate decoction. Snake wines are widely available in China and throughout east Asia.

**Contraindications** Caution in yin and blood deficiency type pain or internal wind.

**Formulae** *Bai Hua She Jiu* (therapeutic wine for chronic wind damp painful obstruction and hemiplegia following wind stroke); *Can She Tang* (stubborn wind damp painful obstruction); *Ding Ming San* (tetanic spasm and childhood convulsions from wind)

## Xú Cháng Qīng (Cynanchi paniculati Radix) swallow wort root

**Preparation and use** Cook no longer than 10–15 minutes to preserve its acrid dispersing nature. When taken directly as powder the dose is 1.5–3 grams, two or three times daily.

**Contraindications** None noted.

## Qín Jiāo (Gentianae macrophyllae Radix) large gentian root

**Preparation and use** Unprocessed for heat problems; stir frying (*chao qin jiao* 炒秦艽) warms it up a bit and makes it better for wind cold damp painful obstruction.

**Contraindications** Middle burner deficiency with loose stools.

**Formulae** *Qin Jiao Bie Jia Tang* (bone steaming fever and night sweats from yin deficiency); *Qin Jiao Bai Zhu Wan* (chronic constipation with bleeding, itchy hemorrhoids); *Qin Jiao Ji Sheng Tang* (postpartum joint pain from blood deficiency with wind); *Da Qin Jiao Tang* (hemiplegia with blood deficiency); *Du Huo Ji Sheng Tang* (wind damp painful obstruction with Kidney deficiency); *Shen Tong Zhu Yu Tang* (chronic musculoskeletal pain from blood stasis); & 9 more in Appendix 7.

## Rěn Dōng Téng (Lonicerae Caulis) honeysuckle vine

**Contraindications** Caution in middle burner yang deficiency.

**Formulae** *Sang Luo Tang* (damp heat painful obstruction); *Zi Cao You* (topical ointment for burns)

## Sāng Zhī (Mori Ramulus) mulberry twigs

**Preparation and use** Neutral in temperature, sang zhi is applicable to heat, cold and deficient conditions. It can be stir fried (*chao sang zhi* 炒桑枝) to warm it up and make it better for cold type pain; processing with wine (*jiu sang zhi* 酒桑枝) enhances its ability to invigorate blood and remove blockages, and is preferred for chronic and stubborn pain.

**Contraindications** None noted.

**Formulae** *Sang Zhi Hu Zhang Tang* (wind damp painful obstruction); *Sang Luo Tang* (damp heat painful obstruction); *Sang Zhi Tang* (shoulder pain and stiffness from wind damp); *Sang Zhi Gao* (a syrup for wind damp heat shoulder pain)

## Xī Xiān Cǎo (Siegesbeckia Herba) common St. Paul's wort

**Preparation and use** Unprocessed xi xian cao is used to clear toxic heat and alleviate wind damp heat pain; processing with wine (*jiu xi xian cao* 酒豨莶草) warms it up and enhances its ability to dispel wind cold damp, strengthen the Liver and Kidneys, and alleviate pain, numbness and hemiplegia. To treat malaria, 60 grams dry weight can be used per day for three days, taken 2 hours before the onset of the fever.

**Contraindications** None noted.

**Formulae** *Xi Xian Jiu* (therapeutic wine for wind damp painful obstruction and hemiplegia); *Xi Tong Wan* (wind damp painful obstruction; hypertension; eczema); *Tou Gu Cao Wan*† (acute and chronic wind damp painful obstruction)

## Chòu Wú Tóng (Clerodendri Folium) clerodendron leaf

**Preparation and use** Used for hypertension from ascendant Liver yang, it should not be cooked for longer than 10–15 minutes. When taken directly in pill or powder form the dose is 3 grams, two or three times daily.

**Contraindications** None noted.

**Formulae** *Sang Zhi Hu Zhang Tang* (wind damp painful obstruction); *Xi Tong Wan* (wind damp painful obstruction; hypertension; eczema)

## Hǎi Tóng Pí (Erythrinae Cortex) coral tree bark

**Preparation and use** Commonly prepared as an alcohol extract for both internal and external use. Can be powdered and mixed with lard or sorbolene for dry itchy skin conditions.

**Contraindications** None noted.

**Formulae** *Hai Tong Pi Jiu* (alcohol extract for wind damp painful obstruction); *Hai Tong Pi Tang* (bruising and pain from trauma, used both internally and as a wash); *Shu Jin Tang* (arm and shoulder pain from wind damp)

## Luò Shí Téng (Trachelospermi Caulis) star jasmine stem

**Contraindications** Caution in middle burner yang deficiency and loose stools.

**Formulae** *Sang Luo Tang* (damp heat painful obstruction); *E Jiao Ji Zi Huang Tang* (tremor and spasm from internal wind generated by yin and blood deficiency); *Luo Shi Tang* (sore throat from heat); *Bai Lian San* (topical powder for chronic ulcers)

## Lǎo Guàn Cǎo (Erodii/Geranii Herba) cranesbill

**Preparation and use** Commonly prepared as an alcohol extract or in syrup form for internal use, and as an ointment for external use.

**Contraindications** None noted.

**Formulae** *Lao Guan Cao Jiu* (alcohol extract for wind damp painful obstruction); *Lao Guan Cao Gao* (syrup for wind damp painful obstruction); *Lao Guan Cao Ruan Gao* (ointment for burns suppurative sores and eczema)

## Chuān Shān Lóng (Dioscoreae nipponicae Rhizoma) Japanese dioscorea rhizome

**Preparation and use** Commonly prepared as an alcohol extract.

**Contraindications** None noted[1].

## Sī Guā Luò (Luffae Fructus) dried vegetable sponge frame; luffa

Placed in the heat clearing group[2] and external use group[3] in other texts.

**Preparation and use** Cooked for 30 minutes[4] prior to the other herbs. The unprocessed form is preferred when there is heat; stir frying (*chao si gua luo* 炒丝瓜络) enhances its ability to invigorate blood, remove obstructions and stop pain; charring (*si gua luo tan* 丝瓜络炭) enhances ability to stop bleeding.

**Contraindications** None noted.

**Formulae** *Shan Qi Nei Xiao Wan* (groin and testicular pain from cold in the Liver channel); *Qing Luo Yin* (summerheat common cold)

## Substances from other groups

Herbs from other groups with some effect on wind damp and wind damp heat painful obstruction include lu lu tong (p.8), cang zhu (p.16), yi yi ren (p.18), han fang ji (p.18), bi xie (p.20), man jing zi (p.26), fang feng (p.28), bai zhi (p.28), hong teng (p.34) and liu yue xue (p.38).

## Endnotes

† These formulae traditionally contain items from endangered animal species and/or obsolete toxic substances, and are unavailable in their original form.

---

1 The slightly toxic designation is noted only in Bensky (2004) 3rd ed. No specific contraindications or cautions appear in any of the texts consulted.
2 Bensky (2004) 3rd ed.
3 *Zhong Yao Xue* (1997)
4 Appendix 6, p.108

| △ Indication ▲ Strong Indication E External Use E Strong External Indication **INDICATIONS** | Wu Jia Pi 五加皮 | Sang Ji Sheng 桑寄生 | Qian Nian Jian 千年健 | Lu Xian Cao 鹿衔草 | Xue Lian Hua 雪莲花 | Shi Nan Ye 石楠叶 | Zhi Chuan Wu 制川乌 | Zhi Cao Wu 制草乌 | | | | | ○ Function ● Strong Function **FUNCTIONS** |
|---|---|---|---|---|---|---|---|---|---|---|---|---|---|
| abscesses & sores – yin type | | ○ | | | | E | | | | | | | calms fetal restlessness |
| amenorrhea – yang deficiency | | | | | △ | | ● | ● | | | | | dispels cold |
| bleeding – hematemesis | ○ | ○ | ○ | △○ | ○ | ○ | ● | ● | | | | | dispels wind damp |
| bleeding – hemoptysis | ○ | | | △ | | | | | | | | | promotes urination |
| bleeding – traumatic | | | E | ○ | | | | | | | | | regulates menstruation |
| bleeding – uterine | | △ | | △○ | △○ | | | | | | | | stops bleeding |
| cough – chronic; Lung def. | | | | △ | | | ● | ● | | | | | stops pain |
| dysmenorrhea – def., cold | ○ | ○ | ○ | ○ | △○ | | | | | | | | strengthens sinew & bone |
| edema | △○ | △○ | | | ○ | ○ | | | | | | | tonifies Liver & Kidneys |
| edema – during pregnancy | | △ | | ○ | | | | | | | | | tonifies Lung & Kidneys |
| headache | | | | | | △ | △● | E● | | | | | warms the channels |
| hemiplegia – cold, bld. stasis | △ | | | | | | △ | △ | | | | | |
| hypertension – Liver & Kid. def. | △ | | | | | | | | | | | | |
| impotence – Kidney yang def. | △ | | | | ▲ | | | | | | | | |
| lactation – insufficient | | △ | | | | | | | | | | | |
| leg qi – cold damp | △ | | | | | | | | | | | | |
| leukorrhea – Sp. & Kid. def. | | | | | △ | | | | | | | | |
| menstruation – irregular | | | | | △ | | | | | | | | |
| miscarriage – threat of; recurrent | | ▲ | | | | | | | | | | | |
| motor development, delayed | △ | | | | | | | | | | | | |
| muscle weakness & atrophy | ▲ | △ | △ | △ | △ | △ | △ | △ | | | | | |
| numbness – extremities | △ | △ | ▲ | | | | ▲ | △ | | | | | |
| osteophytes, bony deformity | | | | ▲ | | | | | | | | | |
| pain – & injury, trauma | △E | | | | | | | | | | | | |
| pain – abdominal, intense cold | | | | | | | △E | E | | | | | |
| pain – chest, angina; cold | | | | | | | △ | | | | | | |
| pain – lower back | ▲ | ▲ | △ | △ | △ | △ | | | | | | | |
| pain – lower body, leg, knee | △ | △ | △ | △ | △ | △ | | | | | | | **Domain (❖)** |
| pain – severe, cold | ❖ | ❖ | ❖ | ❖ | ❖ | ❖ | ▲E❖ | △E❖ | | | | | Kidney |
| painful obst. – Kidney def. | ▲ | ▲ | △ | △ | △ | △ | ❖ | ❖ | | | | | Heart |
| painful obst. – wind cold damp | △❖ | △❖ | △❖ | △❖ | ▲❖ | △❖ | ▲E❖ | ▲E❖ | | | | | Liver |
| painful obst. – wind damp | △ | △ | △ | △ | △ | △ | ❖ | ❖ | | | | | Spleen |
| palpitations | | | | △ | | | | | | | | | |
| pregnancy – back & abd. pain | | ▲ | | | | | | | | | | | |
| pregnancy – bleeding during | | ▲ | | | | | | | | | | | **Flavour, nature (♦)** |
| skin – dry & scaly | | △ | | | | | ♦ | ♦ | | | | | toxic |
| skin – itchy wind rash; urticaria | | | | | | △♦ | | | | | | | slightly toxic |
| spasm & cramp – skeletal mm. | ♦ | | △♦ | | | ♦ | | | | | | | acrid |
| sweating – night sweats | ♦ | ♦ | ♦ | △♦ | ♦ | ♦ | ♦ | ♦ | | | | | bitter |
| toothache – severe cold | | | | ♦ | ♦ | | △ | | | | | | sweet |
| wheezing – Kidney deficiency | ♦ | | ♦ | △♦ | ♦ | | | | | | | | warm |
| | | | | | | | ♦ | ♦ | | | | | hot |
| | | ♦ | | | | ♦ | | | | | | | neutral |
| **Standard dosage range (g)** | 6–9 | 9–18 | 6–9 | 9–30 | 6–12 | 9–15 | 1.5–3 | 1.5–3 | | | | | |

Wŭ Jiā Pí (Acanthopanacis Cortex) eleutherococcus root bark

**Preparation and use**  Commonly prepared in alcohol extract.

**Contraindications**  Yin deficiency with heat.

**Formulae**  *Wu Jia Pi San*[1] (developmental delay in children); *Wu Jia Pi San*[2] (wind damp painful obstruction and spasm); *Wu Pi Yin* (mild lower body edema; wind damp painful obstruction); *Wu Jia Pi Jiu* (alcohol extract for wind damp painful obstruction with Liver and Kidney deficiency); *Jia Wei Di Huang Wan*† (failure to thrive); *Xu Duan Wan* (chronic back pain from Kidney deficiency); *Xi Xian Jiu* (therapeutic wine for wind damp painful obstruction and hemiplegia); *Bai Hua She Jiu* (therapeutic wine for chronic wind damp painful obstruction and post wind stroke hemiplegia)

Sāng Jì Shēng (Taxilli Herba) mistletoe

**Preparation and use**  mostly used unprocessed, but can be processed with wine (*jiu chao sang ji sheng* 酒炒桑寄生) to enhance its ability to dispel wind damp

**Contraindications**  None noted.

**Formulae**  *Du Huo Ji Sheng Tang* (wind damp painful obstruction with Liver and Kidney deficiency); *Qin Jiao Ji Sheng Tang* (postpartum joint pain from blood deficiency); *Shou Tai Wan* (threatened or habitual miscarriage from Kidney deficiency); *Shou Wu He Ji* (hypertension, dizziness and numb extremities from Liver blood deficiency with ascendant yang); *Tian Ma Gou Teng Yin* (headache and dizziness from ascendant Liver yang)

Qiān Nián Jiàn (Homalomenae Rhizoma) homalomena rhizome

**Preparation and use**  Commonly prepared in alcohol extract.

**Contraindications**  Caution in patients with yin deficiency and heat.

Lù Xián Căo (Pyrolae Herba) pyrola

**Contraindications**  None noted.

**Formulae**  *Gu Zhi Zeng Sheng Wan* (bony proliferation, osteophytes)

Xuě Lián Huā (Saussurea laniceps Flos) Himalayan snow lotus

**Contraindications**  Pregnancy.

Shí Nán Yè (Photinia Folium) Chinese photinia

**Contraindications**  Do not exceed the recommended dosage range.

**Formulae**  *Shi Nan Wan* (chronic wind damp painful obstruction and Kidney deficiency type backache and leg pain); *Shi Nan Jiu* (itchy wind rash)

Zhì Chuān Wū (Aconitii Radix preparata) processed aconite main root

Also known as wū tóu 乌头.

**Preparation and use**  This herb is toxic[3] and rarely used outside China, but it does possess unparalleled pain relieving ability in the correct and tightly controlled circumstances. When used in decoction, only the processed herb is used and it must be boiled for at least 30–60 minutes[4] prior to the other herbs, the longer the better. <u>Do not</u> take with alcohol as it facilitates absorption of the toxic alkaloids and increases the potential for side effects.

**Contraindications**  Pregnancy, patients with yin deficiency, heat of any type or ascendant yang. Not suitable for prolonged use. Do not exceed the recommended dosage range. Incompatible[5] with bai ji (p.14), bai lian (p.38), zhi ban xia (p.54), chuan bei mu (p.56), zhe bei mu (p.56) and gua lou (p.56).

**Formulae**  *Wu Tou Tang* (severe joint pain and stiffness from cold damp painful obstruction); *Xiao Huo Luo Dan* (stubborn painful obstruction, loss of function and numbness from cold, phlegm and blood stasis); *Wu Tou Chi Shi Zhi Wan* (severe chest pain from cold accumulation)

Zhì Căo Wū (Aconitii kusnezoffii Radix preparata) processed wild aconite root

**Preparation and use**  This herb is toxic[6] and usually only used externally in prepared liniments and plasters. It is found in one very hot prepared medicine (*Xiao Huo Luo Dan*, below), which comes in small pills, so the dose can be tightly controlled.

**Contraindications**  Pregnancy, in patients with yin deficiency, heat of any type or ascendant yang. Incompatible[7] with bai ji (p.14), bai lian (p.38), zhi ban xia (p.54), chuan bei mu (p.56), zhe bei mu (p.56) and gua lou p.(56).

**Formulae**  *Xiao Huo Luo Dan* (stubborn painful obstruction, loss of function and numbness from cold, phlegm and blood stasis)

Substances from other groups

Herbs from other groups with some effect on wind damp painful obstruction ba ji tian (p.82), xian ling pi (p.82), xian mao (p.82), gou ji (p.84), du zhong (p.84), xu duan (p.84), and gu sui bu (p.84).

Endnotes

† These formulae traditionally contain items from endangered animal species and/or obsolete toxic substances, and are unavailable in their original form.

---

1 *Shen Shi Zun Sheng Shu* (Master Shen's Book for Revering Life)
2 *Bao Ying Cuo Yao* (Outline of Infant Care)

3 Appendix 3.1, p.102
4 Appendix 6, p.108
5 Appendix 2, p.100
6 Appendix 3.1, p.102
7 Appendix 2, p.100

| INDICATIONS | Ling Yang Jiao 羚羊角 | Shan Yang Jiao 山羊角 | Niu Huang 牛黄 | Zhen Zhu 珍珠 | Gou Teng 钩藤 | Tian Ma 天麻 | Di Long 地龙 | Quan Xie 全蝎 | Wu Gong 蜈蚣 | Bai Jiang Can 白僵蚕 | FUNCTIONS |
|---|---|---|---|---|---|---|---|---|---|---|---|
| abscesses & sores – skin | | | ▲ | | | | ○ | E | E | △E | alleviates wheezing |
| abscess – breast, mastitis | ○ | | | ○ | | | | | | △E | brightens the eyes |
| cervical lymphadenitis (*luo li*) | ○ | ○ | | | ○ | ○ | | △E | △E | △ | calms the Liver |
| chloasma, facial pigmentation | | | | △E○ | | | | | | | calms & sedates the shen |
| convulsions – chronic childhood | ○ | | ● | △ | △ | ▲ | | △○ | △○ | ▲○ | clears toxic heat |
| convulsions – febrile | ▲○ | △○ | △ | ○ | ▲○ | | △○ | △ | | △ | cools the Liver |
| cough – whooping | ● | | ○ | | ○ | ○ | ▲ | ○ | ○ | ○ | extinguishes wind |
| delirium – in high fever | △○ | △○ | △ | | | | ○ | △ | | | pacifies ascendant yang |
| dizziness, vertigo | △ | △ | | | △ | ▲ | ○ | | | | promotes urination |
| dysuria – damp heat, stone | | | | | | | △ | ● | ● | ○ | stops pain |
| eclampsia | △ | △ | ○ | | △○ | △● | | ● | ● | ○ | stops spasm & tremor |
| eyes – weak, from deficiency | | | ○ | △E | | | | | | | transforms phlegm heat |
| eyes – corneal opacity, cataract | △ | | | △E | | | ○ | ○ | ○ | | unblocks collaterals |
| eyes – red, sore, blurry | △ | △ | | △E | △ | △ | | | | △ | |
| fever – high | ▲ | ▲ | ▲ | | △ | | △ | | | | |
| headache – ascendant yang | △ | △ | | | △ | ▲ | | | | | |
| headache – migraine, vascular | | | | | △ | ▲ | △ | △ | △ | | |
| headache – stubborn | | | | | | | △ | ▲ | ▲ | | |
| headache – wind heat | | | | | △ | | | | | △ | |
| hemiplegia | | | | | | | △ | ▲ | △ | △ | |
| hypertension – Liv. fire, yang↑ | △ | △ | △ | | ▲ | ▲ | △ | | | | |
| impotence – blood stasis | | | | | | | | | △ | | |
| nodules & masses – phlegm | | | | | | | | △E | △E | △E | |
| numbness – extremities | | | | | | △ | ▲ | △ | △ | | |
| pain – neuropathic | | | | | | | | △ | △ | | **Domain (❖)** |
| pain – stubborn; joint, muscle | | | | | | | ❖ | △ | △ | ❖ | Lung |
| painful obst. – wind damp | | | | | △ | △❖ | △ | △ | | | Bladder |
| painful obst. – wind damp heat | △❖ | ❖ | ❖ | ❖ | ❖ | ❖ | △❖ | ❖ | ❖ | ❖ | Liver |
| palpitations with anxiety | ❖ | | ❖ | ▲❖ | | | | | | | Heart |
| paralysis – facial | | | | | ❖ | △ | △ | ▲ | ▲ | ▲ | Pericardium |
| paralysis – spastic; yang type | | | | | | | △❖ | △ | △ | | Spleen |
| seizures, epilepsy | △ | △ | △ | △ | △ | ▲ | △ | ▲ | △ | △ | |
| skin – itching; eczema | | | | | | | | | | △ | |
| skin – rash, purpura; hot blood | △ | | | | | | | | | | **Flavour, nature (♦)** |
| skin – damp rashes; nappy rash | | | E | | | | | ♦ | ♦ | | toxic |
| spasm – tetanic | △ | | △ | | △ | △ | | △♦ | ▲♦ | △♦ | acrid |
| spasm & tremor – heat, wind | △ | △ | △♦ | | | ▲ | △ | | | | bitter |
| throat – sore; acute, with pus | ♦ | ♦ | ▲ | ♦ | | | ♦ | | | △♦ | salty |
| ulcers – skin, chronic | | | | E♦ | ♦ | ♦ | | | | | sweet |
| ulcers – mouth | ♦ | ♦ | △ | E♦ | | | ♦ | | | | cold |
| wheezing – Lung heat; phlegm | | | ♦ | | ♦ | | ▲ | | | | cool |
| wind stroke – prevention of | △ | △ | △ | | | | △♦ | △♦ | △ | ♦ | neutral |
| withdrawal mania (*dian kuang*) | | | △ | | | | △ | | ♦ | | warm |
| **Standard dosage range (g)** | 1-3 | 9-15 | *see p.97* | 0.3-1 | 9-15 | 3-9 | 6-15 | 2-5 | 1-3 | 3-9 | |

△ Indication
▲ Strong Indication
E External Use
E Strong External Indication

○ Function
● Strong Function

### Líng Yáng Jiǎo (Saigae tataricae Cornu) saiga antelope horn

The saiga antelope is listed in CITES[1] Appendix 2. Limited trade is permitted with appropriate documentation, but its status is questionable and may be on the verge of being seriously endangered, so should not be used. The horn of the mountain goat (shan yang jiao, below), is an adequate substitute.

**Preparation and use** When decocted, the shaved horn is cooked for at least 2 hours[2] before the other herbs. When taken directly in powder or pill form, the dose is 0.3–0.6 grams, two or three times daily.

**Contraindications** Chronic convulsions from Spleen deficiency. Caution in patients with an allergic or atopic constitution.

**Formulae** *Ling Yang Gou Teng Tang*† (tremors and convulsions from wind generated by heat in the Liver); *Ling Yang Jiao San*[3]† (eclampsia); *Ling Yang Jiao San*[4]† (eye pain and visual disorders from Liver fire); *Zi Xue Dan*† (febrile convulsions)

### Shān Yáng Jiǎo (Naemorhedi Cornu) goral goat horn

**Preparation and use** When decocted the shaved horn is cooked for 1–2 hours[5] prior to the other herbs. When taken directly in powder or pill form, the dose is 3–5 grams, two or three times daily.

**Contraindications** Chronic convulsions from Spleen deficiency. Caution in patients with an allergic or atopic constitution.

### Niú Huáng (Bovis Calculus) cattle gallstone

Placed in the toxic heat clearing group[6] and orifice opening group[7] in other texts.

**Preparation and use** Not suitable for decoction, only used in pill and powder form at doses of 0.2-0.5 grams.

**Contraindications** Pregnancy; in patients without clear excess heat and/or phlegm conditions; middle burner yang deficiency.

**Formulae** *Niu Huang Jie Du Wan* (toxic heat sores, ulcers and throat pain); *Niu Huang Shang Qing Wan*† (ulceration and pain of the oral cavity, eyes and throat from fire); *Zhi Bao Dan*† (impaired consciousness or coma); *An Gong Niu Huang Wan*† (delirium, loss of consciousness and high fever from heat affecting the Pericardium); *Niu Huang San*† (wind stroke and hemiplegia from phlegm heat); *Liang Jing Wan*† (childhood febrile convulsions); *Liu Shen Wan*† (sore swollen throat and boils from toxic heat); *Zhu Huang San* (oral ulceration)

### Zhēn Zhū (Margarita) pearl

**Preparation and use** Mostly used in pill or powder form, in doses of 0.3–1 gram, taken two or three times daily. When used in decoction, the powdered pearl is added to the warm strained decoction.

**Contraindications** Caution during pregnancy.

**Formulae** *Jin Bo Zhen Xin Wan*† (infantile convulsions and seizures from heat in the Liver and Heart); *Zhen Zhu San* (painful eyes and visual disturbances from Liver deficiency with heat); *Zhu Huang San* (oral ulceration); *Sheng Ji San*† (chronic non healing ulcers and sores); *Xing Jun San*† (severe sudden turmoil disorder)

### Gōu Téng (Uncariae Ramulus cum Uncis) uncaria stem with hooks

**Preparation and use** Cook no longer than 10–15 minutes[8].

**Contraindications** Caution in patients without excess heat patterns.

**Formulae** *Ling Yang Gou Teng Tang*† (tremors and convulsions from wind generated by heat in the Liver); *Gou Teng Yin Zi*† (childhood convulsions from heat); *Tian Ma Gou Teng Yin* (headache and dizziness from ascendant Liver yang); *Gou Teng Di Long Tang* (chronic migraine headaches from Liver heat); *E Jiao Ji Zi Huang Tang* (spasms and tremors from yin and blood deficiency); *Niu Huang San*† (wind stroke and hemiplegia from phlegm heat)

### Tiān Má (Gastrodiae Rhizoma) gastrodia orchid rhizome

Listed in Appendix 2 of CITES[9] which permits limited trade with appropriate documentation.

**Preparation and use** When taken directly in pill or powder form, the dose is 1–1.5 grams, two or three times daily.

**Contraindications** None noted.

**Formulae** *Ban Xia Bai Zhu Tian Ma Tang* (dizziness and headache from wind phlegm); *Tian Ma Gou Teng Yin* (dizziness and headache from ascendant Liver yang); *Gou Teng Yin Zi*† (childhood convulsions from heat); *Xing Pi Wan* (chronic childhood convulsions from Spleen deficiency); *Ding Xian Wan*† (seizures from wind phlegm)

### Dì Lóng (Pheretima) earthworm

**Preparation and use** If fresh worms are used, the dose is 10–20 grams and they are cooked to a syrup with sugar or honey. This preparation is used for wheezing from Lung heat. When powdered and taken directly the dose is 1–2 grams, two or three times daily.

**Contraindications** Middle burner deficiency, when used alone in patients without excess heat patterns.

**Formulae** *Di Long Jie Jing Tang* (febrile convulsions); *Gou Teng Di Long Tang* (chronic migraine headaches from Liver heat); *Bu Yang Huan Wu Tang* (hemiplegia from qi deficiency with blood stasis); *Xiao Huo Luo Dan* (stubborn painful obstruction, loss of function and numbness from cold, phlegm and blood stasis); *Sang Luo Tang* (damp heat painful obstruction)

### Quán Xiē (Scorpio) scorpion

**Preparation and use** When taken directly in pill or powder form, the dose is 0.6–1 gram, two or three times daily.

**Contraindications** Pregnancy; internal wind generated by blood or yin deficiency. Not suitable for prolonged use. Do not exceed the recommended dosage range or symptoms of toxicity[10] may occur.

**Formulae** *Zhi Jing San* (spasms, tremors, convulsions, stubborn headache); *Qian Zheng San* (facial paralysis and fasciculation); *Wu Hu Zhui Feng San* (tetanic spasm); *Quan Xie Ru Xiang San*† (chronic painful obstruction); *Quan Xie Xiao Feng San* (mumps and toxic swellings)

### Wú Gōng (Scolopendra) centipede

**Preparation and use** When taken directly in pill or powder form, the dose is 0.6–1 gram, two or three times daily.

**Contraindications** Pregnancy; internal wind generated by blood or yin deficiency; chronic childhood convulsions. Not suitable for prolonged use. Do not exceed the recommended dosage range or symptoms of toxicity[11] may occur.

**Formulae** *Zhi Jing San* (spasms, tremors, convulsions, stubborn headache); *Cuo Feng San*† (opisthotonos and muscle rigidity); *Wu Hu Zhui Feng San* (tetanic spasm); *Luo Li San* (tuberculous lymphadenitis); *Kang Wei Ling* (erectile dysfunction from blood stasis)

### Bái Jiāng Cán (Bombyx Batryticatus) mummified silkworm

**Preparation and use** Taken directly in pills or powder, the dose is 1–1.5 grams, two or three times daily. For wind heat eye problems, itching, sore throat and headaches, the unprocessed substance is used; for all other problems the stir fried form (*chao jiang can* 炒僵蚕) is preferred.

**Contraindications** None noted.

**Formulae** *Qian Zheng San* (facial paralysis and fasciculation); *Qian Jin San*† (chronic childhood convulsions from phlegm heat); *Cuo Feng San*† (opisthotonos and muscle rigidity); *Wu Hu Zhui Feng San* (tetanic spasm); *Bai Jiang Can San* (wind heat headache, throat and eye problems); *Pu Ji Xiao Du Yin* (toxic heat in the throat and head)

### Substances from other groups

Substances from other groups that can extinguishing wind include ci ji li (p.48), mu li (p.48), long gu (p.72) and dan nan xing (p.58).

### Endnotes

† These formulae traditionally contain items from endangered animal species and/or obsolete toxic substances, and are unavailable in their original form.

1 Appendix 5, p.106
2 Appendix 6, p.108
3 *Ji Sheng Fang* (Formulas to Aid the Living)
4 *He Ji Ju Fang* (Imperial Grace Formulary of the Tai Ping Era)
5 Appendix 6, p.108
6 *Zhong Yao Xue* (1997)
7 Bensky et al (2004) 3rd ed.; *Shi Yong Zhong Yao Xue* (1985)
8 Appendix 6, p.108

9 Appendix 4, p.105
10 Appendix 3.1, p.101
11 Ibid.

## 1.1 HERBS CONTRAINDICATED DURING PREGNANCY

The main action of herbs likely to cause problems during pregnancy falls into three groups: 1. Blood stasis dispersing and blood breaking; 2. Bitter, cold purgatives, or those with a descending effect on qi and blood; 3. Herbs that promote urination and potentially diminish amniotic fluid and damage yin. The first trimester is the most sensitive time, and when problems are likely to occur as a result of herb ingestion.

The issue of herbs during pregnancy is complicated. There is a surprising diversity of opinion amongst the main sources, even on the status of some of the more common herbs. Texts asserting a contraindication are footnoted in red; those asserting a caution, in black. When a text is not represented it does not have an opinion one way or the other. Contraindications for herbs without footnotes are derived from secondary sources. The final number is the page reference.

1 *Zhong Yao Xue* (2000)
2 *Zhong Yao Xue* (1997)
3 *Shi Yong Zhong Yao Xue* (1985)
4 Bensky et al. (2004) 3rd ed.
5 Chen (2004)
6 Xu & Wang (2002)

**Bā Dòu Shuāng**[1, 2, 3, 4, 5, 6] (Crotonis Fructus Pulveratum) 62

**Bái Huā Shé Shé Cǎo**[4, 6] (Hedyotis diffusae Herba) 36
- None of the Chinese sources consulted note either a caution or contraindication. A caution may be more appropriate.

**Bān Máo**[1, 2, 3, 4, 5, 6] (Mylabris) 24

**Biē Jiǎ**[1, 2, 4, 5, 6] (Trionycis Carapax) 80

**Bīng Piàn**[1, 2, 4, 5, 6] (Borneol) 50

**Chán Sū**[1, 2, 3, 4, 5, 6] (Bufonis Venenum) 50

**Cháng Shān**[1, 4, 6] (Dichroeae Radix) 22

**Chǎo Pú Huáng**[1, 2, 4, 5, 6] (Typhae Pollen preparata) 12

**Chē Qián Zǐ**[4, 6] (Plantaginis Semen) 18
- None of the Chinese sources consulted note either a caution or contraindication. A caution may be more appropriate.

**Chóng Lóu**[1, 2, 4, 5, 6] (Paridis Rhizoma) 36

**Chuān Niú Xī**[1, 2, 3, 4, 5, 6] (Cyathulae Radix) 8

**Cì Jí Lí**[1, 2, 4, 5, 6] (Tribuli Fructus) 48

**Dà Fēng Zǐ**[1, 4] (Hydnocarpi Semen) 24

**Dà Huáng**[1, 2, 3, 4, 5, 6] (Rhei Radix et Rhizoma) 60

**Dà Suàn**[2, 4, 5] (Alli sativi Bulbus) 52
- Contraindicated as a retention enema.

**Dǎn Nán Xīng**[5] (Arisaema cum Bile) 58
- Although no source explicitly states a contraindication and this substance is not considered toxic, a contraindication is prudent due to the toxic status of the parent herb (tian nan xing).

**Dān Shēn**[4] (Salviae miltiorrhizae Radix) 6
- None of the Chinese sources consulted note either a caution or contraindication. Large doses should be avoided, but a caution may be more appropriate.

**Dì Biē Chóng**[1, 2, 3, 4, 5, 6] (Eupolyphaga/Steleophaga) 10

**Ē Wèi**[1] (Ferulae Resina) 30

**É Zhú**[1, 2, 4, 5, 6] (Curcumae Rhizoma) 10

**Fān Xiè Yè**[1, 2, 3, 4, 5, 6] (Senna Folium) 60

**Gān Jiāng**[3, 4, 5, 6] (Zingiberis Rhizoma) 88

**Gān Qī**[2, 5] (Toxicodendri Resina) 10

**Gān Suì**[1, 2, 3, 4, 5, 6] (Kansui Radix) 62

**Gūa Dì**[4] (Melo Pedicellus) 22

**Guàn Zhòng**[2, 3, 4, 5, 6] (Dryopteridis crassirhizomae Rhizome) 52

**Guī Bǎn**[1, 2, 4, 5, 6] (Testudinis Plastrum) 80
- The processed resin, gui ban jiao, is not contraindicated.

**Guì Zhī**[1, 2, 3, 4, 5, 6] (Cinnamomi Ramulus) 28

**Hè Shī**[1, 4] (Carpesii abrotanoidis Fructus) 52

**Hóng Dà Jǐ**[1, 2, 3, 5] (Knoxiae Radix) 62

**Hóng Huā**[1, 2, 3, 4, 5, 6] (Carthami Flos) 6

**Hú Jiāo**[4, 5] (Piperis Fructus) 88
- Not used in therapeutic doses, but considered safe in the quantities used to season food.

**Hǔ Zhàng**[1, 2, 4, 5, 6] (Polygoni cuspidati Rhizoma) 8

**Huā Ruǐ Shí**[1, 2, 4, 5, 6] (Ophicalcitum) 12

**Huá Shí**[4, 6] (Talcum) 20
- None of the Chinese sources consulted note either a caution or contraindication. A caution may be more appropriate.

**Huái Jiǎo**[1, 2, 4, 5, 6] (Sophorae Fructus) 13

**Huái Niú Xī**[1, 2, 3, 4, 5, 6] (Achyranthis bidentatae Radix) 6

**Jí Xìng Zǐ** (Impatiens balsamina Semen) 10

**Jī Xuè Téng**[5] (Spatholobi Caulis) 6
- The blood invigorating action of this herb is mild and well balanced by its tonic effect, so a caution may be more appropriate.

**Jiāng Huáng**[4, 5] (Curcumae longae Rhizoma) 8

**Kǔ Liàn Pí**[4] (Meliae Cortex) 52

**Lí Lú**[1, 2, 3, 4, 5] (Veratri nigri Radix et Rhizoma) 22

**Liú Huáng**[1, 2, 3, 4, 5, 6] (Sulphur) 24

**Liú Jì Nú**[1, 2, 4, 5, 6] (Artemesiae anomalae Herba) 8

**Lóng Kuí**[4] (Solani nigri Herba) 86

**Lòu Lú**[1, 3, 4, 6] (Rhapontici Radix) 38

**Lú Huì**[1, 2, 3, 4, 5, 6] (Aloe) 60

**Lù Lù Tōng**[3, 4, 5, 6] (Liquidambaris Fructus) 8

**Mǎ Chǐ Xiàn**[4] (Portulacae Herba) 34
- This plant is consumed in parts of China as a vegetable. A caution may be more appropriate.

**Máng Xiāo**[1, 2, 4, 5, 6] (Natrii Sulfas) 60

**Méng Chóng**[1, 2, 3, 4, 5] (Tabanus) 10

**Míng Dǎng Shēn**[4] (Changii Radix) 58

**Mò Yaò**[1, 2, 4, 5, 6] (Myrrha) 6

**Mù Biē Zǐ**[1, 2, 4, 5] (Momordicae Semen) 24

**Mǔ Dān Pí**[1, 2, 3, 4, 5, 6] (Moutan Cortex) 40

**Niú Huáng**[1, 2, 4, 5, 6] (Bovis Calculus) 96

**Páo Jiāng** (Zingiberis Rhizoma preparata) 14
- Not a traditional contraindication, but included here because the parent herb, gan jiang, is contraindicated.

**Pú Huáng**[1, 2, 4, 5, 6] (Typhae Pollen) 8

**Qiān Jīn Zǐ**[1, 2] (Euphorbia lathyris Semen) 62

**Qiān Niú Zǐ**[1, 2, 3, 4, 5, 6] (Pharbitidis Semen) 62

**Qīng Méng Shí**[1, 2, 3, 4, 5] (Chloriti Lapis) 58

**Qú Mài**[1, 2, 3, 4, 5, 6] (Dianthi Herba) 20

**Quán Xiē**[1, 4, 5, 6] (Scorpio) 96

**Rén Gōng Shè Xiāng**[1, 2, 3, 4, 5, 6] (Synthetic muscone) 50

**Ròu Guì**[1, 2, 3, 4, 5, 6] (Cinnamomi Cortex) 88

**Rǔ Xiāng**[1, 2, 3, 4, 5, 6] (Olibanum) 6
**Sān Léng**[1, 2, 3, 4, 5, 6] (Sparganii Rhizoma) 10
**Sān Qī**[2, 4, 5, 6] (Notoginseng Radix) 12
**Shān Zhā**[4] (Crataegi Fructus) 30
- This contraindication is specific for large doses. What constitutes a large dose is not stated, but presumably small doses, up to 12 grams, can be used cautiously.
**Shāng Lù**[1, 2, 3, 4, 5] (Phytolaccae Radix) 62
**Shè Gān**[1, 5, 6] (Belamcandae Rhizoma) 36
**Shēn Jīn Cǎo**[1, 4, 5, 6] (Lycopodii Herba) 90
**Shuǐ Zhì**[1, 2, 3, 4, 5, 6] (Hirudo) 10
**Sū Mù**[1, 2, 3, 4, 5, 6] (Sappan Lignum) 8
**Táo Rén**[1, 2, 3, 4, 5, 6] (Persicae Semen) 6
**Tiě Xiàn Cài**[2] (Acalyphae Herba) 14
**Tōng Cǎo**[1, 4, 5, 6] (Tetrapanacis Medulla) 20
**Tòu Gǔ Cǎo** (Speranskia Herba) 90
**Wáng Bù Liú Xíng**[1, 2, 4, 5, 6] (Vaccariae Semen) 8
**Wú Gōng**[1, 2, 4, 5, 6] (Scolopendra) 96
**Wǔ Líng Zhī**[1, 2, 4, 5, 6] (Trogopterori Faeces) 6
**Xià Tiān Wú** (Corydalis decumbens Rhizoma) 90
- No specific contraindications could be found for this herb, but it has a similar composition and therapeutic profile to yan hu suo, so a contraindication would seem warranted.
**Xuè Jié**[1, 2, 4, 5, 6] (Daemonoropis Resina) 24
**Xuě Lián Huā** (Saussurea laniceps Flos) 94
**Yā Dǎn Zǐ**[3, 5, 6] (Bruceae Fructus) 36

**Yán Hú Suǒ**[1, 2, 4, 5, 6] (Corydalis Rhizoma) 6
**Yì Mǔ Cǎo**[1, 4, 5, 6] (Leonurus Herba) 6
**Yì Yǐ Rén**[5, 6] (Coicis Semen) 18
- None of the Chinese sources consulted support this assertion. An extensive search failed to uncover any rationale for the contraindication, although the root of this plant is clearly contraindicated. Bensky (2004) states that 'Long term consumption during pregnancy can lead to miscarriage', but evidence for contraindication is tenuous. These seeds appear in food items routinely available in China and Japan. A caution may be more appropriate.
**Yīng Sù Ké**[1, 4] (Papaveris Pericarpium) 4
**Yù Lǐ Rén**[1, 3, 4, 6] (Pruni Semen) 60
**Yù Jīn**[4, 5, 6] (Curcumae Radix) 8
- None of the Chinese sources consulted asserted either a caution or contraindication. Large doses should be avoided, but a caution may be more appropriate.
**Yuán Huā**[1, 2, 3, 4, 5, 6] (Genkwa Flos) 62
**Zào Jiá**[1, 2, 3, 4, 5, 6] (Gleditsiae Fructus) 54
**Zào Jiǎo Cì**[2, 3, 4, 5] (Gleditsiae Spina) 54
**Zhāng Nǎo**[1, 2, 3, 4, 5] (Camphora) 50
**Zhì Bái Fù Zǐ**[1, 2, 3, 4, 5, 6] (Typhonii Rhizoma preparata) 54
**Zhì Cǎo Wū**[1, 2, 3, 5, 6] (Aconitii kusnezoffii Radix preparata) 94
**Zhì Chuān Wū**[1, 2, 3, 4, 5, 6] (Aconitii Radix preparata) 94
**Zhì Fù Zǐ**[1, 2, 3, 4, 5, 6] (Aconiti Radix lateralis preparata) 88
**Zhì Tiān Nán Xīng**[1, 2, 3, 4, 5, 6] (Arisaematis Rhizoma preparata) 54

## 1.2 HERBS TO BE USED CAUTIOUSLY DURING PREGNANCY

**Bā Yuè Zhá**[4] (Akebiae Fructus) 66
**Bài Jiàng Cǎo**[4] (Patriniae Herba) 34
**Bàn Zhī Lián**[4] (Scutellariae barbate Herba) 86
**Bīng Láng**[1, 5, 6] (Arecae Semen) 52
**Chán Tuì**[1, 2, 4, 5, 6] (Cicadae Periostracum) 26
**Chì Shí Zhī**[1, 4, 5, 6] (Halloysitum rubrum) 4
**Chì Xiǎo Dòu**[4] (Phaseoli Semen) 18
- The caution is due to the claim in Bensky (2004) that 'overdose can induce miscarriage'. This assertion is not supported by any other source. In addition, they are a common food item in China and Japan, and appear in many traditional foods, without apparent deleterious effects.
**Chuān Xiōng**[4, 6] (Chuanxiong Rhizoma) 6
**Dà Fù Pí**[4, 5] (Arecae Pericarpium) 64
**Dài Zhě Shí**[1, 2, 4, 5, 6] (Haematitum) 48
**Dōng Kuí Zǐ**[1, 2, 3, 4, 5] (Malvae Semen) 20
**Hé Huān Pí**[1, 4, 5] (Albizziae Cortex) 70
**Hóng Téng**[1, 4, 6] (Sargentodoxae Caulis) 34
**Hòu Pò**[1, 2, 4, 5, 6] (Magnoliae officinalis Cortex) 16
**Hú Lú Bā**[5] (Trigonellae Semen) 84

**Huā Jiāo**[1, 2, 4, 5, 6] (Zanthoxyli Pericarpium) 88
**Jì Huā**[2] (Loropetalum chinensis Flos) 14
**Jué Míng Zǐ**[5] (Cassiae Semen) 48
**Mǎ Biān Cǎo**[1, 2, 4, 5] (Verbenae Herba) 10
**Mù Tōng**[1, 2, 3, 4] (Akebiae Caulis) 20
**Mù Zéi**[4, 5] (Equiseti hiemalis Herba) 26
**Shén Qū**[2, 5] (Massa medicata fermentata) 30
**Sū Hé Xiāng**[4] (Styrax Liquidis) 50
**Suān Zǎo Rén**[5] (Ziziphi spinosae Semen) 70
**Wēi Líng Xiān**[5] (Clematidis Radix) 90
**Xiāng Yuán**[2, 5] (Citri Fructus) 66
**Xiǎo Huí Xiāng**[5] (Foeniculi Fructus) 88
**Xīn Yí Huā**[4] (Magnoliae Flos) 28
**Yǔ Yú Liáng**[1, 3, 4, 6] (Limonitum) 4
**Zé Lán**[4] (Lycopi Herba) 6
**Zhēn Zhū**[4] (Margarita) 96
**Zhēn Zhū Mǔ**[1, 4] (Margaritiferae Concha usta) 48
**Zhǐ Ké**[1, 2, 4, 5, 6] (Aurantii Fructus) 64
**Zhǐ Shí**[1, 2, 4, 5, 6] (Aurantii Fructus immaturus) 64

| ANTAGONISTIC (xiāng wù 相恶) | |
|---|---|
| These are herbs that counteract or neutralize each others positive effects if used together. Some of these substances are now obsolete. Traditionally these were known as the 'nineteen antagonisms'. | |
| **Bā Dòu** (Crotonis Fructus)      – – antagonizes – – | **Qiān Niú Zǐ** (Pharbitidis Semen) |
| **Dīng Xiāng** (Caryophylli Flos) | **Yù Jīn** (Curcumae Radix) |
| **Rén Shēn** (Ginseng Radix) | **Wǔ Líng Zhī** (Trogopterori Faeces)<br>**Zào Jiá** (Gleditsiae Fructus) |
| **Dǎng Shēn** (Codonopsis Radix) | **Wǔ Líng Zhī** (Trogopterori Faeces) |
| **Ròu Guì** (Cinnamomi Cortex) | **Chì Shí Zhī** (Halloysitum rubrum) |
| **Láng Dú** 狼毒 (Euphorbia fisheriana Radix)[1] | **Mì Tuó Sēng** 密陀僧 (Lythargyrum)[2] |
| **Liú Huáng** (Sulphur) and | **Pò Xiāo** (Sal Glauberis)[3] |
| **Shuǐ Yín** 水银 (Hydragyrum)[4] | **Pī Shí** 砒石 (Arsenolite)[5] |
| **Yā Xiāo** 牙硝 (Nitrum)[6] | **Sān Léng** (Sparganii Rhizoma) |
| **Zhì Chuān Wū** (Aconitii Radix preparata)<br>**Zhì Cǎo Wū** (Aconitii kusnezoffii Radix preparata) | **Xī Jiǎo** (Rhinocerotis Cornu)[7] |
| **Lái Fú Zǐ** (Raphani Semen)[8] | **Rén Shēn** (Ginseng Radix)<br>**Shú Dì Huáng** (Rehmanniae Radix preparata)<br>**Zhì Hé Shǒu Wū** (Polygoni multiflori Radix preparata) |
| **Fěi Zǐ** (Torreyae Semen)[9] | **Lǜ Dòu** (Phaseoli radiati Semen) |

1 Obsolete due to toxicity.
2 Obsolete; a form of lead oxide.
3 An unrefined form of mang xiao p.60.
4 Obsolete; a form of mercury.
5 Obsolete; a form of arsenic.
6 A form of sodium nitrite (NaNo$_3$).
7 Obsolete due to endangered status.
8 An addition to the traditional antagonists. The powerful pungent dispersing action of lai fu zi counteracts the supplementing effect of these herbs, so benefit is negated. According to Chen (2004), however this effect can be harnessed to counteract an overdose of ren shen and settle the resulting over-stimulation.
9 An addition to the traditional antagonists.

| INCOMPATIBLE (xiāng fǎn 相反) | |
|---|---|
| These are herbs which, if used together, may cause toxic or other unwanted effects. Some of the traditional incompatibilities have been challenged by modern research and have been found to have little basis. Traditionally these were known as the 'eighteen incompatibilities'. | |
| **Gān Cǎo** (Glycyrrhizae Radix) | **Gān Suì** (Kansui Radix)<br>**Hǎi Zǎo** (Sargassum)[10]<br>**Hóng Dà Jǐ** (Knoxiae Radix)<br>**Kūn Bù** (Eckloniae Thallus)[10]<br>**Yuán Huā** (Genkwa Flos) |
| **Zhì Cǎo Wū** (Aconitii kusnezoffii Radix preparata)<br>**Zhì Chuān Wū** (Aconitii Radix preparata)<br>**Zhì Fù Zǐ** (Aconiti Radix lateralis preparata) | **Bái Jí** (Bletillae Rhizoma)<br>**Bái Liàn** (Ampelopsis Radix)<br>**Chuān Bèi Mǔ** (Fritillariae cirrhosae Bulbus)<br>**Guā Lóu** (Trichosanthis Fructus)<br>**Zhè Bèi Mǔ** (Fritillariae thunbergii Bulbus)<br>**Zhì Bàn Xià** (Pinelliae Rhizoma preparata) |
| **Lí Lú** (Veratri nigri Radix et Rhizoma) | **Bái Sháo** (Paeoniae Radix alba)<br>**Běi Shā Shēn** (Glehniae Radix)<br>**Chì Sháo** (Paeoniae Radix rubra)<br>**Dān Shēn** (Salviae miltiorrhizae Radix)<br>**Dǎng Shēn** (Codonopsis Radix)<br>**Kǔ Shēn** (Sophorae flavescentis Radix)<br>**Nán Shā Shēn** (Adenophorae Radix)<br>**Rén Shēn** (Ginseng Radix)<br>**Xì Xīn** (Asari Herba)<br>**Xuán Shēn** (Scrophulariae Radix) |

10 Gan cao is often combined with hai zao and kun bu (e.g. Hai Zao Yu Hu Tang), so this incompatibility is redundant and has been removed from the official pharmacopeia.

| 3.1 TOXIC HERBS | |
|---|---|
| These are powerful medicines that have the potential to cause significant toxic effects if improperly used. Doses and time limits must be strictly observed and the use of the substance closely monitored. | |
| **Herb** | **Symptoms of toxicity** |
| **Bā Dòu Shuāng** (Crotonis Fructus Pulveratum) | Stomatitis, burning of the esophagus, salivation, watery or bloody diarrhea, albuminuria, cyanosis, delirium, hypotension, miscarriage and shock. Oral doses of 10–20 unprocessed seeds can be fatal. |
| **Bái Huā Shé** (Agistrokodon/ Bungarus) | Headache, dizziness, hypertension, palpitations. |
| **Bān Máo** (Mylabris) | Nausea and vomiting, salivation, hematemesis, bloody diarrhea, ulceration and burning of the oral cavity, proteinuria. |
| **Chán Sū** (Bufonis Venenum) | Nausea and vomiting, abdominal pain, diarrhea, numbness of the mouth and lips, sweating, arrhythmia, decreased tendon reflexes, cyanosis. |
| **Cháng Chūn Huā** (Catharanthus roseus Flos) | Nausea and vomiting, constipation, abdominal pain, hair loss, weakness, numbness in the extremities, myalgia, oliguria, blurring vision. |
| **Cháng Shān** (Dichroeae Radix) | Vomiting, abdominal pain, bloody diarrhea, dizziness, arrhythmia, cyanosis, hypotension. |
| **Dà Fēng Zǐ** (Hydnocarpi Semen) | Nausea and vomiting, abdominal pain, dizziness, fever, proteinuria. |
| **Fēng Fáng** (Vespae Nidus) | Kidney damage with edema, backache and oliguria. |
| **Gān Suì** (Kansui Radix) | Nausea and vomiting, abdominal pain, diarrhea, dizziness, headache, palpitations, hypotension, hypothermia, impaired consciousness. |
| **Gūa Dì** (Melo Pedicellus) | Nausea and vomiting, abdominal pain, diarrhea, palpitations, hypotension, cyanosis, respiratory depression. |
| **Huáng Yào Zǐ** (Dioscoreae bulbiferae Rhizoma) | Dry mouth, burning in the mouth and throat, salivation, anorexia, nausea and vomiting, diarrhea, abdominal pain, jaundice, hepatitis, liver damage. |
| **Kǔ Liàn Pí** (Meliae Cortex) | Nausea and vomiting, abdominal pain, diarrhea, drowsiness, dizziness, tachycardia, sweating, cyanosis, hepatitis, gastrointestinal bleeding, rashes. |
| **Lí Lú** (Veratri nigri Radix et Rhizoma) | Tingling and numbness of the mouth and tongue, nausea and vomiting, salivation, burning epigastric pain, dizziness, sweating, hypotension, respiratory depression. |
| **Liú Huáng** (Sulphur) | Dizziness, headache, photophobia, catarrh, burning sensation of the mucous membranes, weakness, nausea and vomiting, abdominal pain, bloody diarrhea, fever, hypotension and shock. |
| **Mù Biē Zǐ** (Momordicae Semen) | Nausea and vomiting, abdominal pain, diarrhea, headache, dizziness, tinnitus, weakness. |
| **Nóng Jí Lì** (Crotalariae Herba) | Nausea and vomiting, abdominal pain, bradycardia, hypotension. |
| **Qiān Jīn Zǐ** (Euphorbia lathyris Semen) | Nausea and vomiting, abdominal pain, diarrhea, dizziness, tachycardia, fever, hematuria. |
| **Quán Xiē** (Scorpio) | Itching of the genitals and anus, urinary pain and retention, dizziness, hypertension, bradycardia, hemolysis and jaundice, respiratory depression. |
| **Shāng Lù** (Phytolaccae Radix) | Nausea and vomiting, abdominal pain, diarrhea, hematemesis, bloody diarrhea, dizziness, headache, slurred speech, bradycardia, hypotension, incontinence. |
| **Tǔ Jīng Pí** (Pseudolaricis Cortex) | Nausea and vomiting, abdominal pain, diarrhea. |
| **Wú Gōng** (Scolopendra) | Nausea and vomiting, abdominal pain, diarrhea, bradycardia, respiratory depression. |
| **Xǐ Shù** (Camptotheca acuminata Fructus et Radix) | Nausea and vomiting, diarrhea, abdominal pain, mouth ulcers, weakness, anorexia, edema, anemia and leukocytosis. |
| **Yā Dǎn Zǐ** (Bruceae Fructus) | Nausea and vomiting, abdominal pain, diarrhea, bloody diarrhea, urticaria, dizziness, liver and kidney damage, somnolence, convulsion, impaired consciousness. |
| **Yīng Sù Ké** (Papaveris Pericarpium) | Vomiting, drowsiness, weakness, anorexia, constipation, sweating, hypotension, respiratory depression. |
| **Yuán Huā** (Genkwa Flos) | Nausea and vomiting, abdominal pain, diarrhea, hematemesis, bloody diarrhea, dizziness, headache, blurred vision, spasms, respiratory failure, anuria, hematuria. |
| **Zhāng Nǎo** (Camphora) | Dizziness, headache, agitation, fever, delirium. |

| Herb | | Symptoms of toxicity |
| --- | --- | --- |
| **Zhì Bái Fù Zǐ** (Typhonii Rhizoma preparata) | Toxic effects occur when the unprocessed herb is ingested, but some effects may be seen if a herb is poorly or incompletely processed. | Numbness, tingling, burning and swelling of the mouth, tongue and throat, slurred speech, oral ulceration, salivation, nausea and vomiting, numb extremities, dizziness, blurred vision. |
| **Zhì Bàn Xià** (Pinelliae Rhizoma preparata) | | Numbness, tingling, burning and swelling of the mouth, tongue and throat, hoarse voice, slurred speech, salivation, abdominal pain, diarrhea, sweating, dyspnea, respiratory depression. |
| **Zhì Cǎo Wū** (Aconitii kusnezoffii Radix preparata) | | As for zhi fu zi, below. Not used internally, but may be inadvertently ingested due to misidentification. |
| **Zhì Chuān Wū** (Aconitii Radix preparata) | | As for zhi fu zi, below. |
| **Zhì Fù Zǐ** (Aconiti Radix lateralis preparata) | | Numbness and burning of the mouth, tongue and throat, slurred speech, numbness of the extremities, salivation, nausea and vomiting, diarrhea, dyspnea, dizziness, blurred vision, arrhythmia, hypotension. The toxic dose depends on degree of processing, the dose relative to the mass of the patient, and the delivery medium, and varies between 15–60 grams. |
| **Zhì Tiān Nán Xīng** (Arisaematis Rhizoma preparata) | | Numbness and paralysis of the mouth and tongue, edema, salivation, oral ulceration, numb extremities, dizziness, respiratory depression, impaired consciousness. |

| 3.2 SLIGHTLY TOXIC / POTENTIAL FOR SIDE EFFECTS | |
|---|---|
| Most substances used in medicine have the potential to cause unwanted effects, gastric upsets and so on when used inappropriately or in excessively high doses. The substances listed here are those that clinical experience has found most likely to produce mild toxic or unwanted effects when used incorrectly. Incorrect use means in excessive doses, used for too long, or when the unprocessed or poorly processed product is used. Although the list of possible side effects may appear somewhat daunting, it should be approached with some perspective. The doses that cause unwanted symptoms are typically far in excess of the normal therapeutic dose, and significant side effects occur in only a small percentage of patients. When used appropriately these substances are very unlikely to cause problems. In general, however, dosage range and recommended treatment times (where noted) should be adhered to, and the patient closely monitored. | |

| Herb | Symptoms of toxicity |
|---|---|
| **Ài Yè** (Artemisiae argyi Folium) | Dry mouth, nausea and vomiting, weakness, dizziness, tinnitus, tremors. Repeated overdose can lead to acute gastroenteritis, hepatitis, jaundice and miscarriage. |
| **Bái Fán** (Alumen) | Nausea and vomiting, gastritis, abdominal pain, ulceration of the gums, dizziness, headache, hematuria. |
| **Bái Guǒ** (Ginkgo Semen) | Fever, vomiting, abdominal pain, diarrhea, salivation, hypersensitivity, cyanosis, dyspnea, convulsions, respiratory failure. |
| **Bái Zhǐ** (Angelicae dahuricae Radix) | Nausea and vomiting, dizziness, palpitations, dyspnea, sweating, hypertension, chest pain, rash. |
| **Cāng Ěr Zǐ** (Xanthii Fructus) | Nausea and vomiting, anorexia, abdominal pain, diarrhea, drowsiness, lack of strength, dizziness, dilated pupils, urticaria, jaundice, arrhythmia, hematuria. |
| **Chóng Lóu** (Paridis Rhizoma) | Nausea and vomiting, diarrhea, dizziness, headache, blurred vision, pallor, dyspnea, arrhythmia, cyanosis. |
| **Chuān Liàn Zǐ** (Toosendan Fructus) | Nausea and vomiting, abdominal pain, bloody diarrhea, jaundice, hepatitis, blurred vision, tremor, numbness, arrhythmia, hypotension, shock. |
| **Chuān Shān Lóng** (Dioscoreae nipponicae Rhizoma) | Nausea and vomiting, stomatitis, diarrhea, abdominal discomfort, dizziness, blurred vision. |
| **Dà Huáng** (Rhei Radix et Rhizoma) | Diarrhea, colicky abdominal pain, nausea and vomiting, jaundice, damage to the intestines and liver, electrolyte imbalance. |
| **Dǎn Nán Xīng** (Arisaema cum Bile) | This substance is not considered toxic if processing is complete. Poor or incomplete processing may potentially leave mild residual toxicity. See Zhi Tian Nan Xing for symptoms of toxicity. |
| **Dì Biē Chóng** (Eupolyphaga/ Steleophaga) | Weakness, nausea, vertigo, gastrointestinal discomfort, papular rash, pruritus. |
| **Fān Xiè Yè** (Senna Folium) | Nausea and vomiting, colicky abdominal pain, urinary retention, damage to the intestines and liver, electrolyte imbalance. |
| **Gān Qī** (Toxicodendri Resina) | Stomatitis, oral ulceration, vomiting, diarrhea, nephropathy, hematuria, erythema, pruritus, urticaria. |
| **Guàn Zhòng** (Dryopteridis crassirhizomae Rhizome) | Nausea and vomiting, abdominal pain, diarrhea, visual disturbance, optic nerve damage, tremor, convulsions, miscarriage. |
| **Hè Shī** (Carpesii abrotanoidis Fructus) | Dizziness, nausea, tinnitus, abdominal pain, diarrhea, weakness, clonic spasms. |
| **Hóng Dà Jǐ** (Knoxiae Radix) | Watery diarrhea, colicky abdominal pain. |
| **Hǔ Ěr Cǎo** (Saxifraga stolonifera Herba) | Unknown. Although classified as slightly toxic, this plant is apparently eaten as a vegetable in parts of China and Japan. |
| **Huā Jiāo** (Zanthoxyli Pericarpium) | Nausea and vomiting, diarrhea, dry mouth, dizziness, spasms, impaired consciousness, dyspnea, urticaria, anaphylaxis. |
| **Jí Xìng Zǐ** (Impatiens balsamina Semen) | Vomiting, diarrhea. |
| **Léi Wán** (Omphalia) | The traditional designation of slight toxicity is disputed on the basis of modern research (Bensky [2004] 3rd. ed., p.1004). No adverse effects are noted. |
| **Lóng Kuí** (Solani nigri Herba) | Nausea and vomiting, diarrhea, burning throat, restlessness, hypotension, spasms, dyspnea. |
| **Lú Huì** (Aloe) | Diarrhea, colicky abdominal pain, nausea and vomiting, jaundice, damage to the intestines and liver, electrolyte imbalance. |

| Herb | Symptoms of toxicity |
|------|----------------------|
| **Má Huáng** (Ephedrae Herba) | Hypertension, cardiac arrhythmia, chest pain, sweating, insomnia, restlessness, rash, fever, tremor; in severe cases ventricular fibrillation and coma. |
| **Mǎn Shān Hóng** (Rhododendron daurici Folium) | Epigastric pain, headache, dizziness and dry mouth, nausea, vomiting, dizziness, chest pain, sweating, skin rash, weakness. |
| **Méng Chóng** (Tabanus) | Miscarriage. |
| **Qiān Niú Zǐ** (Pharbitidis Semen) | Nausea and vomiting, abdominal pain, bloody diarrhea, dizziness, headache, tachycardia, hematuria, cyanosis. |
| **Qīng Dài** (Indigo Naturalis) | Nausea and vomiting, abdominal pain, diarrhea, rectal bleeding. |
| **Qīng Fēng Téng** (Sinomenii Caulis) | Gastrointestinal discomfort, rash, sweating, dyspnea, hypotension, tachycardia. |
| **Rén Shēn** (Ginseng Radix) | Hypertension, headache, dizziness, insomnia, irritability, edema, weight loss, increased bleeding tendency, maculopapular rash, pruritus. |
| **Ròu Dòu Kòu** (Myristicae Semen) | Nausea, vertigo, incoherent speech, delirium, hallucinations. |
| **Shān Cí Gū** (Cremastrae/Pleiones Pseudobulbus) | Nausea and vomiting, diarrhea, abdominal pain, weakness, lethargy, hair loss, myalgia. |
| **Shān Dòu Gēn** (Sophorae tonkinensis Radix) | Nausea and vomiting, epigastric pain and fullness, heartburn, vertigo, sweating, chest oppression, loss of balance, hypotension. |
| **Shǐ Jūn Zǐ** (Quisqualis Fructus) | Nausea and vomiting, diarrhea, abdominal pain, dizziness. |
| **Shí Liú Pí** (Granati Pericarpium) | Nausea and vomiting, diarrhea, abdominal pain, vertigo, headache, blurred vision, tinnitus, weakness, tremor. |
| **Shí Nán Yè** (Photinia Folium) | Unknown. |
| **Shuǐ Zhì** (Hirudo) | Nausea, vomiting, abdominal pain, increased bleeding. |
| **Táo Rén** (Persicae Semen) | Nausea and vomiting, a bitter and astringent taste, salivation, abdominal pain, diarrhea, bleeding, headache, dizziness, restlessness and agitation, ptosis, hypotension, palpitations, weakness, dyspnea, cyanosis, respiratory depression. Toxicity is associated with the amygdalin component, a glycoside common to plants of the Prunus genus (almond, apricot, peach and cherry). Amygdalin is converted into hydrogen cyanide in the gut. |
| **Wǔ Bèi Zǐ** (Galla Chinensis) | Vomiting, diarrhea, epigastric pain, constipation; in severe cases liver damage. |
| **Wú Zhū Yú** (Evodiae Fructus) | Headache, vertigo, abdominal pain, diarrhea, chest oppression, rash, visual disturbances, hallucinations. |
| **Xì Xīn** (Asari Herba) | Headache, nausea, sweating, restlessness, panting, tachycardia and arrhythmia, hypertension, impaired consciousness, respiratory failure. |
| **Xiān Máo** (Curculiginis Rhizoma) | Swollen tongue, numbness in the extremities, restlessness and agitation, sweating, impairment of consciousness. |
| **Xìng Rén** (Armeniacae Semen) | Nausea and vomiting, bitter and astringent taste, salivation, abdominal pain, diarrhea, headache, dizziness, restlessness and agitation, ptosis, hypotension, palpitations, weakness, dyspnea, cyanosis, respiratory depression. The toxic dose for children is 10–20 kernels, for adults 40–60. |
| **Zào Jiá** (Gleditsiae Fructus) | Dry mouth, abdominal distension and pain, nausea and vomiting, watery diarrhea, headache, weakness, numbness, palpitations, jaundice. |

## ANIMALS

| CITES[1] APPENDIX 1[2] – CRITICALLY ENDANGERED, NO TRADE PERMITTED<br>CITES APPENDIX 2[3] – LIMITED TRADE PERMITTED WITH APPROPRIATE DOCUMENTATION |
| --- |
| See obsolete herbs and substances (Appendix 5, p.106) |

| CITES APPENDIX 3[4] – LIMITED TRADE PERMITTED WITH APPROPRIATE DOCUMENTATION | | |
| --- | --- | --- |
| | Comments | Possible substitutions |
| **Guī Bǎn** (Testudinis Plastrum) | Both these turtles are farmed extensively for food in China. High demand, however, propels wild harvesting throughout South East Asia leading to rapidly diminishing wild stocks. | **Mǔ Lì** (Ostreae Concha) to enrich yin and anchor the yang.<br>**Nǚ Zhēn Zǐ** (Ligustri Fructus) plus **Mò Hàn Lián** (Ecliptae Herba) to nourish yin. |
| **Biē Jiǎ** (Trionycis Carapax) | | **Sān Léng** (Sparganii Rhizoma) plus **Mǔ Lì** (Ostreae Concha) to dissipate masses.<br>**Qīng Hāo** (Artemisiae annuae Herba) to clear deficient heat. |

## PLANTS

The status of the plants listed below is current at the time of publication (2016) but is subject to revision from time to time. With all of these plants it is only the wild stocks that are subject to the convention. For the most up to date listings see the CITES website (www.cites.org). The actual abundance of any particular species can be difficult to ascertain precisely, as farm cultivation and tissue culturing of many plants is extensive.

| CITES APPENDIX 1 – ENDANGERED[5], NO TRADE IN WILD PLANTS PERMITTED[6] | | |
| --- | --- | --- |
| | Comments | Possible substitutions |
| **Mù Xiāng** (Aucklandiae Radix) | Farmed for medical use in China. | **Tǔ Mù Xiāng** (Inulae Radix) |

| CITES APPENDIX 2 – LIMITED TRADE PERMITTED WITH APPROPRIATE DOCUMENTATION[7] | | |
| --- | --- | --- |
| **Bái Jí** (Bletillae Rhizoma) | | **Ǒu Jié** (Nelumbinis Nodus rhizomatis) |
| **Chén Xiāng** (Aquilariae Lignum resinatum) | An extensive fake market exists due to rarity and expense. | **Hòu Pò** (Magnoliae officinalis Cortex)<br>**Wū Yào** (Linderae Radix) |
| **Gān Suì** (Kansui Radix) | | **Tíng Lì Zǐ** (Lepidii/Descurainiae Semen) |
| **Gǒu Jǐ** (Cibotii Rhizoma) | | **Xù Duàn** (Dipsaci Radix) |
| **Lú Huì** (Aloe) | Aloe vera, one of the species that is used to produce this herb, is not subject to the convention. All other Aloe species are listed. | |
| **Qiān Jīn Zǐ** (Euphorbia lathyris Semen) | | **Tíng Lì Zǐ** (Lepidii/Descurainiae Semen) |
| **Rén Shēn** (Ginseng Radix) | Only the plants of the Russian federation are included in the convention. Ginseng is widely cultivated and available in many grades and prices. | **Dǎng Shēn** (Codonopsis Radix) Popular as an inexpensive substitute for general qi deficiency conditions, but not suitable for severe conditions or bleeding. |
| **Ròu Cōng Róng** (Cistanches Herba) | | **Suǒ Yáng** (Cynomorii Herba) |
| **Shān Cí Gū** (Cremastrae/Pleiones Pseudobulbus) | | **Xuán Shēn** (Scrophulariae Radix) for hot nodules. |
| **Shí Hú** (Dendrobi Herba) | | **Yù Zhú** (Polygonati odorati Rhizoma) |
| **Tiān Má** (Gastrodiae Rhizoma) | | **Gōu Téng** (Uncariae Ramulus cum Uncis) |
| **Xī Yáng Shēn** (Panacis quinquefolii Radix) | | **Tài Zǐ Shēn** (Pseudostellariae Radix) |

1 Convention on International Trade of Endangered Species of fauna and flora.
2 Appendix I lists species that are threatened with extinction and are, or may be, affected by trade.
3 Appendix 2 lists species that are not necessarily threatened with extinction, but may become so unless trade is subject to strict regulation.
4 The species in Appendix 3 are listed after a member country has requested assistance from CITES in controlling their trade. The species are not necessarily threatened with extinction globally, but may be threatened locally. In all member countries trade in these species is only permitted with an appropriate export permit and a certificate of origin.
5 Endangered with respect to plants means wild stocks. Most if not all the endangered plants are cultivated extensively, either in commercial farms or from tissue culture.
6 Trade of cultivated plants is permitted but strictly controlled and certificates of cultivation can be difficult to obtain.
7 Although these herbs are legally available, some may be hard to obtain.

These items are derived from endangered animal species, are considered too toxic, are illegal or unethical. A few of the items listed are still legal and available in some countries, but their use in a modern clinical setting is indefensible.

| ANIMALS | | |
|---|---|---|
| Substance | Comments | Possible substitutes |
| **Chuān Shān Jiǎ** (Manitis Squama) pangolin scales | Listed in Appendix 2 of CITES, but the Chinese pangolin is significantly endangered, and a zero annual export quota is in force. It is used as a food item in Southern China, but is now considered too endangered to be used and is therefore obsolete. | **Wáng Bù Liú Xíng** (Vaccariae Semen, p.8): an adequate substitute for blood stasis and to promote lactation. **Zào Jiǎo Cì** (Gleditsiae Spina, p.54): for contained toxic lesions. |
| **Dài Mào** (Eretmochelydis Carapax) Hawksbill turtle shell | Listed in Appendix 1 of CITES. | **Shuǐ Niú Jiǎo** (Bubali Cornu, p.40) to clear heat and extinguish wind **Mǔ Lì** (Ostreae Concha, p.48) or **Dài Zhě Shí** (Haematitum, p.48) for ascendant yang |
| **Hǎi Gǒu Shèn** Callorhini Testes et Penis) male seal genitals | Use is unethical and unjustified. Seals are poached and killed to obtain the genitals. | **Suǒ Yáng** (Cynomorii Herba, p.82) **Xiān Líng Pí** (Epimedii Herba, p.82) |
| **Hǎi Lóng** (Syngnathus) pipefish | Heavily overexploited for the aquarium and medicine trade. | **Xiān Líng Pí** (Epimedii Herba, p.82) |
| **Hǎi Mǎ** (Hippocampus) seahorse | Listed in Appendix 2 of CITES, and heavily overexploited for the aquarium and medicine trade. | **Xiān Líng Pí** (Epimedii Herba, p.82) for impotence **Yì Zhì Rén** (Alpiniae oxyphyllae Fructus, p.82) and **Bǔ Gǔ Zhī** (Psoraleae Fructus, p.82) for urinary frequency and incontinence |
| **Hóu Zǎo** (Macacae mulattae Calculus) macaque gall stone | Use is unethical and unjustified. Macaques are poached and killed to obtain the gall stone. | **Niú Huáng** (Bovis Calculus, p.96) |
| **Hǔ Gǔ** (Tigris Os) Tiger bone | Listed in Appendix 1 of CITES. The tiger is critically endangered and protected worldwide; the illegal demand for the bone is one factor pushing their demise. The traditional substitute, panther, leopard or other wild cat bone, are all threatened in some way and hence also unethical and obsolete. | **Qiān Nián Jiàn** (Homalomenae Rhizoma, p.94) **Zhū Gǔ** (Suis Os) 猪骨, **Māo Gǔ** (Felis Os) 猫骨; **Gǒu Gǔ** (Canis Os) 狗骨 The bones of pig, domestic cat and dog respectively, are seen in some modern prepared medicines in place of Hu Gu. |
| **Líng Yáng Jiǎo** (Saigae tataricae Cornu) Saiga antelope horn | Listed in Appendix 2 of CITES. Although this substance is still available, the saiga antelope is endangered and should be considered obsolete. Good substitutes are available. | **Shān Yáng Jiǎo** (Naemorhedi Cornu, p.96) is best; second best is **Zhēn Zhū Mǔ** (Margaritiferae Concha usta, p.48) |
| **Shè Xiāng** (Moschus) secretion from the scent gland of the musk deer | Listed in Appendix 1 & 2 (depending on species). Farmed in China, however, the musk deer is a shy and skittish creature that does not respond well to captivity. This practice should be condemned. A good synthetic substitute is available, and other herbs can be used for specific purposes. | **Rén Gōng Shè Xiāng** (Synthetic muscone, p.50), a chemical analogue of musk is commercially manufactured and is found in most prepared medicines where musk is required. This has a very similar therapeutic profile. **Bái Zhǐ** (Angelicae dahuricae Radix, p.28) can be used for headaches and pain **Shí Chāng Pú** (Acori tatarinowii Rhizoma, p.50) for disturbances of consciousness |
| **Xī Jiǎo** (Rhinocerotis Cornu) Rhinoceros horn | Listed in Appendix 1 of CITES. The illegal medicine trade and demand for dagger handles from Yemen and other Arab nations drives poaching. | **Shuǐ Niú Jiǎo** (Bubali Cornu, p.40) |
| **Xióng Dǎn** (Vesica Fellea Ursi) Gallbladder of the asiatic or Himalayan black bear | The Himalayan black bear is listed in Appendix 2 of CITES. Although farmed for its gall, the practice is barbaric and should be condemned. | **Zhū Dǎn Zhī** (Suis Fel, p.58) |

| PLANTS | | |
|---|---|---|
| Substance | Comments | Possible substitutes |
| **Guǎng Fáng Jǐ** 广防己 (Arisolochiae fangchi Radix) | These plants belong to the Aristolochia family and contain aristolochic acid, a nephrotoxin. Used for wind damp bi pain and edema. | **Hàn Fáng Jǐ** (Stephaniae tetrandrae Radix, p.18) |
| **Guān Mù Tōng** 关木通 (Arisolochiae manshuriensis Caulis) | | |
| **Láng Dú** 狼毒 (Euphorbia fisheriana Radix) | Extremely toxic. | |
| **Léi Gōng Téng** 雷公藤 (Tripterygii wilfordii Radix) | Commonly used in China as an anti-inflammatory and immunosuppressive agent for autoimmune conditions. It is toxic and not suitable for use outside the controlled environment of the hospital or specialist centres. Monitoring of blood, and liver and kidney function is necessary during use. | **Qín Jiāo** (Gentianae macrophyllae Radix, p.92) |
| **Mǎ Dōu Líng** 马兜铃 (Aristolochiae Fructus) | Belongs to the Aristolochia family and contains aristolochic acid, a nephrotoxin. Used for phlegm heat cough. | **Qúan Guā Lóu** (Trichosanthis Fructus, p.56) **Pí Pa Yè** (Eriobotryae Folium, p.68) |
| **Mǎ Qián Zǐ** 马钱子 (Strychni Semen) | Extremely toxic. | |
| **Qīng Mù Xiāng** 青木香 (Arisolochiae debelis Radix) | Belongs to the Aristolochia family and contains aristolochic acid, a nephrotoxin. Used for qi stagnation type chest and abdominal pain. | **Chuān Liàn Zǐ** (Toosendan Fructus, p.64) |
| **Xún Gǔ Fēng** 寻骨风 (Arisolochiae fangchi Radix) | Belongs to the Aristolochia family and contains aristolochic acid, a nephrotoxin. Used for joint pain. | **Hàn Fáng Jǐ** (Stephaniae tetrandrae Radix, p.18) |
| **Yīng Sù Ké** 罂粟壳 (Papaveris Pericarpium) | The source of opium and heroin, this plant is illegal in most countries and thus obsolete. This is a shame because when used therapeutically in the appropriate circumstances by an experienced physician this is an exemplary substance with no mind altering or addictive effects. | Chronic cough: **Hē Zǐ** (Chebulae Fructus, p.4) plus **Bái Guǒ** (Ginkgo Semen, p.68) Chronic diarrhea: **Wēi Hē Zǐ** (roasted Chebulae Fructus, p.4) |

| MINERALS | | |
|---|---|---|
| These substances were traditionally used externally for skin diseases. | | |
| **Mì Tuó Sēng** 密陀僧 (Lithargyrum) | Lead oxide. | |
| **Péng Shā** 硼砂 (Borax) | Sodium tetraborate; $Na_2B_4O_7 \cdot 10H_2O$ | |
| **Pī Shí** 砒石 (Arsenolite) | Arsenic. | |
| **Qiān Dān** 铅丹 (Minum) | A form of lead oxide; $Pb_3O_4$ | |
| **Qīng Fěn** 轻粉 (Calomelas) | Mercurous chloride. | |
| **Shuǐ Yín** 水银 (Hydragyrum) | Mercury. | |
| **Xióng Huáng** 雄黄 (Realgar) | Arsenic sulphide. | |
| **Zhū Shā** 朱砂 (Cinnabaris) | Mercuric sulphide. | **Zǐ Shí Yīng** (Fluoritum) for *shen* disturbances. |

| | |
|---|---|
| **Decocted first** (xiān jiān 先煎)<br>These substances require prolonged cooking to extract all therapeutic components, to degrade toxic components or to provide sufficient material to catalyze the reactions and synergies of the remaining ingredients. Minerals or hard animal parts should be broken up in a mortar and pestle, or shaved (horns), before decoction. Specific cooking times are noted in the text. | **Biē Jiǎ** (Trionycis Carapax) 80<br>**Cí Shí** (Magnetitum) 72<br>**Dài Zhě Shí** (Haematitum) 48<br>**Fú Hǎi Shí** (Costaziae Os) 58<br>**Guī Bǎn** (Testudinis Plastrum) 80<br>**Hǎi Gé Qiào** (Meretricis/Cyclinae) 58<br>**Hán Shuǐ Shí** (Glauberitum) 32<br>**Huā Ruǐ Shí** (Ophicalcitum) 12<br>**Huá Shí** (Talcum) 20<br>**Líng Yáng Jiǎo** (Saigae tataricae Cornu) 96<br>**Lóng Chǐ** (Fossilia Dentis Mastodi) 72<br>**Lóng Gǔ** (Fossilia Ossis Mastodi) 72<br>**Mǔ Lì** (Ostreae Concha) 48<br>**Qīng Méng Shí** (Chloriti Lapis) 58<br>**Shān Yáng Jiǎo** (Naemorhedi Cornu) 96<br>**Shēng Tiě Luò** (Ferri Frusta) 72<br>**Shí Gāo** (Gypsum Fibrosum) 32<br>**Shí Jué Míng** (Haliotidis Concha) 48<br>**Shuǐ Niú Jiǎo** (Bubali Cornu) 40<br>**Sī Guā Luò** (Luffae Fructus) 92<br>**Wǎ Léng Zǐ** (Arcae Concha) 10<br>**Zào Xīn Tǔ** (Terra flava usta) 14<br>**Zhēn Zhū Mǔ** (Margaritiferae Concha usta) 48<br>**Zhì Chuān Wū** (Aconitii Radix preparata) 94<br>**Zhì Fù Zǐ** (Aconiti Radix lateralis preparata) 88<br>**Zǐ Bèi Chǐ** (Mauritiae/Cypraeae Concha) 48<br>**Zǐ Shí Yīng** (Fluoritum) 72 |
| **Added near the end of cooking** (hòu xià 后下)<br>These herbs need no more than a minute or two cooking, or are thrown in when the decoction is taken off the heat. Most contain volatile oils which boil away if overcooked. | **Bái Dòu Kòu** (Amomi Fructus rotundus) 16<br>**Bò Hé** (Mentha haplocalycis Herba) 26<br>**Cǎo Dòu Kòu** (Alpiniae katsumadai Semen) 16<br>**Dà Huáng** (Rhei Radix et Rhizoma)[1] 60<br>**Fān Xiè Yè** (Senna Folium) 60<br>**Ròu Guì** (Cinnamomi Cortex)[2] 88<br>**Shā Rén** (Amomi Fructus) 16<br>**Xìng Rén** (Armeniacae Semen) 68 |
| **Requires short cooking**<br>These herbs need only 5–15 minutes of cooking maximum, or their therapeutic action diminishes. | **Chuān Xiōng** (Chuanxiong Rhizoma) 6<br>**Gōu Téng** (Uncariae Ramulus cum Uncis) 96<br>**Jīng Jiè** (Schizonepetae Herba) 28<br>**Mù Xiāng** (Aucklandiae Radix) 64<br>**Qīng Hāo** (Artemisiae annuae Herba) 44<br>**Xiǎo Jì** (Cirsii Herba) 12<br>**Yú Xīng Cǎo** (Houttuyniae Herba) 36<br>**Zhú Yè** (Phyllostachys nigrae Folium) 32<br>**Zǐ Sū Yè** (Perillae Folium) 28 |
| **Dissolved in the strained decoction** (róng huà 溶化)<br>These substances are either unsuitable for cooking, or will stick to the pot and other herbs if decocted. They can be dissolved in the hot strained decoction or taken separately. | **Ē Jiāo** (Asini Corii Colla)[3] 78<br>**Fēng Mì** (Mel) 74<br>**Guī Bǎn Jiāo** (Testudinis Plastrum Colla)[3] 81<br>**Lù Jiǎo Jiāo** (Cervi Cornus Colla)[3] 83<br>**Máng Xiāo** (Natrii Sulfas) 60<br>**Yí Táng** (Maltosum) 74<br>**Zhú Lì** (Bambusae Succus) 56 |

| | |
|---|---|
| **Taken with the strained decoction** (chōng fú 冲服)<br>These substances are taken as powder, added to the strained decoction, or taken separately and washed down by the strained decoction. | **Chuān Bèi Mǔ** (Fritillariae cirrhosae Bulbus) 56<br>**Hǔ Pò** (Succinum) 72<br>**Lù Róng** (Cervi Cornu pantotrichum) 82<br>**Niú Huáng** (Bovis Calculus) 96<br>**Sān Qī** (Notoginseng Radix) 12 |
| **Cooked in a cloth bag** (bāo jiān 包煎)<br>These are substances that have irritant hairs, are tiny seeds or that can muddy a decoction and make it (more) unpalatable. | **Cán Shā** (Bombycis Faeces) 90<br>**Chē Qián Zǐ** (Plantaginis Semen) 18<br>**Chì Shí Zhī** (Halloysitum rubrum) 4<br>**Ér Chá** (Catechu) 24<br>**Hǎi Gé Qiào** (Meretricis/Cyclinae) 58<br>**Hǎi Jīn Shā** (Lygodii Spora) 18<br>**Hè Shī** (Carpesii abrotanoidis Fructus) 52<br>**Huā Ruǐ Shí** (Ophicalcitum) 12<br>**Huá Shí** (Talcum) 20<br>**Mǎ Bó** (Lasiosphaerae/Calvatiae) 36<br>**Pí Pa Yè** (Eriobotryae Folium) 68<br>**Pú Húang** (Typhae Pollen) 8, 12<br>**Qīng Méng Shí** (Chloriti Lapis) 58<br>**Wǔ Líng Zhī** (Trogopterori Faeces) 6<br>**Xīn Yí Huā** (Magnoliae Flos) 28<br>**Xuán Fù Huā** (Inulae Flos) 54<br>**Zào Xīn Tǔ** (Terra flava usta) 14 |
| **Cooked in a double boiler** (líng jiān 另煎)<br>These are expensive herbs that require prolonged and gentle extraction. The technique involves cooking the herb for several hours in a sealed container placed within another container of boiling water. This enables maximum extraction and no loss of active components. | **Rén Shēn** (Ginseng Radix) 74<br>**Xī Yáng Shēn** (Panacis quinquefolii Radix) 74 |

1 The cooking time required for da huang varies depending on its intended use. When strong purgation is required steeping in the hot decoction or cooking for only a minute or two enhances its purgative action; longer cooking (over 20 minutes) reduces the purgative effect and enhances its blood activating action.
2 Some sources state that rou gui is best taken separately as powder.
3 Easier when pulverized in a coffee grinder first.

# APPENDIX 7. FORMULAE NOTED IN THE TEXT

Formulae that are obsolete in their original form due to the presence of endangered species or toxic substances are marked by †, with the obsolete items in red.

| Formula | Source text | Ingredients |
|---|---|---|
| **Ai Fu Nuan Gong Wan** 艾附暖宫丸<br>Mugwort & Cyperus Pill to Warm the Uterus | Ren Zhai Zhi Zhi | ai ye, xiang fu, wu zhu yu, chuan xiong, bai shao, huang qi, xu duan, sheng di huang, rou gui, dang gui |
| **An Gong Niu Huang Wan**† 安宫牛黄丸<br>Calm the Palace Pill with Cow Gallstone | Wen Bing Tiao Bian | niu huang, yu jin, huang lian, shan zhi zi, huang qin, bing pian, zhen zhu, gold leaf, zhu sha, xiong huang, xi jiao (now shui niu jiao), she xiang (now ren gong she xiang) |
| **An Shen Bu Xin Wan** 安神补心丸<br>Calm the Shen & Supplement the Heart Pill | Zhong Yao Zhi Shi Shou Ce | zhen zhu mu, ye jiao teng, nu zhen zi, mo han lian, he huan pi, dan shen, tu si zi, sheng di huang, wu wei zi, shi chang pu |
| **An Shen Ding Zhi Wan** 安神定志丸<br>Calm the Shen & Settle the Zhi Pill | Yi Xue Xin Wu | fu ling, fu shen, ren shen, yuan zhi, shi chang pu, long chi |
| **An Shen Wan** 安神丸<br>Calm the Shen Pill | Zhong Yi Zhi Ji Shou Ce | he huan hua, sheng di huang, xuan shen, nu zhen zi, he huan pi, dan shen, ye jiao teng, sang shen |
| **An Tai Yin** 安胎饮<br>Calm Fetus Drink | Zheng Zhi Zhun Sheng | shu di huang, dang gui, bai shao, chuan xiong, bai zhu, fu ling, gan cao, di yu, ban xia qu, e jiao, huang qin, ai ye |
| **An Zhong San** 安中散<br>Calm the Middle Powder | He Ji Ju Fang | gan cao, yan hu suo, xiao hui xiang, gao liang jiang, gan jiang, rou gui, mu li |
| **Ba Ji Wan** 巴戟丸<br>Morinda Pill | He Ji Ju Fang | ba ji tian, gao liang liang, rou gui, wu zhu yu |
| **Ba Ji Wan** 巴戟丸<br>Morinda Pill | Tai Ping Sheng Hui Fang | ba ji tian, huai niu xi, du zhong, wu jia pi, qiang huo, rou gui, gan jiang |
| **Ba Li San** 八厘散<br>Eight Thousandths of a Tael Powder | Yi Zong Jin Jian | duan zi ran tong, ru xiang, mo yao, xue jie, hong hua, su mu, ding xiang, mu bie zi, she xiang (now ren gong she xiang) |
| **Ba Zhen Tang** 八珍汤<br>Eight Treasure Decoction | Zheng Ti Lei Yao | ren shen, bai zhu, gan cao, fu ling, dang gui, shu di huang, bai shao, chuan xiong |
| **Ba Zheng San** 八正散<br>Eight Herb Powder for Rectification | He Ji Ju Fang | che qian zi, qu mai, bian xu, hua shi, shan zhi zi, mu tong, zhi gan cao, da huang, deng xin cao |
| **Bai Bu Ding** 百部酊<br>Stemona Tincture | Zhong Yi Pi Fu Bing Xue Jian Bian | bai bu, grain alcohol |
| **Bai Bu Gao** 百部膏<br>Stemona Ointment | Yi Xue Xin Wu | bai bu, bai xian pi, he shi |
| **Bai Bu Tang** 百部汤<br>Stemona Decoction | Ben Cao Hui Yan | bai bu, bei sha shen, mai dong, sang bai pi, di gu pi, bai he, yi yi ren, huang qi, fu ling |
| **Bai Dou Kou Tang** 白豆蔻汤<br>Cardamon Decoction | Shen Shi Zun Sheng Shu | bai dou kou, huo xiang, chen pi, sheng jiang |
| **Bai Dou Kou Wan** 白豆蔻丸<br>Cardamon Pill | Qi Xiao Liang Fang | bai dou kou, chen pi, hou po, ren shen (or dang shen), bai zhu, mu xiang, mu gua |
| **Bai He Di Huang Tang** 百合地黄汤<br>Lily Bulb & Rehmannia Decoction | Jin Gui Yao Lüe | bai he, sheng di huang, mai dong, wu wei zi, gan cao |
| **Bai He Gu Jin Tang** 百合固金汤<br>Lily Bulb Decoction to Preserve metal | Yi Fang Ji Jie | bai he, shu di huang, sheng di huang, xuan shen, chuan bei mu, jie geng, gan cao, mai dong, bai shao, dang gui |
| **Bai He Hua Shi San** 百合滑石汤<br>Lily Bulb & Talcum Powder | Jin Gui Yao Lüe | bai he, hua shi |
| **Bai Hu Jia Cang Zhu Tang** 白虎加苍术汤<br>White Tiger plus Atractylodes Decoction | Lei Zheng Huo Ren Shu | shi gao, cang zhu, zhi mu, gan cao, jing mi |
| **Bai Hu Jia Ren Shen Tang** 白虎加人参汤<br>White Tiger plus Ginseng Decoction | Shang Han Lun | shi gao, ren shen, zhi mu, gan cao, jing mi |
| **Bai Hu Tang** 白虎汤<br>White Tiger Decoction | Shang Han Lun | shi gao, zhi mu, gan cao, jing mi |
| **Bai Hua Gao** 百花膏<br>Stemona & Coltsfoot Syrup | Ji Sheng Fang | bai bu, kuan dong hua |
| **Bai Hua She Jiu** 白花蛇酒<br>White Flower Snake Wine | Yan Fang | bai hua she, qiang huo, qin jiao, wu jia pi, tian ma, fang feng, bai jiu (rice or sorghum wine) |
| **Bai Ji Li San** 白蒺藜散<br>Tribulus Powder | Zhang Shi Yi Tong | ci ji li, ju hua, jue ming zi, qing xiang zi, man jing zi, lian qiao, gan cao |
| **Bai Ji Pi Pa Wan** 白及枇杷丸<br>Bletilla & Loquat Pill | Zheng Zhi Zhun Sheng | bai ji, pi pa ye, ou jie, e jiao, sheng di huang |
| **Bai Ji San** 白及散<br>Bletilla Powder | Pu Ji Ben Shi Fang | bai ji, bai wei, hai piao xiao, huang qin, long gu |
| **Bai Jiang Can San** 白僵蚕散<br>Silkworm Powder | Zheng Zhi Zhun Sheng | bai jiang can, jing jie, sang ye, mu zei, xi xin, gan cao, xuan fu hua |
| **Bai Jie Zi San** 白芥子散<br>Mustard Seed Powder | Zheng Zhi Zhun Sheng | bai jie zi, mu bie zi, mo yao, rou gui, mu xiang |
| **Bai Jin Wan** 白金丸<br>White Gold Pill | Yi Fang Kao | bai fan, yu jin |
| **Bai Lian San** 白蔹散<br>Ampelopsis Powder | Ji Feng Pu Ji Fang | bai lian, bai ji, luo shi teng |

| Formula | Source text | Ingredients |
|---|---|---|
| **Bai Ling Tiao Gan Tang** 百灵调肝汤<br>Bai Lings' Decoction to Regulate the Liver | Bai Ling Fu Ke | wang bu liu xing, zao jiao ci, tong cao, dang gui, chi shao, chuan niu xi, chuan lian zi, quan gua lou, zhi shi, qing pi, gan cao |
| **Bai Qian Tang** 白前汤<br>Cynanchum Decoction | Qian Jin Yao Fang | bai qian, zhi ban xia, zi wan, hong da ji |
| **Bai Ri Ke Ke Li Ji** 百日咳颗粒剂<br>Whooping Cough Granules | Prepared medicine | zhu dan zhi, bai bu, zi wan |
| **Bai Tong Tang** 白通汤<br>White Penetrating Decoction | Shang Han Lun | zhi fu zi, gan jiang, cong bai |
| **Bai Tou Weng Jia Gan Cao E Jiao Tang**<br>白头翁加甘草阿胶汤<br>Pulsatilla plus Licorice & Ass Hide Gelatine Decoction | Jin Gui Yao Lüe | bai tou weng, huang bai, huang lian, qin pi, gan cao, e jiao |
| **Bai Tou Weng Tang** 白头翁汤<br>Pulsatilla Decoction | Shang Han Lun | bai tou weng, huang bai, huang lian, qin pi |
| **Bai Wei Tang** 白薇汤<br>Cynanchum Atratum Decoction | Pu Ji Ben Shi Fang | bai wei, ren shen (or dang shen), dang gui, gan cao |
| **Bai Ye Tang** 柏叶汤<br>Arborvitae Leaf Decoction | Jin Gui Yao Lüe | ce bai ye, gan jiang, ai ye |
| **Bai Zhi San** 白芷散<br>Angelica Dahurica Powder | Jiao Zhu Fu Ren Liang Fang | bai zhi, hai piao xiao, xue yu tan |
| **Bai Zi Yang Xin Tang** 柏子养心汤<br>Arborvitae Seed Dec. to Nourish the Heart | Ti Ren Hui Bian | bai zi ren, gou qi zi, shu di huang, xuan shen, dang gui, mai dong, fu ling, shi chang pu, gan cao |
| **Ban Liu Wan** 半硫丸<br>Pinellia & Sulphur Pill | He Ji Ju Fang | zhi ban xia, liu huang |
| **Ban Mao Ding** 斑蝥酊<br>Blister Beetle Tincture | Jing Yan Fang | ban mao, grain alcohol |
| **Ban Xia Bai Zhu Tian Ma Tang** 半夏白术天麻汤<br>Pinellia, Atractylodes & Gastrodia D. | Yi Xue Xin Wu | zhi ban xia, chao bai zhu, tian ma, fu ling, ju hong (or chen pi), gan cao, sheng jiang, da zao |
| **Ban Xia Hou Po Tang** 半夏厚朴汤<br>Pinellia & Magnolia Decoction | Jin Gui Yao Lüe | zhi ban xia, hou po, fu ling, sheng jiang, zi su ye |
| **Ban Xia Xie Xin Tang** 半夏泻心汤<br>Pinellia Decoction to Purge the Heart | Shang Han Lun | zhi ban xia, huang qin, huang lian, gan jiang, zhi gan cao, ren shen (or dang shen), da zao |
| **Bao He Wan** 保和丸<br>Preserve Harmony Pill | Dan Xi Xin Fa | shan zha, shen qu, lai fu zi, chen pi, zhi ban xia, lian qiao, fu ling |
| **Bao Long Wan**† 抱龙丸<br>Embrace the Dragon Pill | Wei Sheng Bao Jian | dan nan xing, tian zhu huang, she xiang (now ren gong she xiang), xiong huang, zhu sha |
| **Bei Mu Gua Lou San** 贝母栝楼散<br>Fritillaria & Trichosanthes Powder | Yi Xue Xin Wu | zhe bei mu, quan gua lou, tian hua fen, fu ling, jie geng, ju hong (or chen pi) |
| **Bi He Yin** 比和饮<br>Comparative Harmony Drink | Lei Zheng Zhi Cai | zao xin tu, ren shen (or dang shen), fu ling, bai zhu, gan cao, chen pi, sha ren, huo xiang, shen qu, sheng jiang, da zao, rice |
| **Bi Huo Dan** 避火丹<br>Evade Fire Special Pill | Zhong Yao Fang Ji Xue | liu ji nu, di yu, du yu tan, da huang, sesame oil |
| **Bi Min Gan Wan** 鼻敏感丸<br>Allergic Rhinitis Pill | Prepared medicine | e bu shi cao, jin yin hua, cang er zi, ye ju hua, bai zhi, bo he |
| **Bi Xie Fen Qing Tang** 萆薢分清饮<br>Fish Poison Yam Drink to Separate The Clear | Dan Xi Xin Fa | bi xie, yi zhi ren, wu yao, shi chang pu |
| **Bi Xie Shen Shi Tang** 萆薢渗湿汤<br>Fish Poison Yam Decoction to Leach Damp | Yang Ke Xin De Ji | bi xie, yi yi ren, huang bai, chi fu ling, mu dan pi, ze xie, tong cao, hua shi |
| **Bi Yan Ning** 鼻咽宁<br>Calm the Nose & Throat | Prepared medicine | cang er zi, xin yi hua, zhu dan zhi, e bu shi cao, chan tui, huo xiang, bing pian, huang qin, dang gui, huang qi |
| **Bi Yun San** 碧云散<br>Blue Cloud Powder | Yi Zong Jin Jian | chuan xiong, e bu shi cao, xi xin, xin yi hua, qing dai |
| **Bie Jia Wan** 鳖甲丸<br>Turtle Shell Pill | Gu Shi Yi Jing | zhi bie jia, duan wa leng zi, chao mai ya, cu san leng, cu e zhu, di bie chong, xiang fu, qing pi |
| **Bu Dai Wan** 布袋丸<br>Cloth Sack Pill | Bu Yao Xiu Zhen Xiao Er Fang Lun | wu yi, shi jun zi, ye ming sha, fu ling, ren shen (or dang shen), lu hui, gan cao |
| **Bu Fei E Jiao Tang**† 补肺阿胶汤<br>Ass Hide Gelatin Dec. to Supplement Lungs | Xiao Er Yao Zheng Zhi Jue | e jiao, niu bang zi, xing ren, zhi gan cao, rice, ma dou ling |
| **Bu Fei Tang** 补肺汤<br>Supplement Lung Decoction | Yong Lei Qian Fang | ren shen (or dang shen), huang qi, shu di huang, wu wei zi, zi wan, sang bai pi |
| **Bu Gu Zhi Wan** 补骨脂丸<br>Psoralea Pill | Ben Cao Gang Mu | bu gu zhi, tu si zi, hu tao ren, chen xiang |
| **Bu Yang Huan Wu Tang** 补阳还五汤<br>Supplement Yang to Restore Five Tenths Dec. | Yi Lin Gai Cuo | huang qi, dang gui wei, chi shao, di long, chuan xiong, tao ren, hong hua |

| Formula | Source text | Ingredients |
|---|---|---|
| **Bu Zhong Yi Qi Tang** 补中益气汤<br>Supplement the Middle & Augment Qi Dec. | Pi We Lun | huang qi, ren shen (or dang shen), bai zhu, dang gui, chen pi, zhi gan cao, chai hu, sheng ma |
| **Can She Tang** 蚕蛇汤<br>Silkworm Droppings & Snake Decoction | Xin Fang | can sha, bai hua she, tou gu cao, shen jin cao, di bie chong, quan xie, wu gong, gan cao |
| **Can Shi Tang** 蚕矢汤<br>Silkworm Droppings Decoction | Huo Luan Lun | can sha, yi yi ren, dou juan, mu gua, huang lian, zhi ban xia, jiu huang qin, tong cao, chao shan zhi zi, wu zhu yu |
| **Cang Er Zi San** 苍耳子散<br>Xanthium Powder | Ji Sheng Fang | chao cang er zi, xin yi hua, bai zhi, bo he |
| **Cang Fu Dao Tan Tang** 苍附导痰汤<br>Atractylodes & Cyperus D. to Guide Phlegm | Ye Tian Shi Nu Ke Zhen Zhi Mi Fang | cang zhu, xiang fu, zhi ban xia, chen pi, fu ling, gan cao, dan nan xing, zhi ke, sheng jiang, shen qu |
| **Cao Guo Ping Wei San** 草果平胃散<br>Tsaoko Fruit Powder to Calm the Stomach | He Ji Ju Fang | cao guo, cang zhu, hou po, chen pi, gan cao, sheng jiang, da zao |
| **Cao Guo Yin** 草果饮<br>Tsaoko Drink | Zheng Zhi Zhun Sheng | cao guo, gao liang jiang, qing pi, huo xiang, zhi ban xia, hou po, ding xiang, sheng jiang, da zao |
| **Chai Ge Jie Ji Tang** 柴葛解肌汤<br>Bupleurum & Kudzu Dec. to Ease Muscles | Shang Han Liu Shu | chai hu, ge gen, huang qin, jie geng, bai shao, shi gao, qiang huo, bai zhi, gan cao, sheng jiang, da zao |
| **Chai Hu Gui Zhi Gan Jiang Tang** 柴胡桂枝干姜汤<br>Bupleurum, Cinnamon & Ginger Dec. | Shang Han Lun | chai hu, gui zhi, gan jiang, tian hua fen, huang qin, duan mu li, zhi gan cao |
| **Chai Hu Jia Long Gu Mu Li Tang**<br>柴胡加龙骨牡蛎汤<br>Bupleurum plus Dragon Bone & Oyster Shell Dec. | Shang Han Lun | chai hu, huang qin, zhi ban xia, ren shen (or dang shen), sheng jiang, fu ling, gui zhi, da huang, long gu, mu li, sheng tie luo, da zao |
| **Chai Hu Shu Gan San** 柴胡疏肝散<br>Bupleurum Powder to Dredge the Liver | Jing Yue Quan Shu | chai hu, chen pi, chuan xiong, xiang fu, zhi ke, bai shao, zhi gan cao |
| **Chan Ju San** 蝉菊散<br>Cicada & Chrysanthemum Power | Xiao Er Dou Zhen Fang Lun | chan tui, ju hua, mu zei |
| **Chan Su Gao** 蟾酥膏<br>Toad Venom Ointment | Yi Xue Zheng Chuan | chan su, ding xiang, han shui shi, ba dou, feng mi |
| **Chang Pu San** 菖蒲散<br>Acorus Powder | Shi Yong Zhong Yao Xue | shi chang pu, tan xiang, ding xiang, mu xiang, ren shen (or dang shen) |
| **Chang Pu Yu Jin Tang** 菖蒲郁金汤<br>Acorus & Turmeric Decoction | Wen Bing Quan Shu | shi chang pu, yu jin, shan zhi zi, mu dan pi, lian qiao, ju hua, dan zhu ye, niu bang zi, hua shi, zhu li, sheng jiang, Zi Jin Ding (below) |
| **Chang Yong Tang** 肠痈汤<br>Intestinal Abscess Decoction | Xin Fang | bai jiang cao, yi yi ren, dong gua zi, jin yin hua, zi hua di ding, mu dan pi, lian qiao, tao ren, qin pi, yan hu suo |
| **Chen Ding Er Xiang San** 沉丁二香散<br>Aquillaria & Clove Powder | Shi Yong Zhong Yao Xue | chen xiang, ding xiang, bai dou kou, zi su ye, shi di |
| **Chen Xiang Hua Qi Wan** 沉香化气丸<br>Aquillaria Pill to Transform Qi | Shi Yong Zhong Yao Xue | chen xiang, mu xiang, hou po, zhi shi, zhi ban xia, fu ling, huo xiang, yu jin, bai shao |
| **Chen Xiang Jiang Qi San** 沉香降气散<br>Aquillaria Powder to Descend Qi | Zhang Shi Yi Tong | chen xiang, xiang fu, sha ren, gan cao, chuan lian zi, yan hu suo |
| **Chi Shi Zhi Yu Yu Liang Tang** 赤石脂禹余粮汤<br>Hallyosite & Limonite Decoction | Shang Han Lun | chi shi zhi, yu yu liang |
| **Chi Xiao Dou Tang** 赤小豆汤<br>Adzuki Bean Decoction | Sheng Ji Zong Lu | chi xiao dou, sang bai pi, zi su ye |
| **Chou Ling Dan†** 臭灵丹<br>Miraculous (but Smelly) Special Pill | Yi Zong Jin Jian | liu huang, ban mao, bing pian, qing fen |
| **Chuan Xin Lian Kang Yan Pian** 穿心莲抗炎片<br>Andrographis Anti-Inflammatory Pill | Prepared medicine | chuan xin lian, pu gong ying, ban lan gen |
| **Chuan Xiong Cha Tiao San** 川芎茶调散<br>Chuanxiong Powder to be Taken with Tea | He Ji Ju Fang | chuan xiong, bai zhi, qiang huo, xi xin, jing jie, bo he, gan cao, fang feng |
| **Ci Shi Liu Wei Wan** 磁石六味丸<br>Magnetite & Six Ingredient Pill | Za Bing Yuan Liu Xi Zhu | ci shi, shu di huang, shan zhu yu, shan yao, mu dan pi, fu ling, ze xie |
| **Ci Zhu Wan†** 磁朱丸<br>Magnetite & Cinnabar Pill | Qian Jin Yao Fang | ci shi, shen qu, zhu sha |
| **Cong Chi Tang** 葱豉汤<br>Shallot & Prepared Soybean Decoction | Zhou Hou Bei Ji Fang | cong bai, dan dou chi |
| **Cuo Feng San†** 撮风散<br>Scoop Up Wind Powder | Zheng Zhi Zhun Sheng | wu gong, quan xie, gou teng, bai jiang can, zhu sha, she xiang |
| **Da Bu Yin Wan** 大补阴丸<br>Great Yin Supplementing Pill | Dan Xi Xin Fa | chao huang bai, jiu zhi mu, shu di huang, gui ban |
| **Da Chai Hu Tang** 大柴胡汤<br>Major Bupleurum Decoction | Shang Han Lun | chai hu, huang qin, zhi ban xia, bai shao, zhi shi, da huang, sheng jiang, da zao |
| **Da Cheng Qi Tang** 大承气汤<br>Major Order the Qi Decoction | Shang Han Lun | da huang, hou po, zhi shi, mang xiao |
| **Da Ding Feng Zhu** 大定风珠<br>Major Arrest Wind Pearls | Wen Bing Tiao Bian | sheng di huang, bai shao, mai dong, mu li, bie jia, gui ban, zhi gan cao, e jiao, huo ma ren, wu wei zi, ji zi huang (egg yolk) |

| Formula | Source text | Ingredients |
|---|---|---|
| **Da Fu Pi San** 大腹皮散<br>Areca Peel Powder | Zheng Zhi Zhun Sheng | da fu pi, bing lang, mu gua, wu yao, sang bai pi, zi su ye, lai fu zi, chen pi, zhi ke, sheng jiang, jing jie, chen xiang |
| **Da Huang Mu Dan Tang** 大黄牡丹汤<br>Rhubarb & Moutan Decoction | Jin Gui Yao Lüe | da huang, mu dan pi, tao ren, dong gua zi, mang xiao |
| **Da Huang Zhe Chong Wan** 大黄䗪虫丸<br>Rhubarb & Field Cockroach Pill | Jin Gui Yao Lüe | da huang, di bie chong, sheng di huang, tao ren, chi shao, xing ren, gan cao, huang qin, meng chong, shui zhi, qi cao, gan qi |
| **Da Jian Zhong Tang** 大建中汤<br>Major Construct the Middle Decoction | Jin Gui Yao Lüe | hua jiao, gan jiang, ren shen (or dang shen), yi tang |
| **Da Qi Xiang Wan** 大七香丸<br>Major Seven Fragrance Pill | He Ji Ju Fang | gan song, ding xiang, xiang fu, rou gui, chao mai ya, chen pi, gan cao, sha ren, huo xiang, wu yao, feng mi |
| **Da Qin Jiao Tang** 大秦艽汤<br>Major Large Gentian Decoction | Yi Xue Fa Ming | qin jiao, shi gao, gan cao, chuan xiong, dang gui, qiang huo, du huo, fang feng, huang qin, bai shao, bai zhi, bai zhu, sheng di huang, shu di huang, fu ling, xi xin |
| **Da Qing Long Tang** 大青龙汤<br>Major Blue Dragon Decoction | Shang Han Lun | ma huang, gui zhi, shi gao, xing ren, gan cao, sheng jiang, da zao |
| **Da Xian Xiong Wan** 大陷胸丸<br>Major Pill for Pathogens Stuck in the Chest | Shang Han Lun | da huang, mang xiao, chao ting li zi, chao xing ren, gan sui, feng mi |
| **Da Yi Han Wan** 大已寒丸<br>Major Stop Cold Pill | He Ji Ju Fang | bi ba, gao liang jiang, pao jiang, rou gui |
| **Da Yuan Yin** 达原饮<br>Reach the Source Drink | Wen Yi Lun | bing lang, hou po, cao guo, zhi mu, bai shao, huang qin, gan cao |
| **Dai Ge San** 黛蛤散<br>Indigo & Clam Shell Powder | Yi Zong Jin Jian | qing dai, hai ge qiao, chao pu huang |
| **Dan Bai Zhi Ke Pian** 胆百止咳片<br>Pig Bile & Stemona Antitussive Pill | Prepared medicine | zhu dan zhi, bai bu, chen pi |
| **Dan Dao Pai Shi Tang** 胆道排石汤<br>Discharge Stones from the Bile Duct Dec. | Zhong Xi Yi Jie He Zhi Liao Ji Fu Zheng | yu jin, jin qian cao, yin chen hao, zhi ke, mu xiang, da huang |
| **Dan Shen Yin** 丹参饮<br>Salvia Drink | Shi Fang Ge Kuo | dan shen, tan xiang, sha ren |
| **Dan Zhi Xiao Yao San** 丹栀逍遥散<br>Rambling Powder plus Moutan & Gardenia | Nei Ke Zhai Yao | mu dan pi, shan zhi zi, chai hu, dang gui, chao bai shao, chao bai zhu, fu ling, zhi gan cao, bo he, pao jiang |
| **Dang Gui Bu Xue Tang** 当归补血汤<br>Angelica Decoction to Supplement Blood | Nei Wai Shang Bian Huo Lun | zhi huang qi, jiu dang gui |
| **Dang Gui Hong Hua Yin** 当归红花饮<br>Angelica & Safflower Drink | Ma Ke Huo Ren Qian Shu | dang gui, hong hua, niu bang zi, lian qiao, ge gen, gan cao |
| **Dang Gui Liu Huang Tang** 当归六黄汤<br>Angelica & Six Yellow Herb Decoction | Lan Shi Mi Cang | dang gui, sheng di huang, shu di huang, huang qi, huang lian, huang qin, huang bai |
| **Dang Gui Long Hui Wan†** 当归龙会丸<br>Angelica & Aloe Pill | Xuan Ming Fang Lun | jiu dang gui, jiu long dan cao, chao shan zhi zi, huang qin, huang lian, huang bai, jiu da huang, lu hui, qing dai, mu xiang, she xiang |
| **Dang Gui Nian Tong Tang**<br>当归拈痛汤<br>Angelica Decoction to Pry Out Pain | Lan Shi Mi Cang | dang gui, qiang huo, cang zhu, fang feng, ku shen, huang qin, yin chen hao, sheng ma, ge gen, zhi mu, ze xie, zhu ling, bai zhu, ren shen, zhi gan cao |
| **Dang Gui San** 当归散<br>Angelica Powder | Jin Gui Yao Lüe | dang gui, bai shao, chuan xiong, huang qin, bai zhu |
| **Dang Gui Sheng Jiang Yang Rou Tang**<br>当归生姜羊肉汤<br>Angelica, Ginger & Mutton Stew | Jin Gui Yao Lüe | dang gui, sheng jiang, sheep or goat meat |
| **Dang Gui Shao Yao San** 当归芍药散<br>Angelica & Peony Powder | Jin Gui Yao Lüe | dang gui, bai shao, chuan xiong, bai zhu, ze xie, fu ling |
| **Dang Gui Si Ni Tang** 当归四逆汤<br>Angelica Decoction for Frigid Extremities | Shang Han Lun | dang gui, gui zhi, bai shao, xi xin, zhi gan cao, tong cao, da zao |
| **Dang Gui Yin Zi** 当归饮子<br>Angelica Drink | Ji Sheng Fang | dang gui, bai shao, sheng di huang, chuan xiong, ci ji li, fang feng, jing jie sui, zhi he shou wu, huang qi, zhi gan cao |
| **Dao Chi San** 导赤散<br>Guide Out the Red Powder | Xiao Er Yao Zheng Zhi Jue | sheng di huang, mu tong, zhu ye, gan cao shao |
| **Dao Qi Tang** 导气汤<br>Guide Qi Decoction | Shen Shi Zun Sheng Shu | wu zhu yu, chuan lian zi, mu xiang, xiao hui xiang |
| **Dao Tan Tang** 导痰汤<br>Guide Out Phlegm Decoction | Ji Sheng Fang | zhi shi, dan nan xing, zhi ban xia, chen pi, fu ling, zhi gan cao |
| **Di Dang Tang** 抵当汤<br>Appropriate Decoction | Shang Han Lun | shui zhi, meng chong, tao ren, jiu da huang |
| **Di Fu Zi Tang** 地肤子汤<br>Kochia Fruit Decoction | Ji Sheng Fang | di fu zi, dong kui zi, qu mai, mu tong, zhu ling, gan cao |

| Formula | Source text | Ingredients |
|---|---|---|
| **Di Gu Pi San** 地骨皮散<br>Lycium Bark Powder | Xiao Er Yao Zheng Zhi Jue | di gu pi, yin chai hu, zhi mu, zhi ban xia, ren shen (or dang shen), gan cao, chi fu ling, sheng jiang |
| **Di Long Jie Jing Tang** 地龙解痉汤<br>Earthworm Decoction to Ease Spasm | Xin Fang | di long, lian qiao, gou teng, jin yin hua, shi gao, quan xie |
| **Di Tan Tang** 涤痰汤<br>Scour Out Phlegm Decoction | Ji Sheng Fang | zhi ban xia, zhu ru, fu ling, dan nan xing, chen pi, zhi shi, shi chang pu, ren shen (or dang shen), gan cao, sheng jiang, da zao |
| **Di Yu Gan Cao Tang** 地榆甘草汤<br>Sanguisorba & Licorice Decoction | Za Bing Yuan Liu Xi Zhu | di yu, gan cao, sha ren |
| **Di Yu Wan** 地榆丸<br>Sanguisorba Pill | Zheng Zhi Zhun Sheng | chao di yu, huang lian, mu xiang, wu mei, wei he zi, chao dang gui, e jiao |
| **Ding Chuan Tang** 定喘汤<br>Alleviate Wheezing Decoction | She Sheng Zhong Miao Fang | bai guo, zhi ma huang, zhi ban xia, su zi, kuan dong hua, sang bai pi, xing ren, huang qin, gan cao |
| **Ding Kou Li Zhong Wan** 丁蔻理中丸<br>Regulate the Middle Pill with Clove & Cardamon | Zhong Guo Zhong Yao Cheng Yao Chu Fang Ji | ding xiang, bai dou kou, ren shen (or dang shen), bai zhu, gan jiang, zhi gan cao |
| **Ding Ming San** 定命散<br>Settle Life Powder | Sheng Ji Zong Lu | bai hua she, wu gong |
| **Ding Xian Wan†** 定痫散<br>Arrest Seizures Pill | Yi Xue Xin Wu | tian ma, chuan bei mu, zhi ban xia, fu ling, fu shen, dan nan xing, shi chang pu, yuan zhi, quan xie, bai jiang can, hu po, deng xin cao, chen pi, dan shen, mai dong, gan cao, zhu li, zhu sha |
| **Ding Xiang Shi Di Tang** 丁香柿蒂汤<br>Clove & Persimmon Calyx Decoction | Zheng Yin Mai Zhi | ding xiang, shi di, ren shen (or dang shen), sheng jiang |
| **Dong Chong Ji Jing** 冬虫鸡精<br>Essence of Chicken with Cordyceps | Prepared medicine | dong chong xia cao, shu di huang, yu zhu, rou cong rong, huang qi, black boned chicken |
| **Du Huo Ji Sheng Tang** 独活寄生汤<br>Pubescent Angelica & Mistletoe Decoction | Qian Jin Yao Fang | du huo, sang ji sheng, qin jiao, fang feng, dang gui, bai shao (or chi shao), du zhong, huai niu xi, fu ling, ren shen (or dang shen), xi xin, rou gui, chuan xiong, sheng di huang (or shu di huang), zhi gan cao |
| **Du Huo Xi Xin Tang** 独活细辛汤<br>Pubescent Angelica & Asarum Decoction | Zheng Yin Mai Zhi | du huo, xi xin, chuan xiong, qiang huo, qin jiao, sheng di huang, fang feng, gan cao |
| **Du Qi Wan** 都气丸<br>Capital Qi Pill | Zheng Yin Mai Zhi | wu wei zi, shu di huang, shan zhu yu, shan yao, mu dan pi, fu ling, ze xie |
| **Du Sheng San** 独圣散<br>Solitary Sage Powder | Yi Zong Jin Jian | shan zha tan, yi tang |
| **Du Zhong Wan** 杜仲丸<br>Eucommia Pill | Sheng Ji Zong Lu | du zhong, xu duan |
| **E Jiao Ji Zi Huang Tang** 阿胶鸡子黄汤<br>Ass Hide Gelatin & Egg Yolk Decoction | Tong Su Shang Han Lun | e jiao, bai shao, shi jue ming, sheng di huang, gou teng, mu li, luo shi teng, fu shen, zhi gan cao, ji zi huang (egg yolk) |
| **E Wei Hua Pi Gao†** 阿魏化痞膏<br>Asafoetida Ointment to Transform Masses | Bei Jing Bu Zhong Yao Cheng Fang Xuan Ji | e wei, san leng, e zhu, da huang, dang gui, xiang fu, chuan wu, cao wu, da suan, bai zhi, shi jun zi, hou po, mu bie zi, hu huang lian, ru xiang, mo yao, xue jie, zhang nao, rou gui, chuan shan jia |
| **E Wei Wan** 阿魏丸<br>Asafoetida Pill | Zheng Zhi Zhun Sheng | e wei, shan zha, huang lian, lian qiao |
| **Er Chen Tang** 二陈汤<br>Two Aged [Herb] Decoction | He Ji Ju Fang | zhi ban xia, chen pi, fu ling, zhi gan cao |
| **Er Dong Tang** 二冬汤<br>Two 'Dong' Decoction | Yi Xue Xin Wu | tian dong, mai dong, tian hua fen, zhi mu, huang qin |
| **Er Jing Wan** 二精丸<br>Two 'Jing' Pill | Yi Bu Jin Lu | huang jing, gou qi zi |
| **Er Long Zuo Ci Wan** 耳聋左慈丸<br>Pill for Deafness that is Kind to the Left | Wen Yi Lun | shu di huang, shan zhu yu, shan yao, mu dan pi, fu ling, ze xie, shi chang pu, wu wei zi, duan ci shi |
| **Er Miao San** 二妙散<br>Two Marvel Powder | Dan Xi Xin Fa | chao huang bai, chao cang zhu |
| **Er Mu Ning Sou San** 二母宁嗽丸<br>Two 'Mu' Pills to Stop Cough | Gu Jin Yi Jian | chuan bei mu, zhi mu, shi gao, huang qin, shan zhi zi, sang bai pi, gua lou ren, fu ling, zhi shi, chen pi, wu wei zi, gan cao |
| **Er Mu San** 二母散<br>Two 'Mu' Powder | Yi Fang Ji Jie | chuan bei mu, zhu mu |
| **Er Qian Tang** 二前汤<br>Two 'Qian' Decoction | Jing Yan Fang | qian hu, bai qian, sang ye, xing ren, jie geng, bo he, niu bang zi, gan cao |
| **Er Xian Tang** 二仙汤<br>Two Immortals Decoction | Shang Hai Shu Guang Yi Yuan Jing Yan Fang | xian mao, xian ling pi, dang gui, ba ji tian, huang bai, zhi mu |
| **Er Yan San** 耳炎散<br>Otitis Powder | Zhong Yao Zhi Shi Shou Ce | bai fan, zhu dan zhi, huang lian, zhang nao |

| Formula | Source text | Ingredients |
|---|---|---|
| **Er Zhi Wan** 二至丸<br>Two Solstice Pill | Yi Fang Ji Jie | mo han lian, nu zhen zi |
| **Fang Feng Tang** 防风汤<br>Saposhnikovia Decoction | Xuan Ming Fang Lun | fang feng, dang fui, xing ren, fu ling, qin jiao, ge gen, gui zhi, ma huang, qiang huo, huang qin, gan cao, sheng jiang, da zao |
| **Fang Feng Tong Sheng San** 防风通圣散<br>Saposhnikovia Powder that Sagely Unblocks | Xuan Ming Fang Lun | fang feng, jing jie, lian qiao, ma huang, bo he, dang gui, chuan xiong, chao bai shao, bai zhu, chao shan zhi zi, jiu da huang, mang xiao, shi gao, huang qin, jie geng, hua shi, gan cao |
| **Fang Ji Fu Ling Tang** 防己茯苓汤<br>Stephania & Poria Decoction | Jin Gui Yao Lüe | han fang ji, fu ling, huang qi, gui zhi, gan cao |
| **Fang Ji Huang Qi Tang** 防己黄芪汤<br>Stephania & Astragalus Decoction | Jin Gui Yao Lüe | han fang ji, huang qi, bai zhu, zhi gan cao, sheng jiang, da zao |
| **Fei Er Wan** 肥儿丸<br>Fat Baby Pill | Yi Zong Jin Jian | ren shen (or dang shen), chao bai zhu, fu ling, huang lian, hu huang lian, shi jun zi, chao shen qu, mai ya, shan zha, zhi gan cao, lu hui |
| **Fei Zi Guan Zhong Tang** 榧子贯众汤<br>Torreya Seed & Shield Fern Root Decoction | Fang Ji Xue | fei zi, bing lang, hong teng, guan zhong |
| **Feng Fang Gao†** 蜂房膏<br>Wasp Nest Ointment | Tai Ping Sheng Hui Fang | feng fang, she tui, huang qi, xuan shen, qian dan |
| **Feng Tan Yin** 风痰饮<br>Wind Phlegm Drink | Jing Yan Fang | li lu, yu jin |
| **Feng Yin Tang** 风引汤<br>Wind Drawing Decoction | Jin Gui Yao Lüe | zi shi ying, da huang, gan jiang, long gu, mu li, gui zhi, gan cao, han shui shi, hua shi, shi gao, chi shi zhi |
| **Fu Fang Ai Di Cha Pian** 复方矮地茶片<br>Compound Ardisia Pill | Prepared medicine | ai di cha, gang mei gen (岗梅根 Ilex asprella Radix), ye ju hua, pi pa ye, gan cao |
| **Fu Fang Man Shan Hong Jiao Nang**<br>复方满山红胶囊<br>Compound Rhododendron Capsule | Prepared medicine | man shan hong, jie geng, ci wu jia (刺五加 siberian ginseng) |
| **Fu Fang Nan Ban Lan Gen Pian** 复方南板蓝根片<br>Compound Isatis Root Pill | Prepared medicine | ban lan gen, zi hua di ding, pu gong ying |
| **Fu Fang Yu Xing Cao Pian** 复方鱼腥草片<br>Compound Houttuynia Pill | Prepared medicine | yu xing cao, huang qin, ban lan gen, lian qiao, jin yin hua |
| **Fu Fang Zhang Nao Ding** 复方樟脑酊<br>Compound Camphor Tincture | Prepared medicine | zhang nao, ba jiao hui xiang you (star anise oil) |
| **Fu Tu Dan** 茯菟丹<br>Poria & Cuscuta Special Pill | He Ji Ju Fang | fu ling, tu si zi, lian zi, wu wei zi, shan yao |
| **Fu Yuan Huo Xue Tang†** 复元活血汤<br>Revive Health by Activating Blood Decoction | Yi Xue Fa Ming | chai hu, dang gui, tian hua fen, tao ren, hong hua, jiu da huang, gan cao, chuan shan jia (now wang bu liu xing) |
| **Fu Zi Li Zhong Wan** 附子理中丸<br>Prepared Aconite Pill to Regulate the Middle | He Ji Ju Fang | zhi fu zi, ren shen (or dang shen), bai zhu, gan jiang, zhi gan cao |
| **Fu Zi Tang** 附子汤<br>Prepared Aconite Decoction | Shang Han Lun | zhi fu zi, fu ling, ren shen (or dang shen), bai zhu, bai shao |
| **Gan Lu Xiao Du Dan** 甘露消毒丹<br>Sweet Dew Special Pill to Eliminate Toxins | Wen Re Jing Wei | hua shi, yin chen hao, shi chang pu, mu tong, huang qin, chuan bei mu, huo xiang, bo he, bai dou kou, lian qiao, she gan |
| **Gan Mai Da Zao Tang** 甘麦大枣汤<br>Licorice, Wheat & Jujube Decoction | Jin Gui Yao Lüe | gan cao, xiao mai, da zao |
| **Gan Sui Tong Jie Tang** 甘遂通解汤<br>Euphorbia Root Dec. to Unblock & Disperse | Zhong Xi Yi Jie He Zhi Liao Ji Fu Zheng | gan sui, da huang, hou po, mu xiang, tao ren, chi shao, huai niu xi |
| **Gao Lin Tang** 膏淋汤<br>Turbid Dysuria Decoction | Yi Xue Zhong Zhong Can Xi Lu | shan yao, qian shi, long gu, mu li, sheng di huang, ren shen (or dang shen), bai shao |
| **Ge Gen Qin Lian Tang** 葛根芩连汤<br>Kudzu, Scutellaria & Coptis Decoction | Shang Han Lun | ge gen, huang qin, huang lian, gan cao |
| **Ge Gen Tang** 葛根汤<br>Kudzu Decoction | Shang Han Lun | ge gen, ma huang, gui zhi, bai shao, gan cao, sheng jiang, da zao |
| **Ge Xia Zhu Yu Tang** 膈下逐瘀汤<br>Disperse Stasis from Below the Diaphragm D. | Yi Lin Gai Cuo | dang gui, chuan xiong, tao ren, hong hua, mu dan pi, chi shao, yan hu suo, chao wu ling zhi, wu yao, xiang fu, zhi ke, gan cao |
| **Gou Ji Yin** 狗脊饮<br>Cibotium Drink | Jing Yan Fang | gou ji, du zhong, xu duan, chuan niu xi, gui zhi, qin jiao, hai feng teng, mu gua, sang zhi, song jie, dang gui wei, shu di huang |
| **Gou Teng Di Long Tang** 钩藤地龙汤<br>Uncaria & Earthworm Decoction | Xin Fang | gou teng, sang ye, xia ku cao, di long, ju hua, huang qin, bo he |
| **Gou Teng Yin Zi†** 钩藤饮子<br>Uncaria Drink | Xiao Er Yao Zheng Zhi Jue | gou teng, tian ma, chan tui, fang feng, ren shen (or dang shen), ma huang, bai jiang can, quan xie, zhi gan cao, chuan xiong, she xiang |

| Formula | Source text | Ingredients |
|---|---|---|
| **Gu Ben Suo Jing Wan** 固本锁精丸 <br> Pill to Secure the Base & Lock up Jing | Zheng Zhi Zhun Sheng | suo yang, shan zhu yu, huang qi, huang bai |
| **Gu Chang Wan†** 固肠丸 <br> Secure the Intestines Pill | Zheng Zhi Zhun Sheng | wu mei, ren shen (or dang shen), cang zhu, fu ling, mu xiang, wei he zi, rou dou kou, ying su ke |
| **Gu Chong Tang** 固冲汤 <br> Secure the Chong Mai Decoction | Yi Xue Zhong Zhong Can Xi Lu | shan zhu yu, sang piao xiao, bai zhu, huang qi, duan long gu, duan mu li, bai shao, qian cao gen, zong lu tang, wu bei zi |
| **Gu Jing Cao Tang** 谷精草汤 <br> Pipewort Flower Decoction | Shen Shi Yao Han | gu jing cao, bai shao, jing jie sui, xuan shen, niu bang zi, lian qiao, jue ming zi, ju hua, long dan cao, jie geng, deng xin cao |
| **Gu Jing Wan** 固经丸 <br> Secure Menses Pill | Yi Xue Ru Men | zhi gui ban, chao huang qin, chao bai shao, chao pu huang, chun pi, xiang fu |
| **Gu Sui Bu San†** 骨碎补散 <br> Drynaria Powder | Tai Ping Sheng Hui Fang | gu sui bu, zi ran tong, gui ban, mo yao, hu tao ren, hu gu (now gou gu) |
| **Gu Zhi Zeng Sheng Wan** 骨质增生丸 <br> Bony Proliferation Pills | Ji Lin Di Si Lin Chuang Xue Yuan Gu Ke Jing Yan Fang | shu di huang, rou cong rong, lu xian cao, xian ling pi, gu sui bu, ji xue teng, lai fu zi |
| **Gua Di San** 瓜蒂散 <br> Melon Pedicle Powder | Shang Han Lun | gua di, chi xiao dou |
| **Gua Ding San** 瓜丁散 <br> Melon Pedicle Powder | Qian Jin Yi Fang | gua di |
| **Gua Lou Niu Bang Tang** 栝楼牛蒡汤 <br> Trichosanthes Seed & Burdock Seed Dec. | Yi Zong Jin Jian | gua lou ren, niu bang zi, tian hua fen, huang qin, shan zhi zi, jin yin hua, lian qiao, zao jiao ci, qing pi, chen pi, chai hu, gan cao |
| **Gua Lou Xie Bai Bai Jiu Tang** 栝楼薤白白酒汤 <br> Trichosanthes, Chive & Wine Dec. | Jin Gui Yao Lüe | quan gua lou, xie bai, bai jiu (rice or sorghum wine) |
| **Gua Lou Xie Bai Ban Xia Tang** 栝楼薤白半夏汤 <br> Trichosanthes, Chive & Pinellia D. | Jin Gui Yao Lüe | quan gua lou, xie bai, zhi ban xia, bai jiu (rice or sorghum wine) |
| **Guan Xin Su He Xiang Wan†** 冠心苏合香丸 <br> Liquid Styrax Pill for Coronary Arteries | Zhong Guo Yao Dian | su he xiang, bing pian, ru xiang, tan xiang, qing mu xiang, zhu sha |
| **Gui Lu Er Xian Jiao** 龟鹿二仙胶 <br> Turtle Shell & Deer Antler Syrup | Yi Fang Kao | gui ban, lu jiao, ren shen, gou qi zi |
| **Gui Pi Tang** 归脾汤 <br> Restore the Spleen Decoction | Ji Sheng Fang | ren shen (or dang shen), zhi huang qi, chao bai zhu, fu ling, dang gui, chao suan zao ren, long yan rou, yuan zhi, mu xiang, zhi gan cao, sheng jiang, da zao |
| **Gui Zhi Fu Ling Wan** 桂枝茯苓丸 <br> Cinnamon Twig & Poria Pill | Jin Gui Yao Lüe | gui zhi, fu ling, mu dan pi, tao ren, chi shao |
| **Gui Zhi Fu Zi Tang** 桂枝附子汤 <br> Cinnamon Twig & Aconite Decoction | Shang Han Lun | gui zhi, zhi fu zi, zhi gan cao, sheng jiang, da zao |
| **Gui Zhi Jia Fu Zi Tang** 桂枝加附子汤 <br> Cinnamon Twig plus Aconite Decoction | Shang Han Lun | gui zhi, bai shao, zhi gan cao, sheng jiang, da zao, zhi fu zi |
| **Gui Zhi Jia Long Gu Mu Li Tang** <br> 桂枝加龙骨牡蛎汤 <br> Cinnamon Twig Decoction plus Dragon Bone & Oyster Shell | Jin Gui Yao Lüe | gui zhi, bai shao, zhi gan cao, sheng jiang, da zao, long gu, mu li |
| **Gui Zhi Shao Yao Zhi Mu Tang** 桂枝芍药知母汤 <br> Cinnamon Twig, Peony & Anemarrhena Decoction | Jin Gui Yao Lüe | gui zhi, bai shao (or chi shao), zhi mu, fang feng, zhi fu zi, bai zhu, ma huang, zhi gan cao, sheng jiang |
| **Gui Zhi Tang** 桂枝汤 <br> Cinnamon Decoction | Shang Han Lun | gui zhi, bai shao, zhi gan cao, sheng jiang, da zao |
| **Hai Tong Pi Jiu** 海桐皮酒 <br> Erythrina Wine | Chuan Xin Shi Yong Fang | hai tong pi, wu jia pi, di gu pi, chuan niu xi, sheng di huang, chao yi ren, du huo, chuan xiong, gan cao, grain alcohol |
| **Hai Tong Pi Tang** 海桐皮汤 <br> Erythrina Decoction | Yi Zong Jin Jian | hai tong pi, tou gu cao, ru xiang, mo yao, dang gui, hua jiao, chuan xiong, hong hua, wei ling xian, fang feng, bai zhi, gan cao |
| **Hai Zao Yu Hu Tang** 海藻玉壶汤 <br> Sargassum Decoction for the Jade Flask | Wai Ke Zheng Zong | hai zao, kun bu, hai dai, zhe bei mu, zhi ban xia, qing pi, chen pi, chuan xiong, dang gui, du huo, lian qiao, gan cao |
| **Han Hua Wan** 含化丸 <br> Pill that Contains Transformative [Power] | Zheng Zhi Zhun Sheng | wa leng zi, hai ge qiao, hai zao, kun bu, he zi, chao wu ling zhi, wu bei zi |
| **Han Jiang Tang** 寒降汤 <br> Cold Descending Decoction | Yi Xue Zhong Zhong Can Xi Lu | dai zhe shi, bai shao, zhi ban xia, zhu ru, gua lou ren, niu bang zi, gan cao |
| **Hao Qin Qing Dan Tang** 蒿芩清胆汤 <br> Artemesia & Scutellaria D. to Clear Gallbladder | Chong Ding Tong Su Shang Han Lun | qing hao, huang qin, zhu ru, zhi ban xia, chi fu ling, chen pi, zhi ke, hua shi, qing dai, gan cao |
| **He Che Da Zao Wan** 河车大造丸 <br> Great Creation Pill with Placenta | Jin Yue Quan Shu | zi he che, shu di huang, tian dong, mai dong, yan du zhong, yan huai niu xi, yan huang bai, zhi gui ban |
| **He Ren Yin** 何人饮 <br> Fleeceflower Root & Ginseng Drink | Jin Yue Quan Shu | he shou wu, ren shen (or dang shen), dang gui, chen pi, pao jiang |

| Formula | Source text | Ingredients |
|---|---|---|
| **He Shou Wu Tang** 何首乌汤<br>Fleeceflower Root Decoction | Yang Yi Da Quan | he shou wu, fang feng, jin yin hua, jing jie, cang zhu, bai xian pi, ku shen, lian qiao, mu tong, deng xin cao, gan cao |
| **He Zi Pi San**† 诃子皮散<br>Terminalia & Citrus Peel Powder | Lan Shi Mi Cang | wei he zi, chen pi, gan jiang, ying su ke |
| **He Zi Qing Yin Tang** 诃子清音汤<br>Terminalia Decoction to Clear the Voice | Zhong Yao Xue | he zi, jie geng, gan cao |
| **He Zi San** 诃子散<br>Terminalia Powder | Su Wen Bing Ji Qi Yi Bao Ming Ji | he zi, wei he zi, huang lian, mu xiang, gan cao, bai zhi, bai shao |
| **Hei Shen San** 黑神散<br>Black Magic Powder | He Ji Ju Fang | pu huang, chao pu huang, shu di huang, sheng di huang, dang gui, rou gui, pao jiang, zhi gan cao, bai shao |
| **Hei Sheng San** 黑圣丹<br>Black Sage Special Pill | Ren Zhai Zhi Zhi | zong lu tang, ai ye tan, di yu, huai hua mi, fu ling, dang gui, bai cao shuang (百草霜 activated charcoal from plants) |
| **Hong Teng Jian** 红藤煎<br>Sargentodoxa Decoction | Zhong Yi Fang Yao Shou Ce | hong teng, zi hua di ding, lian qiao, jin yin hua, da huang, mo yao, ru xiang, mu dan pi, yan hu suo, gan cao |
| **Hou Po Cao Guo Tang** 厚朴草果汤<br>Magnolia Bark & Tsaoko Decoction | Wen Bing Tiao Bian | hou po, xiang ren, cao guo, zhi ban xia, fu ling, chen pi |
| **Hou Po Wen Zhong Tang** 厚朴温中汤<br>Magnolia Bark Dec. to Warm the Middle | Nei Wai Shang Bian Huo Lun | hou po, chen pi, gan jiang, zhi gan cao, fu ling, mu xiang, cao dou kou |
| **Hu Lu Ba Wan** 葫芦巴丸<br>Fenugreek Pill | He Ji Ju Fang | hu lu ba, xiao hui xiang, ba ji tian, chuan lian zi, wu zhu yu, zhi chuan wu |
| **Hu Po Bao Long Wan**† 琥珀抱龙丸<br>Amber Pill to Embrace the Dragon | Yu Ying Jia Mi Fang | hu po, tian zhu huang, dan nan xing, tan xiang, fu ling, ren shen (or dang shen), zhi shi, zhi ke, shan yao, gan cao, zhu sha |
| **Hu Po Ding Zhi Wan**† 琥珀定志丸<br>Amber Pill to Settle the Zhi | Shen Shi Zun Sheng Shu | hu po, shi chang pu, yuan zhi, ren shen, fu ling, fu shen, zhi tian nan xing, zhu sha |
| **Hu Po San** 琥珀散<br>Amber Powder | Zheng Zhi Zhun Sheng | hu po, hai jin sha, mo yao, chao pu huang |
| **Hu Qian Wan**† 虎潜丸<br>Hidden Tiger Pill | Dan Xi Xin Fa | huang bai, gui ban, zhi mu, shu di huang, chen pi, bai shao, suo yang, gan jiang, hu gu (now gou gu) |
| **Hua Ban Tang**† 化斑汤<br>Transform Macules Decoction | Wen Bing Tiao Bian | shi gao, zhi mu, gan cao, xuan shen, rice, xi jiao (now shui niu jiao) |
| **Hua Chong Wan**† 化虫丸<br>Dissolve Parasites Pill | He Ji Ju Fang | he shi, bing lang, ku lian pi, bai fan, qian dan |
| **Hua Rui Shi Bai Ji San** 花蕊石白及散<br>Ophicalcite & Bletilla Powder | Jing Yan Fang | duan hua rui shi, bai ji, xue yu tan |
| **Hua Rui Shi San** 花蕊石散<br>Ophicalcite Powder | He Ji Ju Fang | duan hua rui shi, liu huang |
| **Hua Xue Dan** 化血丹<br>Transform Bleeding Special Pill | Yi Xue Zhong Zhong Can Xi Lu | duan hua rui shi, san qi, xue yu tan |
| **Huai Hua San** 槐花散<br>Sophora Japonica Flower Powder | Pu Ji Ben Shi Fang | chao huai hua mi, ce bai ye tan, jing jie tan, chao zhi ke |
| **Huai Jiao Wan** 槐角丸<br>Sophora Japonica Fruit Pill | He Ji Ju Fang | chao huai jiao, di yu, chao zhi ke, jiu dang gui, fang feng, huang qin |
| **Huang Lian E Jiao Tang** 黄连阿胶汤<br>Coptis & Ass Hide Gelatin Decoction | Shang Han Lun | huang lian, e jiao, huang qin, bai shao, ji zi huang (egg yolk) |
| **Huang Lian Jie Du Tang** 黄连解毒汤<br>Coptis Decoction to Resolve Toxin | Wai Tai Mi Yao | huang lian, huang qin, huang bai, shan zhi zi |
| **Huang Lian Tang** 黄连汤<br>Coptis Decoction | Qian Jin Yao Fang | huang lian, huang bai, shi liu pi, dang gui, e jiao, gan jiang, gan cao |
| **Huang Lian Zhu Ru Ju Pi Ban Xia Tang**<br>黄连竹茹橘皮半夏汤<br>Coptis, Bamboo Shavings, Tangerine Peel & Pinellia Dec. | Wen Re Jing Wei | huang lian, zhu ru, chen pi, zhi ban xia |
| **Huang Qi Gui Zhi Wu Wu Tang** 黄芪桂枝五物汤<br>Astragalus & Cinnamon Twig Five Substance Decoction | Jin Gui Yao Lüe | huang qi, gui zhi, bai shao, sheng jiang, da zao |
| **Huang Qi Tang** 黄芪汤<br>Astragalus Decoction | Pu Ji Ben Shi Fang | zhi huang qi, shu di huang, bai shao, wu wei zi, mai dong, fu ling, zhi gan cao, sheng jiang, da zao, wu mei |
| **Huang Qin Hua Shi Tang** 黄芩滑石汤<br>Scutellaria & Talcum Decoction | Wen Bing Tiao Bian | huang qin, hua shi, fu ling pi, da fu pi, bai dou kou, tong cao, zhu ling |
| **Huang Tu Tang** 黄土汤<br>Yellow Earth Decoction | Jin Gui Yao Lüe | zao xin tu, sheng di huang, bai zhu, zhi fu zi, huang qin, e jiao, zhi gan cao |
| **Hui Chun Dan**† 回春丹<br>Return to Spring Special Pill | Jing Xiu Tang Yao Shuo | dan nan xing, niu huang, tian zhu huang, bai jiang can, quan xie, tian ma, gou teng, chuan bei mu, zhi ban xia, chen pi, mu xiang, bai dou kou, zhi ke, chen xiang, tan xiang, da huang, gan cao, she xiang (now ren gong she xiang), zhu sha |

| Formula | Source text | Ingredients |
|---------|-------------|-------------|
| **Huo Dan Wan** 藿胆丸<br>Patchouli & Pig Bile Pill | Yi Zong Jin Jian | huo xiang, zhu dan zhi |
| **Huo Luo Xiao Ling Dan** 活络效灵丹<br>Especially Effective Pill to Activate Collaterals | Yi Xue Zhong Zhong Can Xi Lu | dang gui, dan shen, ru xiang, mo yao |
| **Huo Po Xia Ling Tang** 藿朴夏苓汤<br>Patchouli, Magnolia Bark, Pinellia & Poria D. | Yi Yuan | huo xiang, hou po, zhi ban xia, fu ling, xing ren, dan dou chi, yi yi ren, zhu ling, ze xie, bai dou kou |
| **Huo Xiang Zheng Qi San** 藿香正气散<br>Patchouli Powder to Rectify Qi | He Ji Ju Fang | huo xiang, hou po, ban xia qu, fu ling, chao bai zhu, chen pi, jie geng, da fu pi, zi su ye, bai zhi, zhi gan cao |
| **Ji Chuan Jian** 济川煎<br>Benefit the River [Flow] Decoction | Jing Yue Quan Shu | rou cong rong, dang gui, huai niu xi, ze xie, sheng ma, zhi ke |
| **Ji Jiao Li Huang Wan** 己椒苈黄丸<br>Stephania, Zanthoxylum, Lepidium & Rhubarb P. | Jin Gui Yao Lüe | han fang ji, jiao mu, chao ting li zi, da huang |
| **Ji Li Ju Hua Tang** 蒺藜菊花汤<br>Tribulus & Chrysanthemum Decoction | Shi Yong Meng Yao Xue | ci ji li, ju hua, jue ming zi, gan cao |
| **Ji Ming San** 鸡鸣散<br>Powder to Take at Cock Crow | Zheng Zhi Zhun Sheng | bing lang, mu gua, chen pi, wu zhu yu, zi su ye, jie geng, sheng jiang, sheng jiang pi |
| **Ji Sheng Shen Qi Wan** 济生肾气丸<br>Kidney Qi Pill (from the Ji Sheng Fang) | Ji Sheng Fang | che qian zi, huai niu xi, fu ling, ze xie, shu di huang, shan zhu yu, shan yao, mu dan pi, rou gui, zhi fu zi |
| **Jia Jian Wei Rui Tang** 加减葳蕤汤<br>Modified Solomon's Seal Decoction | Tong Su Shang Han Lun | yu zhu, cong bai, jie geng, bai wei, dan dou chi, bo he, da zao, zhi gan cao |
| **Jia Jian Zheng Qi San** 加减正气散<br>Modified Rectify Qi Powder | Xin Fang | da fu pi, huo xiang, xing ren, chao mai ya, chao shen qu, fu ling pi, yin chen hao, hou po, chen pi |
| **Jia Wei Di Huang Wan†** 加味地黄丸<br>Augmented Rehmannia Pill | Yi Zong Jin Jian | shu di huang, shan yao, shan zhu yu, fu ling, mu dan pi, ze xie, lu rong, wu jia pi, she xiang |
| **Jia Wei Si Wu Tang** 加味四物汤<br>Augmented Four Ingredient Decoction | Fu Qing Zhu Nu Ke | shu di huang, dang gui, bai shao, chuan xiong, bai zhu, shan zhu yu, jing jie sui, xu duan, gan cao |
| **Jia Yi Gui Zang Tang** 甲乙归藏汤<br>Ist & 2nd Decoction for Restoring Organs | Yi Chun Sheng Yi | zhen zhu mu, bai shao, sheng di huang, long chi, ye jiao teng, chai hu, bo he, dang gui, dan shen, bai zi ren, he huan hua, chen xiang, da zao |
| **Jian Pi Chu Shi Wan** 健脾除湿汤<br>Strengthen Spleen to Get Rid of Damp Dec. | Zhong Guo Yao Wu Da Quan | tu fu ling, ze xie, bai zhu, fu ling pi |
| **Jian Pi Wan** 健脾丸<br>Strengthen the Spleen Pill | Zheng Zhi Zhun Sheng | bai zhu, mu xiang, huang lian, gan cao, fu ling, ren shen (or dang shen), shen qu, chen pi, sha ren, mai ya, shan yao, rou dou kou |
| **Jiang Huang San** 姜黄散<br>Turmeric Powder | Zheng Zhi Zhun Sheng | jiang huang, e zhu, hong hua, rou gui, dang gui, chuan xiong, bai shao, yan hu suo, mu dan pi, |
| **Jiao Ai Tang** 胶艾汤<br>Ass Hide Gelatin & Mugwort Decoction | Jin Gui Yao Lüe | e jiao, ai ye, shu di huang, dang gui, bai shao, chuan xiong, zhi gan cao |
| **Jie Geng Tang** 桔梗汤<br>Platycodon Decoction | Shang Han Lun | jie geng, gan cao |
| **Jie Gu Dan** 接骨丹<br>Special Pill to Knit Bones | Za Bing Yuan Liu Xi Zhu | gu sui bu, xu duan, zi ran tong, ru xiang, mo yao, long gu, dang gui, chuan xiong, chi shao, gui ban, bai zhi, yu li ren |
| **Jie Nüe Qi Bao Yin** 截疟七宝饮<br>Seven Treasure Drink to Check Malaria | Yang Shi Jia Zang Fang | jiu chang shan, bing lang, cao guo, hou po, qing pi, chen pi, zhi gan cao |
| **Jin Bo Zhen Xin Wan†** 金箔镇心丸<br>Gold Leaf Pill to Settle the Heart | Za Bing Yuan Liu Xi Zhu | zhen zhu, hu po, dan nan xing, tian zhu huang, niu huang, gold leaf, xiong huang, she xiang, zhu sha |
| **Jin Fei Cao San** 金沸草散<br>Inula Powder | He Ji Ju Fang | xuan fu hua, sheng jiang, zhi ban xia, xi xin, qian hu, jing jie, chi shao, gan cao, da zao |
| **Jin Gang Wan** 金刚丸<br>Indomitable Gold Pill | Bao Ming Ji | ba ji tian, bi xie, rou cong rong, du zhong, tu si zi |
| **Jin Gui Shen Qi Wan** 金匮肾气丸<br>Kidney Qi Pill (from the Jin Gui Yao Lüe) | Jin Gui Yao Lüe | shu di huang, shan zhu yu, shan yao, mu dan pi, fu ling, ze xie, rou gui, zhi fu zi |
| **Jin Huang San** 金黄散<br>Gold & Yellow Powder | Yi Zong Jin Jian | da huang, huang bai, jiang huang, bai zhi, chen pi, cang zhu, hou po, gan cao, tian hua fen, tian nan xing |
| **Jin Ling Zi San** 金铃子散<br>Melia Toosendan Powder | Su Wen Bing Ji Qi Yi Bao Ming Ji | chuan lian zi, yan hu suo |
| **Jin Shui Liu Jun Jian** 金水六君煎<br>Six Gentlemen of Metal & Water Decoction | Jing Yue Quan Shu | shu di huang, dang gui, chen pi, zhi ban xia, fu ling, gan cao, sheng jiang |
| **Jin Suo Gu Jing Wan** 金锁固精丸<br>Metal Lock Pill to Stabilize Jing | Yi Fang Ji Jie | sha yuan zi, qian shi, lian xu, duan long gu, duan mu li |
| **Jing Fang Bai Du San** 荆防败毒散<br>Schizonepeta & Saposhnikovia Powder to Overcome Toxin | She Sheng Zhong Miao Fang | jing jie, fang feng, qiang huo, du huo, chuan xiong, bo he, chai hu, qian hu, jie geng, zhi ke, fu ling, gan cao, sheng jiang |
| **Jing Wan Hong** 京万红<br>Capital Ten Thousand Red [Ointment] | Prepared medicine | ban bian lian, di yu, mo yao, ru xiang, dang gui, hong hua, mu gua, bing pian |
| **Jiu Wei Qiang Huo Tang** 九味羌活汤<br>Nine Herb Decoction with Notopterygium | Ci Shi Nan Zhi | qiang huo, fang feng, cang zhu, xi xin, chuan xiong, bai zhi, sheng di huang, huang qin, gan cao |

| Formula | Source text | Ingredients |
|---|---|---|
| **Jiu Xian San**† 九仙散<br>Nine Immortal Powder | Yi Xue Xin Wu | ren shen (or dang shen), e jiao, chuan bei mu, kuan dong hua, sang bai pi, wu wei zi, wu mei, jie geng, zhi ying su ke |
| **Ju He Wan** 橘核丸<br>Tangerine Seed Pill | Ji Sheng Fang | ju he, chuan lian zi, hai zao, kun bu, tao ren, yan hu suo, hou po, zhi shi, mu tong, rou gui, mu xiang |
| **Ju Pi Tang** 橘皮汤<br>Tangerine Peel Decoction | Jin Gui Yao Lüe | chen pi, sheng jiang |
| **Ju Pi Zhu Ru Tang** 橘皮竹茹汤<br>Tangerine Peel & Bamboo Shavings Decoction | Jin Gui Yao Lüe | chen pi, zhu ru, ren shen (or dang shen), zhi gan cao, sheng jiang, da zao |
| **Juan Bi Tang** 蠲痹汤<br>Remove Painful Obstruction Decoction | Yang Shi Jia Zang Fang | qiang huo, dang gui, jiang huang, chi shao, huang qi, fang feng, gan cao, sheng jiang |
| **Juan Bi Tang** 蠲痹汤<br>Remove Painful Obstruction Decoction | Yi Xue Xin Wu | qiang huo, du huo, qin jiao, dang gui, chuan xiong, rou gui, mu xiang, ru xiang, zhi gan cao, sang zhi, hai feng teng |
| **Juan Tong San** 蠲痛散<br>Remove Pain Powder | Jiao Zhu Fu Ren Liang Fang | li zhi he, xiang fu |
| **Jue Ming Wan** 决明丸<br>Cassia Seed Pill | Zheng Zhi Zhun Sheng | jue ming zi, chao shan yao, sheng di huang, gou qi zi, ju hua, fang feng, che qian zi, man jing zi, chuan xiong, xi xin, fu ling, shan zhi zi, xuan shen |
| **Jue Ming Zi San** 决明子散<br>Cassia Seed Powder | Shen Shi Zun Sheng Shu | jue ming zi, shi jue ming, ju hua, man jing zi, huang qin, chi shao, mu zei, chuan xiong, qiang huo, shi gao, gan cao |
| **Kai Jin San** 开噤散<br>Anorectic [Dysenteric Disorder] Powder | Yi Xue Xin Wu | shi chang pu, shi lian zi, chen pi, ren shen (or dang shen), dan shen, fu ling, he ye, huang lian, dong gua zi |
| **Kai Xin San** 开心散<br>Happiness Powder | Qian Jin Yao Fang | ren shen, fu ling, shi chang pu, yuan zhi |
| **Kang Wei Ling** 亢痿灵<br>Effective [Formula] for Impotence | Prepared medicine | wu gong, dang gui, bai shao, zhi gan cao |
| **Ke Xue Fang** 咳血方<br>Hemoptysis Formula | Dan Xi Xin Fa | qing dai, gua lou ren, fu hai shi, shan zhi zi tan, he zi |
| **Kong Xian Dan** 控涎丹<br>Control Mucus Special Pill | San Yin Ji Yi Bing Zheng Fang Lun | gan sui, hong da ji, bai jie zi |
| **Ku Shen Di Huang Tang** 苦参地黄汤<br>Sophora Flavescens & Rehmannia Decoction | Wai Ke Da Cheng | ku shen, sheng di huang |
| **Kuan Dong Hua Tang** 款冬花汤<br>Coltsfoot Decoction | Sheng Ji Zong Lu | kuan dong hua, xing ren, chuan bei mu, zhi mu, sang bai pi, wu wei zi, zhi gan cao |
| **Kui Zi Fu Ling San** 葵子茯苓丸<br>Malva & Poria Powder | Jin Gui Yao Lüe | dong kui zi, fu ling |
| **Lai Fu Tang** 来复汤<br>Return Trip Decoction | Yi Xue Zhong Zhong Can Xi Lu | shan zhu yu, ren shen, long gu, mu li, bai shao, zhi gan cao |
| **Lan Wei Jie Du Tang** 阑尾解毒汤<br>Eliminate Toxin from the Appendix Decoction | Qing Dao Tai Xi Yi Yuan Jing Yan Fang | hong teng, bai jiang cao, jin yin hua, pu gong ying, dong gua zi, chi shao, da huang, mu xiang, huang qin, tao ren, chuan lian zi |
| **Lao Guan Cao Gao** 老鹳草膏<br>Cranesbill Syrup | Shi Yong Zhong Yao Xue | lao guan cao, ji xue teng, dang gui, sang zhi, feng mi |
| **Lao Guan Cao Jiu** 老鹳草酒<br>Cranesbill Wine | Shi Yong Zhong Yao Xue | lao guan cao, gui zhi, dang gui, bai shao, hong hua, alcohol |
| **Lao Guan Cao Ruan Gao** 老鹳草软膏<br>Cranesbill Ointment | Zhong Guo Yao Dian | lao guan cao, sorbolene or lanolin |
| **Lei Wan San** 雷丸散<br>Omphalia Powder | Yang Shi Jia Zang Fang | lei wan, shi jun zi, he shi, fei zi, bing lang |
| **Li Zhong Wan** 理中丸<br>Regulate the Middle Pill | Shang Han Lun | ren shen (or dang shen), bai zhu, gan jiang, zhi gan cao |
| **Lian Pi Sha Chong Yin** 楝皮杀虫饮<br>Melia Drink to Kill Parasites | Zhong Yao Xue | ku lian pi, bai bu, wu mei |
| **Lian Po Yin** 连朴饮<br>Coptis & Magnolia Bark Drink | Huo Luan Lun | huang lian, hou po, shi chang pu, zhi ban xia, shan zhi zi, dan dou chi, lu gen |
| **Lian Qiao Bai Du San** 连翘败毒散<br>Forsythia Powder to Overcome Toxin | Shi Bing Lun | lian qiao, jin yin hua, jing jie, fang feng, qiang huo, du huo, su mu, chuan xiong, dang gui wei, tian hua fen, chai hu, sheng ma, niu bang zi, jie geng, gan cao |
| **Lian Qiao Jin Bei Jian** 连翘金贝煎<br>Forsythia, Lonicera & Bolbostemma Dec. | Jing Yue Quan Shu | lian qiao, jin yin hua, tu bei mu (土贝母 Bolbostematis Rhizoma; can use zhe bei mu), pu gong ying, xia ku cao, hong teng |
| **Liang Fu Wan** 良附丸<br>Galangal & Cyperus Pill | Liang Fang Ji Ye | gao liang jiang, cu xiang fu |
| **Liang Ge San** 凉膈丸<br>Cool the Diaphragm Powder | He Ji Ju fang | lian qiao, huang qin, shan zhi zi, bo he, da huang, mang xiao, gan cao |
| **Liang Jing Wan**† 凉惊丸<br>Cool Convulsions [from heat] Pill | Xiao Er Yao Zheng Zhi Jue | long dan cao, qing dai, niu huang, gou teng, huang lian, fang feng, jin yin hua, she xiang |

| Formula | Source text | Ingredients |
|---|---|---|
| **Ling Gui Zhu Gan Tang** 苓桂术甘汤<br>Poria, Cinnamon, Atractylodes & Licorice D. | Shang Han Lun | fu ling, gui zhi, bai zhu, zhi gan cao |
| **Ling Yang Gou Teng Tang**† 羚羊钩藤汤<br>Saiga Antelope Horn & Uncaria Dec. | Tong Su Shang Han Lun | ling yang jiao (or shan yang jiao), gou teng, sang ye, chuan bei mu, sheng di huang, zhu ru, ju hua, bai shao, fu ling, gan cao |
| **Ling Yang Jiao San**† 羚羊角散<br>Saiga Antelope Horn Powder | Ji Sheng Fang | ling yang jiao (or shan yang jiao), fang feng, du huo, suan zao ren, wu jia pi, yi yi ren, dang gui, chuan xiong, fu shen, xing ren, mu xiang, zhi gan cao, sheng jiang |
| **Ling Yang Jiao San**† 羚羊角散<br>Saiga Antelope Horn Powder | He Ji Ju Fang | ling yang jiao (or shan yang jiao), sheng ma, long dan cao, shan zhi zi, jue ming zi, che qian zi, gan cao |
| **Liu Huang Ruan Gao** 硫磺软膏<br>Sulphur Ointment | Zhong Yao Xue | liu huang, vaseline |
| **Liu Mo Tang** 六磨汤<br>Six Milled Herbs Decoction | Shi Yi De Xiao Fang | chen xiang, bing lang, wu yao, mu xiang, zhi ke, da huang |
| **Liu Shen Wan**† 六神丸<br>Six Magical Ingredients Pill | Lei Yun Shang Song Feng Tang Fang | chan su, niu huang, bing pian, zhen zhu, she xiang (now ren gong she xiang), xiong huang |
| **Liu Wei Di Huang Wan** 六味地黄丸<br>Six Ingredient Pill with Rehmannia | Xiao Er Yao Zheng Zhi Jue | shu di huang, shan zhu yu, shan yao, mu dan pi, fu ling, ze xie |
| **Liu Yi San** 六一散<br>Six to One Powder | Xuan Ming Fang Lun | hua shi, gan cao |
| **Long Chi San** 龙齿散<br>Dragon Teeth Powder | Zheng Zhi Zhun Sheng | long chi, bai shao, mai dong, da huang, sheng ma |
| **Long Dan Xie Gan Tang** 龙胆泻肝汤<br>Gentiana Decoction to Purge the Liver | Yi Fang Ji Jie | jiu long dan cao, chao huang qin, shan zhi zi, sheng di huang, ze xie, che qian zi, jiu dang gui, chai hu, mu tong, gan cao |
| **Lu Gan Shi San** 炉甘石散<br>Calamine Powder | Zheng Zhi Zhun Sheng | lu gan shi, bing pian, huang lian |
| **Lu Dou Yin** 绿豆饮<br>Mung Bean Drink | Jing Yue Quan Shu | lu dou |
| **Lu Dou Yin** 绿豆饮<br>Mung Bean Drink | Zheng Zhi Zhun Sheng | lu dou, huang lian, ge gen, gan cao |
| **Luo Li San** 瘰疬散<br>Scrofula Powder | Xin Fang | wu gong, quan xie, lu jiao, hu tao ren, yang ti gen |
| **Luo Shi Tang** 络石汤<br>Star Jasmine Decoction | Yan Fang | luo shi teng, jie geng, chi fu ling, zi wan, shi gan, mu tong |
| **Ma Huang Fu Zi Xi Xin Tang** 麻黄附子细辛汤<br>Ephedra, Aconite & Asarum Decoction | Shang Han Lun | ma huang, zhi fu zi, xi xin |
| **Ma Huang Jia Zhu Tang** 麻黄加术汤<br>Ephedra plus Atractylodes Decoction | Jin Gui Yao Lüe | ma huang, gui zhi, xing ren, zhi gan cao, bai zhu |
| **Ma Huang Lian Qiao Chi Xiao Dou Tang** 麻黄连翘赤小豆汤<br>Ephedra, Forsythia Fruit & Adzuki Bean Decoction | Shang Han Lun | ma huang, lian qiao, chi xiao dou, xing ren, sang bai pi, zhi gan cao, sheng jiang, da zao |
| **Ma Huang Tang** 麻黄汤<br>Ephedra Decoction | Shang Han Lun | ma huang, gui zhi, xing ren, gan cao |
| **Ma Ren Cong Rong Tang** 麻仁苁蓉汤<br>Hemp Seed & Cistanches Decoction | Ji Yan Fang | huo ma ren, rou cong rong, dang gui, su zi |
| **Ma Xing Shi Gan Tang** 麻杏石甘汤<br>Ephedra, Apricot Seed, Gypsum & Licorice D. | Shang Han Lun | ma huang, xing ren, shi gao, gan cao |
| **Ma Xing Yi Gan Tang** 麻杏意甘汤<br>Ephedra, Apricot Seed, Coix & Licorice D. | Jin Gui Yao Lüe | ma huang, xing ren, yi yi ren, zhi gan cao |
| **Ma Zi Ren Wan** 麻子仁丸<br>Hemp Seed Pill | Shang Han Lun | huo ma ren, da huang, hou po, chao zhi shi, bai shao, chao xing ren |
| **Mai Men Dong Tang** 麦门冬汤<br>Ophiopogon Decoction | Jin Gui Yao Lüe | mai dong, ren shen (or dang shen), zhi ban xia, gan cao, da zao, rice |
| **Mai Wei Di Huang Wan** 麦味地黄丸<br>Ophiopogon, Schizandra & Rehmannia Pill | Yi Ji Bao Jian | shu di huang, shan zhu yu, shan yao, mu dan pi, fu ling, ze xie, mai dong, wu wei zi |
| **Mao Gen Tang** 茅根汤<br>Imperata Root Decoction | Wai Tai Mi Yao | bai mao gen, ge gen |
| **Mao Gen Yin Zi** 茅根饮子<br>Imperata Root Drink | Wai Tai Mi Yao | bai mao gen, ren shen, sheng di huang, fu ling |
| **Meng Shi Gun Tan Wan** 礞石滚痰丸<br>Chlorite Pill to Roll Away Phlegm | Dan Xi Xin Fa Fu Yu | duan qing meng shi, jiu da huang, jiu huang qin, chen xiang |
| **Mi Meng Hua San** 密蒙花散<br>Buddleia Flower Bud Powder | He Ji Ju Fang | mi meng hua, ci ji li, ju hua, shi jue ming, mu zei, qiang huo |
| **Mu Gua Jian** 木瓜煎<br>Chinese Quince Decoction | Pu Ji Ben Shi Fang | mu gua, sheng di huang, ru xiang, mo yao |

| Formula | Source text | Ingredients |
|---|---|---|
| **Mu Gua Tang** 木瓜汤<br>Chinese Quince Decoction | Ren Zhai Zhi Zhi | mu gua, huo xiang, zi su ye, wu zhu yu, sheng jiang |
| **Mu Li San** 牡蛎散<br>Oyster Shell Powder | He Ji Ju Fang | duan mu li, huang qi, ma huang gen, fu xiao mai |
| **Mu Xiang Bing Lang Wan** 木香槟榔丸<br>Aucklandia & Betel Nut Pill | Ru Men Shi Qin | mu xiang, bing lang, qing pi, chen pi, e zhu, huang lian, huang bai, da huang, xiang fu, qian niu zi |
| **Mu Xiang Shun Qi San** 木香顺气散<br>Aucklandia Powder to Smooth Qi | Yi Xue Tong Zhi | mu xiang, xiang fu, bing lang, qing pi, chen pi, hou po, cang zhu, zhi ke, sha ren, zhi gan cao |
| **Nei Xiao Luo Li Wan** 内消瘰疬丸<br>Internally Resolving Scrofula Pill | Yang Yi Da Quan | xia ku cao, xuan shen, zhi bei mu, hai zao, mang xiao, lian qiao, hai ge qiao, tian hua fen, bai wei, dang gui, zhi ke, jie geng, zhi da huang, bo he, sheng di huang, gan cao |
| **Nei Xiao San†** 内消散<br>Internally Resolving Pill | Wai Ke Zheng Zong | bai ji, jin yin hua, tian hua fen, zao jiao ci, zhe bei mu, zhi mu, zhi ban xia, ru xiang, chuan shan jia |
| **Niu Bang Jie Ji Tang** 牛蒡解肌汤<br>Burdock Seed Decoction to Ease the Muscles | Yang Ke Xin De Ji | niu bang zi, lian qiao, xia ku cao, shan zhi zi, mu dan pi, bo he, jing jie, shi hu, xuan shen |
| **Niu Bang Tang** 牛蒡汤<br>Burdock Seed Decoction | Zheng Zhi Zhun Sheng | niu bang zi, jiu da huang, fang feng, jing jie, bo he, gan cao |
| **Niu Huang Jie Du Wan** 牛黄解毒丸<br>Cattle Gallstone Pill to Resolve Toxin | Zheng Zhi Zhun Sheng | niu huang, jin yin hua, chong lou, gan cao |
| **Niu Huang San†** 牛黄散<br>Cattle Gallstone Powder | Xin Fang | niu huang, tian zhu huang, gou teng, quan xie, zhu sha, she xiang |
| **Niu Huang Shang Qing Wan†** 牛黄上清丸<br>Cattle Gallstone Pill to Clear the Upper [Burner] | Zhong Guo Zhong Yao Cheng Yao Chu Fang Ji | niu huang, bing pian, huang lian, huang qin, huang bai, shan zhi zi, shi gao, bo he, lian zi xin, bai zhi, jie geng, ju hua, chuan xiong, chi shao, dang gui, jing jie, da huang, lian qiao, gan cao, zhu sha, xiong huang |
| **Nuan Gan Jian** 暖肝煎<br>Warm the Liver Decoction | Jing Yue Quan Shu | dang gui, gou qi zi, xiao hui xiang, rou gui, wu yao, chen xiang, fu ling, sheng jiang |
| **Pi Pa Qing Fei Yin** 枇杷清肺饮<br>Loquat Leaf Drink to Clear the Lungs | Yi Zong Jin Jian | pi pa ye, ren shen (or dang shen), gan cao, huang lian, huang bai, sang bai pi |
| **Pi Pa Ye Yin** 枇杷叶饮<br>Loquat Leaf Drink | Pu Ji Ben Shi Fang | pi pa ye, zhi ban xia, fu ling, ren shen (or dang shen), bai mao gen, bing lang, sheng jiang |
| **Pi Shen Shuang Bu Wan** 脾肾双补丸<br>Supplement the Spleen and Kidney Pill | Xian Xing Zhai Yi Xue Guang Bi Ji | ren shen (or dang shen), shan yao, lian zi, shan zhu yu, bu gu zhi, ba ji tian, tu si zi, wu wei zi, rou dou kou, chen pi, che qian zi, sha ren |
| **Ping Wei San** 平胃散<br>Calm the Stomach Powder | He Ji Ju Fang | cang zhu, hou po, chen pi, gan cao, sheng jiang, da zao |
| **Po Gu Zhi Wan** 破故纸丸<br>Psoralea Pill | Ji Sheng Fang | bu gu zhi, xiao hui xiang |
| **Pu Ji Xiao Du Yin** 普济消毒饮<br>Universal Benefit Drink to Eliminate Toxin | Dong Yuan Shi Xiao Fang | jiu huang qin, jiu huang lian, xuan shen, niu bang zi, lian qiao, ban lan gen, jie geng, chai hu, gan cao, chen pi, ma bo, bai jiang can, bo he, sheng ma |
| **Qi Bao Mei Ran Dan** 七宝美髯丹<br>Seven Treasure Pill for Beautiful Whiskers | Ben Cao Gang Mu | zhi he shou wu, fu ling, chi fu ling, huai niu xi, dang gui, gou qi zi, tu si zi, bu gu zhi |
| **Qi Ju Di Huang Wan** 杞菊地黄丸<br>Lycium Fruit, Chrysanthemum & Rehmannia P. | Yi Ji Bao Jian | shu di huang, shan zhu yu, shan yao, mu dan pi, fu ling, ze xie, gou qi zi, ju hua |
| **Qi Li San†** 七厘散<br>Seven Thousandths of a Tael Powder | Liang Fang Ji Ye | xue jie, ru xiang, mo yao, hong hua, bing pian, er cha, she xiang (now ren gong she xiang), zhu sha |
| **Qi Wei Bai Zhu San** 七味白术散<br>Seven Ingredient Powder with Atractylodes | Xiao Er Yao Zheng Zhi Jue | ren shen (or dang shen), bai zhu, fu ling, huo xiang, ge gen, mu xiang, zhi gan cao |
| **Qian Gen San** 茜根散<br>Rubia Root Powder | Lei Zheng Zhi Cai | qian cao gen, e jiao, dang gui, huang qin, ce bai ye, sheng di huang, gan cao |
| **Qian Gen Wan†** 茜根丸<br>Rubia Root Pill | Shi Yi De Xiao Fang | qian cao gen, sheng ma, di yu, huang lian, dang gui, zhi ke, bai shao, xi jiao (now shui niu jiao), |
| **Qian Hu San** 前胡散<br>Peucedanum Powder | Zheng Zhi Zhun Sheng | qian hu, xing ren, sang bai pi, chuan bei mu, mai dong, gan cao |
| **Qian Jin San†** 千金散<br>Powder worth One Thousand Gold Pieces | Shou Shi Bao Yuan | bai jiang can, quan xie, tian ma, dan nan xing, niu huang, huang lian, gan cao, bing pian, zhu sha |
| **Qian Zheng San** 牵正散<br>Lead to Symmetry Powder | Yang Shi Jia Zang Fang | zhi bai fu zi, bai jiang can, quan xie |
| **Qiang Huo Sheng Shi Tang** 羌活胜湿汤<br>Notopterygium Decoction to Overcome Damp | Nei Wai Shang Bian Huo Lun | qiang huo, du huo, gao ben, fang feng, zhi gan cao, chuan xiong, man jing zi |
| **Qin Jiao Bai Zhu Wan** 秦艽白术丸<br>Large Gentian & Atractylodes Pill | Lan Shi Mi Cang | qin jiao, bai zhu, dang gui wei, tao ren, zao jiao ci, di yu, chao zhi ke, ze xie |
| **Qin Jiao Bie Jia Tang** 秦艽鳖甲汤<br>Large Gentian & Turtle Shell Decoction | Wei Sheng Bao Jian | qin jiao, bie jia, di gu pi, qing hao, chai hu, dang gui, wu mei |

| Formula | Source text | Ingredients |
|---|---|---|
| **Qin Jiao Ji Sheng Tang** 秦艽寄生汤<br>Large Gentian & Mistletoe Decoction | Jiao Zhu Fu Ren Liang Fang | qin jiao, sang ji sheng, bai shao (or chi shao if less than 7 days postpartum), dang gui, shu di huang (or sheng di huang if less than 7 days postpartum), pu huang, chao pu huang, xu duan, du huo, chen pi, hong hua, shan zha, xiang fu, wu yao |
| **Qing Chang Yin** 清肠饮<br>Clear the Intestine Drink | Bian Zheng Lu | jin yin hua, di yu, mai dong, xuan shen, yi yi ren, huang qin, dang gui, gan cao |
| **Qing Dai Hai Shi Wan** 青黛海石丸<br>Indigo & Pumice Pill | Zheng Yin Mai Zhi | qing dai, gua lou ren, chuan bei mu, fu hai shi |
| **Qing Dai Shi Gao Tang** 青黛石膏汤<br>Indigo & Gypsum Decoction | Chong Ding Tong Su Shang Han Lun | qing dai, sheng di huang, shi gao, sheng ma, huang qin, chao shan zhi zi, cong bai |
| **Qing E Wan** 青娥丸<br>Young Maiden Pill | He Ji Ju Fang | du zhong, hu tao ren, bu gu zhi, da suan |
| **Qing Fei Hua Tan Wan** 清肺化痰丸<br>Clear the Lungs & Transform Phlegm Pill | Shi Yong Zhong Yao Xue | tian zhu huang, chen pi, zhi ban xia, dan nan xing, huang lian, shi gao, bing pian |
| **Qing Ge Jian** 清膈煎<br>Cool the Diaphragm Decoction | Jing Yue Quan Shu | fu hai shi, chuan bei mu, chen pi, dan nan xing, bai jie zi, mu tong |
| **Qing Gu San** 清骨散<br>Cool the Bones Powder | Zheng Zhi Zhun Sheng | yin chai hu, qing hao, qin jiao, di gu pi, zhi mu, hu huang lian, bie jia, gan cao |
| **Qing Hao Bie Jia Tang** 青蒿鳖甲汤<br>Sweet Wormwood & Turtle Shell Decoction | Wen Bing Tiao Bian | qing hao, bie jia, zhi mu, mu dan pi, sheng di huang |
| **Qing Liang San** 清凉散<br>Clearing & Cooling Powder | Zeng Bu Wan Bing Hui Chun | shan dou gen, lian qiao, jie geng, bai zhi, shan zhi zi, huang qin, huang lian, fang feng, bo he, dang gui, zhi ke, sheng di huang, gan cao, deng xin cao |
| **Qing Luo Yin** 清络饮<br>Clear the Collaterals Drink | Wen Bing Tiao Bian | he ye, xi gua, bian dou, jin yin hua, si gua luo, dan zhu ye (all fresh) |
| **Qing Pi Wan** 青皮丸<br>Green Tangerine Peel Pill | Shen Shi Zun Sheng Shu | qing pi, chao shan zha, chao shen qu, chao mai ya, cao guo |
| **Qing Pi Yin** 清脾饮<br>Clear the Spleen Drink | Ji Sheng Fang | cao guo, chai hu, huang qin, qing pi, hou po, zhi ban xia, bai zhu, fu ling, gan cao, sheng jiang |
| **Qing Qi Hua Tan Wan** 清气化痰丸<br>Clear Qi & Transform Phlegm Pill | Yi Fang Kao | huang qin, gua lou ren, dan nan xing, zhi ban xia, chen pi, xing ren, chao zhi shi, fu ling |
| **Qing Shu Yi Qi Tang** 清暑益气汤<br>Clear Summerheat & Augment Qi Decoction | Wen Re Jing Wei | xi yang shen, shi hu, mai dong, huang lian, zhu ye, bo he geng, zhi mu, gan cao, xi gua pi, rice |
| **Qing Wei San** 清胃散<br>Cool the Stomach Powder | Pi Wei Lun | sheng di huang, dang gui, huang lian, mu dan pi, sheng ma |
| **Qing Wen Bai Du Yin** 清瘟败毒饮<br>Cool Warm Disease & Overcome Toxin Drink | Yi Zhen Yi De | shi gao, sheng di huang, huang qin, shan zhi zi, zhi mu, chi shao, xuan shen, lian qiao, mu dan pi, jie geng, zhu ye, shui niu jiao, huang lian, gan cao |
| **Qing Xin Lian Zi Yin** 清心莲子饮<br>Cool the Heart Drink with Lotus Seed | He Ji Ju Fang | shi lian zi, huang qin, mai dong, di gu pi, che qian zi, gan cao, fu ling, ren shen (or dang shen), huang qi |
| **Qing Yin Wan†** 清音丸<br>Clear the Voice Pill | Lan Shi Mi Cang | jie geng, he zi, gan cao, qing dai, bing pian, feng mi, peng sha |
| **Qing Ying Tang†** 清营汤<br>Clear the Ying Level Decoction | Wen Bing Tiao Bian | sheng di huang, xuan shen, mai dong, jin yin hua, lian qiao, dan shen, huang lian, zhu ye, xi jiao (now shui niu jiao) |
| **Qing Zao Jiu Fei Tang** 清燥救肺汤<br>Clear Dryness & Rescue the Lungs Decoction | Yi Men Fa Lu | shi gao, ren shen (or nan sha shen), sang ye, mai dong, hei zhi ma, xing ren, zhi pi pa ye, e jiao, gan cao |
| **Qu Tao Tang** 驱绦汤<br>Expel Tapeworm Decoction | Fang Ji Xue | nan gua zi, bing lang |
| **Quan Xie Ru Xiang San†** 全蝎乳香散<br>Scorpion & Frankincense Powder | Xin Fang | quan xie, zhi ru xiang, zhi chuan wu, cang zhu, chuan shan jia |
| **Quan Xie Xiao Feng San** 全蝎消风散<br>Scorpion Powder to Eliminate Wind | Xin Fang | quan xie, dang shen, bai zhi |
| **Ren Shen Bai Du San** 人参败毒散<br>Ginseng Powder to Overcome Toxin | Xiao Er Yao Zheng Zhi Jue | ren shen (or dang shen), fu ling, gan cao, qian hu, jie geng, du huo, chai hu, chuan xiong, zhi ke, qiang huo, bo he, sheng jiang |
| **Ren Shen Ge Jie San** 人参蛤蚧散<br>Ginseng & Gecko Powder | Wei Sheng Bao Jian | ren shen (or dang shen), zhi ge jie, xing ren, zhi gan cao, fu ling, zhi mu, chuan bei mu, sang bai pi |
| **Ren Shen Hu Tao Tang** 人参胡桃汤<br>Ginseng & Walnut Kernel Decoction | Ji Sheng Fang | ren shen (or dang shen), hu tao ren, sheng jiang |
| **Ren Shen Lu Rong Wan** 人参鹿茸丸<br>Ginseng & Deer Antler Velvet Pill | Zhong Guo Zhong Yao Cheng Yao Chu Fang Ji | ren shen, lu rong, dang gui, du zhong, bu gu zhi, ba ji tian, tu si zi, huai niu xi, fu ling, huang qi, wu wei zi, long yan rou, xiang fu, dong chong xia cao, huang bai, feng mi |
| **Rou Cong Rong Wan** 肉苁蓉丸<br>Cistanches Pill | Zheng Zhi Zhun Sheng | rou cong rong, shu di huang, tu si zi, wu wei zi, shan yao |
| **Ru Sheng San** 如圣散<br>Sage Like Powder | Zheng Zhi Zhun Sheng | zong lu tan, wu mei tan, pao jiang |

| Formula | Source text | Ingredients |
|---|---|---|
| **Run Chang Wan** 润肠丸<br>Moisten the Intestines Pill | Pi Wei Lun | da huang, dang gui wei, qiang huo, tao ren, huo ma ren |
| **San Bi Tang** 三痹汤<br>Three Painful Obstruction Decoction | Fu Ren Liang Fang | du huo, fang feng, qin jiao, xi xin, du zhong, xu duan, huai niu xi, shu di huang, dang gui, bai shao, chuan xiong, ren shen (or dang shen), huang qi, fu ling, gan cao, rou gui, sheng jiang |
| **San Cai Feng Sui Dan** 三才封髓丹<br>Three Skills Pill to Seal the Marrow | Wei Sheng Bao Jian | tian dong, shu di huang, ren shen, huang bai, sha ren, gan cao |
| **San Jia Fu Mai Tang** 三甲复脉汤<br>Three Shell Decoction to Restore the Pulse | Wen Bing Tiao Bian | gui ban, bie jia, mu li, e jiao, sheng di huang, mai dong, bai shao, zhi gan cao |
| **San Jin Hu Tao Tang** 三金胡桃汤<br>Three Gold [Herb] & Walnut Kernel Dec. | Shi Yong Fang Ji Xue | jin qian cao, hai jin sha, ji nei jin, hu tao ren, sheng di huang, xuan shen, tian dong, shi wei, bian qu, qu mai, huai niu xi, che qian cao, hua shi, mu tong, gan cao |
| **San Jin Tang** 三金汤<br>Three Gold [Herb] Decoction | Fang Ji Xue | jin qian cao, hai jin sha, ji nei jin, dong kui zi, shi wei, qu mai |
| **San Leng Wan** 三棱丸<br>Sparganium Pill | Jing Yan Liang Fang | san leng, e zhu, mu dan pi, yan hu suo, chuan xiong, jiu da huang, chuan niu xi |
| **San Ren Tang** 三仁汤<br>Three Seed Decoction | Wen Bing Tiao Bian | yi yi ren, xing ren, bai dou kou, hou po, tong cao, hua shi, zhi ban xia, zhu ye |
| **San She Dan Chuan Bei Ye** 三蛇胆川贝液<br>Three Snakes Bile & Fritillaria Drink | Prepared medicine | she dan (蛇胆 snake bile), chuan bei mu |
| **San Shi Tang** 三石汤<br>Three Stones Decoction | Wen Bing Tiao Bian | shi gao, han shui shi, hua shi, xing ren, zhu ru, jin yin hua, tong cao |
| **San Wu Bai San** 三物白散<br>Three Ingredient White Powder | Shang Han Lun | ba dou shuang, jie geng, chuan bei mu |
| **San Wu Bei Ji Wan** 三物备急丸<br>Three Ingredient Pill for Emergencies | Jin Gui Yao Lüe | da huang, ba dou shuang, gan jiang |
| **San Xian Yin** 三鲜饮<br>Three Fresh [Herb] Drink | Yi Xue Zhong Zhong Can Xi Lu | fresh juice of xiao ji, bai mao gen and lotus root |
| **San Zhi Yin** 三汁饮<br>Three Juice Drink | Fang Ji Xue | fresh juice of jiu cai and sheng jiang, milk |
| **San Zi Yang Qin Tang** 三子养亲汤<br>Three Seed Decoction to Nourish Ancestors | Han Shi Yi Tong | bai jie zi, su zi, lai fu zi |
| **Sang Ju Yin** 桑菊饮<br>Mulberry Leaf & Chrysanthemum Drink | Wen Bing Tiao Bian | sang ye, ju hua, xing ren, lian qiao, jie geng, bo he, gan cao, lu gen |
| **Sang Luo Tang** 桑络汤<br>Mulberry Twig & Star Jasmine Stem Dec. | Shi Yong Fang Ji Xue | sang zhi, luo shi teng, ren dong teng, qing hao, bai wei, chao tao ren, hong hua, di gu pi, hai tong pi, di long |
| **Sang Pi Bai Qian Tang** 桑皮白前汤<br>Mulberry Bark & Cynanchum Root Dec. | Za Bing Yuan Liu Xi Zhu | sang bai pi, bai qian, xing ren, shi gao |
| **Sang Piao Xiao San** 桑螵蛸散<br>Mantis Egg Case Powder | Ben Cao Yan Yi | sang piao xiao, yuan zhi, shi chang pu, ren shen (or dang shen), fu shen, dang gui, long gu, gui ban |
| **Sang Xing Tang** 桑杏汤<br>Mulberry Leaf & Apricot Kernel Decoction | Wen Bing Tiao Bian | sang ye, xing ren, nan sha shen, zhe bei mu, dan dou chi, shan zhi zi, li pi (pear skin) |
| **Sang Zhi Gao** 桑枝膏<br>Mulberry Twig Syrup | Zui Xin Fang Ji Shou Ce | sang zhi, sugar |
| **Sang Zhi Hu Zhang Tang** 桑枝虎杖汤<br>Mulberry Twig & Bushy Knotweed Decoction | Ji Yan Fang | sang zhi, hu zhang, jin que gen 金雀根 (Caragana sinica Radix), chou wu tong, da zao |
| **Sang Zhi Tang** 桑枝汤<br>Mulberry Twig Decoction | Shi Yong Fang Ji Xue | sang zhi, huang qi, dang gui, wei ling xian, qin jiao, fu ling, han fang ji, chuan xiong, sheng ma |
| **Sha Shen Mai Dong Tang** 沙参麦冬汤<br>Glehnia & Ophiopogon Decoction | Wen Bing Tiao Bian | bei sha shen, mai dong, tian hua fen, sang ye, bian dou, yu zhu, gan cao |
| **Sha Qi Chan Su Wan†** 痧气蟾酥丸<br>Toad Venom Pill for Acute Enteritis | Prepared medicine | chan su, ding xiang, da huang, tian ma, gan cao, she xiang (now ren gong she xiang), xiong huang, zhu sha |
| **Shan Qi Nei Xiao Wan** 疝气内消丸<br>Pill to Eliminate Shan Disorders | Prepared medicine | li zhi he, xiao hui xiang, chuan lian zi, wu zhu yu, chen xiang, rou gui, ju he, bai zhu, gan cao, qing pi, pao jiang, si gua luo, bu gu zhi, ba jiao hui xiang, zhi fu zi |
| **Shao Fu Zhu Yu Tang** 少腹逐瘀汤<br>Dispel Blood Stasis from the Low Abdomen D. | Yi Lin Gai Cuo | xiao hui xiang, gan jiang, yan hu suo, mo yao, dang gui, chuan xiong, rou gui, chi shao, pu huang, chao wu ling zhi |
| **Shao Yao Gan Cao Tang** 芍药甘草汤<br>Peony & Licorice Decoction | Shang Han Lun | bai shao, zhi gan cao |
| **Shao Yao Tang** 芍药汤<br>Peony Decoction | Su Wen Bing Ji Qi Yi Bao Ming Ji | bai shao, huang qin, huang lian, da huang, dang gui, bing lang, mu xiang, rou gui, gan cao |
| **She Chuang Zi San** 蛇床子散<br>Cnidium Fruit Powder | Fu Chan Ke Xue | she chuang zi, hua jiao, bai bu, bai fan, ku shen |
| **She Dan Chuan Bei Mo** 蛇胆川贝末<br>Snake Bile & Fritillary Powder | Prepared medicine | she dan (蛇胆, snake bile), chuan bei mu |

| Formula | Source text | Ingredients |
|---|---|---|
| **She Dan Chuan Bei Pi Pa Gao** 蛇胆川贝枇杷膏<br>Snake Bile, Fritillary & Loquat Syrup | Prepared medicine | she dan (蛇胆, snake bile), chuan bei mu, pi pa ye, jie geng, zhi ban xia, feng mi |
| **She Gan Ma Huang Tang** 射干麻黄汤<br>Belamcanda & Ephedra Decoction | Jin Gui Yao Lüe | she gan, ma huang, xi xin, zhi ban xia, zi wan, kuan dong hua, wu wei zi, sheng jiang, da zao |
| **She Gan Tang** 射干汤<br>Belamcanda Decoction | You You Xin Shu | she gan, sheng ma, ma bo, mang xiao |
| **She Gan Xiao Du Yin** 射干消毒饮<br>Belamcanda Decoction to Eliminate Toxin | Zhang Shi Yi Tong | she gan, xuan shen, lian qiao, jing jie, niu bang zi, gan cao |
| **Shen Fu Tang** 参附汤<br>Ginseng & Prepared Aconite Decoction | Jiao Zhu Fu Ren Liang Fang | ren shen, zhi fu zi |
| **Shen Ling Bai Zhu San** 参苓白术散<br>Ginseng, Poria & Atractylodes Powder | He Ji Ju Fang | ren shen (or dang shen), fu ling, bai zhu, chao bian dou, chao shan yao, yi yi ren, lian zi, chen pi, jie geng, sha ren, zhi gan cao, da zao |
| **Shen Rong Gu Ben Wan** 参茸固本丸<br>Ginseng & Deer Velvet Pill to Secure the Base | Zhong Guo Yi Xue Da Ci Dian | ren shen, lu rong, chao shan yao, bai zhu, fu ling, huang qi, dang gui, shu di huang, bai shao, gou qi zi, ba ji tian, rou cong rong, tu si zi, huai niu xi, rou gui, xiao hui xiang, chen pi, gan cao |
| **Shen Su Yin** 参苏饮<br>Ginseng & Perilla Leaf Drink | He Ji Ju Fang | ren shen (or dang shen), zi su ye, ge gen, qian hu, zhi ke, jie geng, zhi ban xia, fu ling, chen pi, mu xiang, gan cao, sheng jiang, da zao |
| **Shen Tong Zhu Yu Tang** 身痛逐瘀汤<br>Disperse Blood Stasis & Ease Body Pain Dec. | Yi Lin Gai Cuo | tao ren, hong hua, dang gui, qin jiao, huai niu xi, chao wu ling zhi, mo yao, di long, xiang fu, chuan xiong, qiang huo, gan cao |
| **Shen Ying Wan** 神应丸<br>Pill that Should Work like Magic | Zheng Zhi Zhun Sheng | wei ling xian, dang gui, rou gui, ba jiao hui xiang |
| **Shen Zhu San** 神术散<br>Magical Atractylodes Powder | He Ji Ju Fang | cang zhu, gao ben, bai zhi, xi xin, qiang huo, chuan xiong, zhi gan cao, sheng jiang, cong bai |
| **Sheng Hua Tang** 生化汤<br>Generation & Transformation Decoction | Fu Qing Zhu Nu Ke | dang gui, chuan xiong, tao ren, pao jiang, zhi gan cao |
| **Sheng Ji Gan Nong San†** 生肌干脓散<br>Powder to Heal Flesh & Dry Pus | Zheng Zhi Zhun Sheng | bai ji, huang lian, zhi bei mu, jiang xiang, hai piao xiao, wu bei zi, qing fen |
| **Sheng Ji San†** 生肌散<br>Powder to Heal Flesh | Yang Yi Da Quan | zhen zhu, zhi mo yao, zhi ru xiang, er cha, chi shi zhi, xue jie, bing pian, qian dan, qing fen |
| **Sheng Ji Yu Hong Gao†** 生肌玉红膏<br>Red Jade Ointment to Promote Healing | Wai Ke Zheng Zong | bai zhi, gan cao, dang gui, zi cao, xue jie, sesame oil, qing fen |
| **Sheng Jiang Xie Xin Tang** 生姜泻心汤<br>Ginger Decoction to Purge the Heart | Shang Han Lun | sheng jiang, zhi ban xia, huang qin, huang lian, gan cao, ren shen (or dang shen), gan jiang, da zao |
| **Sheng Ma Ge Gen Tang** 升麻葛根汤<br>Cimicifuga & Kudzu Decoction | Xiao Er Yao Zheng Zhi Jue | sheng ma, ge gen, chi shao, gan cao |
| **Sheng Mai San** 生脉散<br>Generate the Pulse Powder | Nei Wai Shang Bian Huo Lun | ren shen (or dang shen), mai dong, wu wei zi |
| **Sheng Tian Qi Pian** 生田七片<br>Raw Tianchi Ginseng Tablets | Prepared medicine | san qi |
| **Sheng Tie Luo Yin†** 生铁落饮<br>Iron Filings Decoction | Yi Xue Xin Wu | sheng tie luo, dan nan xing, zhe bei mu, xuan shen, tian dong, mai dong, lian qiao, dan shen, fu ling, ju hong, shi chang pu, yuan zhi, zhu sha |
| **Sheng Xian Tang** 升陷汤<br>Raise the Sunken Decoction | Yi Xue Zhong Zhong Can Xi Lu | huang qi, zhi mu, jie geng, chai hu, sheng ma |
| **Shi Di Tang** 柿蒂汤<br>Persimmon Calyx Decoction | Ji Sheng Fang | shi di, ding xing, sheng jiang |
| **Shi Hu Qing Wei San** 石斛清胃散<br>Dendrobium Powder to Clear the Stomach | Zhang Shi Yi Tong | shi hu, fu ling, chen pi, zhi ke, bian dou, huo xiang, chi shao, gan cao |
| **Shi Hu Ye Guang Wan†** 石斛夜光丸<br>Dendrobium Pill for Night Vision | Rui Zhu Tang Jing Yan Fang | shi hu, tian dong, mai dong, shu di huang, sheng di huang, ren shen, fu ling, tu si zi, ju hua, jue ming zi, xing ren, shan yao, gou qi zi, huai niu xi, wu wei zi, ci ji li, rou cong rong, chuan xiong, zhi gan cao, zhi ke, qiang xiang zi, fang feng, huang lian, xi jiao (now shui niu jiao), ling yang jiao (now shan yang jiao) |
| **Shi Hui San** 十灰散<br>Powder of Ten Charred [Herbs] | Shi Yao Shen Shu | da ji, xiao ji, he ye, ce bai ye, bai mao gen, qian cao gen, shan zhi zi, da huang, mu dan pi, zong lu pi |
| **Shi Jue Ming Wan** 石决明丸<br>Abalone Shell Pill | Zheng Zhi Zhun Sheng | shi jue ming, tu si zi, shu di huang, zhi mu, shan yao, xi xin, wu wei zi |
| **Shi Nan Jiu** 石楠酒<br>Photinia Tincture | Sheng Ji Zong Lu | shi nan ye, grain alcohol |
| **Shi Nan Wan** 石楠丸<br>Photinia Pill | Sheng Ji Zong Lu | shi nan ye, huai niu xi, bai zhu, huang qi, lu rong, rou gui, gou qi zi, mu gua, fang feng, tian ma |
| **Shi Pi Yin** 实脾饮<br>Bolster the Spleen Drink | Ji Sheng Fang | bai zhu, fu ling, da fu pi, mu gua, zhi fu zi, gan jiang, hou po, cao dou kou, mu xiang, zhi gan cao, sheng jiang, da zao |

| Formula | Source text | Ingredients |
|---|---|---|
| **Shi Quan Da Bu Tang** 十全大补汤<br>All Inclusive Great Supplementing Decoction | He Ji Ju Fang | ren shen, bai zhu, gan cao, fu ling, dang gui, shu di huang, bai shao, chuan xiong, rou gui, huang qi |
| **Shi Wei San** 石苇散<br>Pyrrosia Powder | Pu Ji Ben Shi Fang | shi wei, che qian zi, qu mai, sang bai pi, dong kui zi, hua shi, chi fu ling, mu tong, gan cao |
| **Shi Wei San** 石苇散<br>Pyrrosia Powder | Wai Tai Mi Yao | shi wei, tong cao, wang bu liu xing, hua shi, zhi gan cao, dang gui, bai zhu, qu mai, bai shao (or chi shao), dong kui zi |
| **Shi Xiao San** 失效散<br>Sudden Smile Powder | He Ji Ju Fang | pu huang, cu wu ling zhi |
| **Shi Zao Tang** 十枣汤<br>Ten Jujube Decoction | Shang Han Lun | gan sui, hong da ji, yuan hua, da zao |
| **Shou Nian San** 手拈散<br>Pinch Powder | Dan Xi Xin Fa | yan hu suo, wu ling zhi, cao guo, mo yao |
| **Shou Tai Wan** 寿胎丸<br>Fetus Longevity Pill | Yi Xue Zhong Zhong Can Xi Lu | xu duan, sang ji sheng, tu si zi, e jiao |
| **Shou Wu He Ji** 首乌合剂<br>Fleeceflower Root Mixture | Xin Fang | zhi he shou wu, sheng di huang, xuan shen, bai shao, nu zhen zi, mo han lian, sha yuan zi, xi xian cao, sang ji sheng, huai niu xi |
| **Shou Wu Yan Shou Dan** 首乌延寿丹<br>Fleeceflower Root Special Pill for Long Life | Shi Bu Zhai Yi Shu | zhi he shou wu, nu zhen zi, mo han lian, sang shen, hei zhi ma, sheng di huang, du zhong, tu si zi, huai niu xi, ren dong teng, jin ying zi, sang ye, xi xian cao |
| **Shu Jin Tang** 舒筋汤<br>Relax Sinews Decoction | Jiao Zhu Fu Ren Liang Fang | jiang huang, qiang huo, hai tong pi, bai shao (or chi shao), dang gui, bai zhu, gan cao |
| **Shu Jin Huo Xue Tang** 疏筋活血汤<br>Dredge Sinews & Activate Blood Decoction | Wan Bing Hui Chun | wei ling xian, chuan niu xi, han fang ji, qiang huo, chuan xiong, dang gui, bai shao (or chi shao), tao ren, sheng di huang, fu ling, cang zhu, chen pi, bai zhi, long dan cao, fang feng, zhi gan cao |
| **Shu Jin Huo Xue Fang** 舒筋活血方<br>Relax Sinew & Activate Blood Formula | Zhong Yi Shang Ke Xue Jiang Yi | shen jin cao, hai tong pi, qin jiao, du huo, dang gui, gou teng, hong hua, ru xiang, mo yao |
| **Shu Xue Wan** 疏血丸<br>Blood Dredging Pill | Yi Zong Jin Jian | ou jie, ce bai ye, bai mao gen, e jiao zhu, jiu dang gui, bai cao shuang (百草霜 activated charcoal from plants) |
| **Shu Zao Yin Zi** 疏凿饮子<br>Dispersing Chisel Drink | Ji Sheng Fang | shang lu, qiang huo, qin jiao, bing lang, da fu pi, fu ling pi, sheng jiang pi, chuan jiao mu, ze xie, mu tong, chi xiao dou |
| **Shui Lu Er Xian Dan** 水陆二仙丹<br>Water & Earth Immortals Special Pill | Zheng Zhi Zhun Sheng | qian shi, jin ying zi |
| **Shui Niu Jiao Da Qing Tang** 水牛角大青汤<br>Water Buffalo Horn & Isatis Leaf Decoction | Shang Han Huo Ren Shu Kuo | shui niu jiao, da qing ye, shan zhi zi, dan dou chi (Formulas originally known as Xi Jiao Da Qing Tang, with xi jiao instead of shui niu jiao) |
| **Shui Niu Jiao Di Huang Tang** 水牛角地黄汤<br>Water Buffalo Horn & Rehmannia Decoction | Qian Jin Yao Fang | shui niu jiao, sheng di huang, chi shao, mu dan pi (Formula originally known as Xi Jiao Di Huang Tang, with xi jiao instead of shui niu jiao) |
| **Si Jing Wan** 四精丸<br>Four Jing Wan | Shi Yi De Xiao Fang | rou cong rong, lu rong, shan yao, fu ling, mu xiang, da zao |
| **Si Jun Zi Tang** 四君子汤<br>Four Gentlemen Decoction | He Ji Ju Fang | ren shen (or dang shen), bai zhu, fu ling, zhi gan cao |
| **Si Miao Wan** 四妙散<br>Four Marvel Pill | Cheng Fang Bian Du | cang zhu, huang bai, yi yi ren, huai niu xi |
| **Si Miao Yong An Tang** 四妙勇安汤<br>Four Marvel Decoction for Well Being | Yan Fang Xin Bian | jin yin hua, xuan shen, dang gui, gan cao |
| **Si Ni San** 四逆散<br>Frigid Extremities Powder | Shang Han Lun | chai hu, bai shao, zhi shi, zhi gan cao |
| **Si Ni Tang** 四逆汤<br>Frigid Extremities Decoction | Shang Han Lun | zhi fu zi, gan jiang, zhi gan cao |
| **Si Shen Wan** 四神丸<br>Four Miracle Pill | Fu Ren Liang Fang | bu gu zhi, rou dou kou, wu wei zi, wu zhu yu |
| **Si Sheng San** 四圣散<br>Four Sage Powder | Ren Zhai Zhi Zhi | quan gua lou, gan cao, ru xiang, mo yao |
| **Si Sheng Wan** 四生丸<br>Four Fresh Pill | Fu Ren Liang Fang | sheng ce bai ye, sheng di huang, sheng he ye, sheng ai ye |
| **Si Wu Tang** 四物汤<br>Four Substance Decoction | Xian Shou Li Shang Xu Duan Mi Fang | shu di huang, dang gui, bai shao, chuan xiong |
| **Si Wu Xiao Feng Yin** 四物消风饮<br>Four Substance Drink to Eliminate Wind | Yi Zong Jin Jian | sheng di huang, dang gui, chi shao, chuan xiong, jing jie, fang feng, bai xian pi, chan tui, bo he, du huo, chai hu, da zao |
| **Su He Xiang Wan†** 苏合香丸<br>Liquid Styrax Pill | He Ji Ju Fang | su he xiang, an xi xiang, chen xiang, ding xiang, xiang fu, tan xiang, ru xiang, bai zhu, he zi, bi ba, bing pian, she xiang (now ren gong she xiang), qing mu xiang, xi jiao (now shui niu jiao), zhu sha |

| Formula | Source text | Ingredients |
|---|---|---|
| **Su Zi Jiang Qi Tang** 苏子降气汤<br>Perilla Fruit Decoction for Directing Qi Down | He Ji Ju Fang | su zi, qian hu, zhi ban xia, chen pi, dang gui, hou po, rou gui, zhi gan cao, zi su ye, sheng jiang, da zao |
| **Suan Zao Ren Tang** 酸枣仁汤<br>Zizyphus Decoction | Jin Gui Yao Lüe | chao suan zao ren, fu ling, chuan xiong, zhi mu, gan cao |
| **Suo Quan Wan** 缩泉丸<br>Restrict the Fountain Pill | Fu Ren Liang Fang | shan yao, wu yao, yi zhi ren |
| **Suo Yang Gu Jing Wan** 锁阳固精丸<br>Synomorium Pill to Secure Jing | Prepared medicine | suo yang, lu jiao shuang, du zhong, shan yao |
| **Tao He Cheng Qi Tang** 桃核承气汤<br>Peach Seed Decoction to Order Qi | Shang Han Lun | tao ren, da huang, gui zhi, mang xiao, zhi gan cao |
| **Tao Hong Si Wu Tang** 桃红四物汤<br>Four Substance D. with Peach Seed & Safflower | Yi Zong Jin Jian | tao ren, hong hua, shu di huang, dang gui, bai shao (or chi shao), chuan xiong |
| **Tao Hua Tang** 桃花汤<br>Peach Flower Decoction | Shang Han Lun | chi shi zhi, gan jiang, jing mi |
| **Tian Ma Gou Teng Yin** 天麻钩藤饮<br>gastrodia & Uncaria Drink | Zhong Yi Nei Ke Za Bing Zheng Zhi Xin Yi | tian ma, gou teng, shi jue ming, shan zhi zi, huang qin, chuan niu xi, du zhong, yi mu cao, sang ji sheng, ye jiao teng, fu shen |
| **Tian Tai Wu Yao San** 天台乌药散<br>Top Quality Lindera Powder | Yi Xue Fa Ming | wu yao mu xiang, xiao hui xiang, qing pi, gao liang jiang, bing lang, chuan lian zi, ba dou |
| **Tian Wang Bu Xin Dan** 天王补心丹<br>Emperor of Heaven's Special Pill to Supplement the Heart | Jiao Zhu Fu Ren Liang Fang | sheng di huang, ren shen (or dang shen), xuan shen, dan shen, fu ling, jie geng, yuan zhi, wu wei zi, dang gui, tian dong, mai dong, chao bai zi ren, chao suan zao ren |
| **Tian Zhu Huang San** 天竺黄散<br>Tabasheer Powder | Zheng Zhi Zhun Sheng | tian zhu huang, bai jiang can, chan tui, yu jin, shan zhi zi, gan cao |
| **Ting Li Da Zao Xie Fei Tang** 葶苈大枣泻肺汤<br>Lepidium & Jujube D. to Drain the Lungs | Jin Gui Yao Lüe | ting li zi, da zao |
| **Tong Guan San** 通关散<br>Open the Gate Powder | Dan Xi Xin Fa Fu Yu | xi xin, zao jia |
| **Tong Jing Wan** 通经丸<br>Dysmenorrhea Pill | Lei Zheng Zhi Cai | su mu, hu po, tao ren, chi shao, dang gui wei, chuan xiong, chuan niu xi, sheng di huang, xiang fu, wu ling zhi |
| **Tong Qiao Huo Xue Tang**† 通窍活血汤<br>Unblock the Orifices & Activate Blood Dec. | Yi Lin Gai Cuo | tao ren, hong hua, chi shao, chuan xiong, sheng jiang, da zao, cong bai, she xiang (now ren gong she xiang) |
| **Tong Ru Dan** 通乳丹<br>Special Pill to Promote Lactation | Fu Qing Zhu Nu Ke | tong cao, ren shen (or dang shen), huang qi, dang gui, mai dong, jie geng, pigs foot |
| **Tong Xie Yao Fang** 痛泻要方<br>Important Formula for Painful Diarrhea | Jing Yue Quan Shu | chao bai zhu, chao bai shao, chen pi, fang feng |
| **Tou Gu Cao Wan**† 透骨草丸<br>Speranskia Pill | Yan Fang | tou gu cao, fang feng, hai feng teng, sheng di, bai shao (or chi shao), dang gui, ci ji li, xi xian cao, chen pi, gan cao, chuan shan jia (now sang zhi or ji xue teng) |
| **Tou Nong San**† 透脓散<br>Discharge Pus Powder | Wai Ke Zheng Zong | huang qi, zao jiao ci, dang gui, chuan xiong, chuan shan jia (now bai zhi or wang bu liu xing) |
| **Tu Fu Ling Gao** 土茯苓膏<br>Smilax Syrup | Zhong Yi Fang Ji Shou Ce | tu fu ling, jin yin hua, bi xie, gan cao, ze xie, dang gui |
| **Tu Jin Pi Ding** 土槿皮酊<br>Golden Larch Tincture | Prepared medicine | tu jing pi, grain alcohol |
| **Tu Si Zi San** 菟丝子丸<br>Cuscuta Seed Pill | Shi Yi De Xiao Fang | tu si zi, lu rong, zhi fu zi, rou cong rong, sang piao xiao, wu wei zi, ji nei jin, mu li |
| **Wa Leng Zi Wan** 瓦楞子丸<br>Cockle Shell Pill | Zhong Yao Xue | duan wa leng zi, xiang fu, tao ren, mu dan pi, dang gui, hong hua, da huang, chuan xiong |
| **Wan Dai Tang** 完带汤<br>End Discharge Decoction | Fu Qing Zhu Nu Ke | bai zhu, shan yao, ren shen (or dang shen), bai shao, che qian zi, cang zhu, gan cao, chen pi, jing jie tan, chai hu |
| **Wei Jing Tang** 苇茎汤<br>Reed Decoction | Qian Jin Yao Fang | lu gen, yi yi ren, dong gua zi, tao ren |
| **Wen Dan Tang** 温胆汤<br>Warm Gallbladder Decoction | San Yin Ji Yi Bing Zheng Fang Lun | zhi ban xia, chen pi, fu ling, gan cao, zhu ru, zhi shi, sheng jiang, da zao |
| **Wen Jing Tang** 温经汤<br>Flow Warming Decoction | Jin Gui Yao Lüe | wu zhu yu, gui zhi, dang gui, bai shao, chuan xiong, e jiao, mu dan pi, mai dong, ren shen, sheng jiang, zhi ban xia, gan cao |
| **Wen Pi Tang** 温脾汤<br>Warm the Spleen Decoction | Qian Jin Yao Fang | da huang, zhi fu zi, gan jiang, ren shen (or dang shen), zhi gan cao |
| **Wu Bei San** 乌贝散<br>Black Shell Powder | Bei Jing Zhong Yi | hai piao xiao, zhe bei mu |
| **Wu Fa Wan** 乌发丸<br>Black Hair Pill | Jing Fan Fang | ce bai ye, zhi he shou wu, sheng di huang, nu zhen zi, mo han lian, hei zhi ma, chen pi, hua jiao, hei dou (黑豆 black beans) |

| Formula | Source text | Ingredients |
|---|---|---|
| **Wu Hu Zhui Feng San** 五虎追风散<br>Five Tiger Powder to Pursue Wind | Shan Xi Sheng Zhong Yi Yan Fang Mi Fang Hui Ji | chan tui, zhi tian nan xing, tian ma, quan xie, bai jiang can |
| **Wu Ji Bai Feng Wan** 乌鸡白凤丸<br>Black Chicken White Phoenix Pill | Prepared medicine – this version from Tianjin Darentang Pharmacy | wu ji (black boned chicken), shu di huang, lu jiao jiao, dang gui, bai shao, ren shen, shan yao, xiang fu, dan shen, tian dong, chuan xiong, qian shi, mu li, huang qin, gan cao, yin chai hu [many different versions of this formula, but with similar indications] |
| **Wu Ji San** 五积散<br>Five Accumulation Powder | He Ji Ju Fang | cang zhu, jie geng, chen pi, ma huang, zhi ke, gan jiang, hou po, bai zhi, zhi ban xia, fu ling, dang gui, chuan xiong, bai shao, rou gui, zhi gan cao |
| **Wu Jia Pi Jiu** 五加皮酒<br>Eleutherococcus Wine | Ben Cao Gang Mu | wu jia pi, dang gui, huai niu xi, shen qu, yellow wine |
| **Wu Jia Pi San** 五加皮散<br>Eleutherococcus Powder | Shen Shi Zun Sheng Shu | wu jia pi, song jie, mu gua |
| **Wu Jia Pi San** 五加皮散<br>Eleutherococcus Powder | Bao Ying Cuo Yao | wu jia pi, gui ban, huai niu xi, mu gua |
| **Wu Jing Jian Wan** 五精煎丸<br>Five Jing Concentrated Pill | Sheng Ji Zong Lu | huang jing, sheng di huang, ren shen, bai zhu, tian dong, huia niu xi, fu ling, ju hua, shi chang pu, rou gui |
| **Wu Ling San** 五苓散<br>Five Ingredient Powder with Poria | Shang Han Lun | fu ling, zhu ling, ze xie, bai zhu, gui zhi |
| **Wu Long Gao** 乌龙膏<br>Black Dragon Ointment | Yi Zong Jin Jian | mu bie zi, ban xia, cao wu, bai zhi, chi shao |
| **Wu Mei Wan** 乌梅丸<br>Black Plum Pill | Shang Han Lun | wu mei, gan jiang, zhi fu zi, huang lian, huang bai, gui zhi, ren shen (or dang shen), xi xin, hua jiao, dang gui |
| **Wu Pi Yin** 五皮饮<br>Five Peel Drink | He Ji Ju Fang | sheng jiang pi, wu jia pi, da fu pi, di gu pi, fu ling pi |
| **Wu Pi San** 五皮散<br>Five Peel Powder | Zhong Zang Jing | fu ling pi, sang bai pi, da fu pi, sheng jiang pi, chen pi |
| **Wu Ren Wan** 五仁丸<br>Five Seed Pill | Shi Yi De Xiao Fang | tao ren, xing ren, bai zi ren, yu li ren, chen pi, feng mi |
| **Wu Tou Chi Shi Zhi Wan** 乌头赤石脂丸<br>Aconite & Hallyosite Pill | Jin Gui Yao Lüe | zhi chuan wu, chi shi zhi, hua jiao, zhi fu zi, gan jiang |
| **Wu Tou Tang** 乌头汤<br>Aconite Decoction | Jin Gui Yao Lüe | zhi chuan wu, ma huang, chao bai shao, zhi gan cao, huang qi, feng mi |
| **Wu Wei Xiao Du Yin** 五味消毒饮<br>Five Ingredient Drink to Eliminate Toxin | Yi Zong Jin Jian | jin yin hua, ye ju hua, zi hua di ding, pu gong ying, tian kui zi |
| **Wu Wei Zi San** 五味子散<br>Schizandra Powder | Zheng Zhi Zhun Sheng | wu wei zi, ren shen (or dang shen), mai dong, xing ren, chen pi, sheng jiang, da zao |
| **Wu Yao Tang** 乌药汤<br>Lindera Decoction | Shen Shi Zun Sheng Shu | wu yao, xiang fu, mu xiang, dang gui, gan cao |
| **Wu Yi San** 芜荑散<br>Stinking Elm Paste Powder | Shi Yong Zhong Yao Xue | wu yi, lei wan, gan qi |
| **Wu Zhi An Zhong Yin** 五汁安中饮<br>Five Juice Drink to Calm the Middle | Zhong Yi Nei Ke Jiang Yi | fresh juice of jiu cai, sheng jiang, lotus root and pear, milk |
| **Wu Zhu Yu Tang** 吴茱萸汤<br>Evodia Decoction | Shang Han Lun | wu zhu yu, ren shen (or dang shen), sheng jiang, da zao |
| **Wu Zi Yan Zong Wan** 五子衍宗丸<br>Five Seed Pill to Amplify the Ancestors | She Sheng Zhong Miao Fang | tu si zi, gou qi zi, fu pen zi, che qian zi, wu wei zi |
| **Xi Tong Wan** 豨桐丸<br>Siegesbeckia & Clerodendron Pill | Ji Shi Yang Sheng Ji | xi xian cao, chou wu tong |
| **Xi Xian Jiu** 豨莶酒<br>Siegesbeckia Wine | Shi Yong Zhong Yao Xue | xi xian cao, cang er zi, hu tao ren, wu jia pi, di gu pi, hai feng teng, fang feng, jin yin hua, dang gui, hong hua, grain alcohol |
| **Xia Ku Cao Gao** 夏枯草膏<br>Prunella Syrup | Yi Zong Jin Jian | xia ku cao, zhe bei mu, xuan shen, kun bu, dang gui, bai jiang can, bai shao, wu yao, xiang fu, chen pi, gan cao, jie geng, chuan xiong, hong hua |
| **Xia Ku Cao San** 夏枯草散<br>Prunella Powder | Zhang Shi Yi Tong | xia ku cao, dang gui, bai shao, xuan shen, gan cao |
| **Xia Yu Xue Tang** 下瘀血汤<br>Purge Static Blood Decoction | Jin Gui Yao Lüe | da huang, tao ren, di bie chong |
| **Xian Fang Huo Ming Yin**† 仙方活命饮<br>Immortal's Formula for Sustaining Life | Jiao Zhu Fu Ren Liang Fang | jin yin hua, bai zhi, fang feng, gan cao, chi shao, dang gui wei, ru xiang, mo yao, chao zao jiao ci, zhe bei mu, tian hua fen, chen pi, chuan shan jia (now wang bu liu xing) |
| **Xian Ling Pi San** 仙灵脾散<br>Epimedium Powder | Tai Ping Sheng Hui Fang | xian ling pi, wei ling xian, cang er zi, rou gui, chuan xiong |

128

| Formula | Source text | Ingredients |
|---|---|---|
| **Xiang Lian Wan** 香连丸<br>Aucklandia & Coptis Pill | He Ji Ju Fang | huang lian (processed with wu zhu yu), mu xiang |
| **Xiang Ru San** 香薷散<br>Mosla Powder | He Ji Ju Fang | xiang ru, chao bian dou, hou po |
| **Xiang Sha Liu Jin Zi Tang** 香砂六君子汤<br>Six Gentlemen D. with Aucklandia & Amomum | He Ji Ju Fang | mu xiang, sha ren, ren shen (or dang shen), bai zhu, fu ling, zhi gan cao, zhi ban xia, chen pi |
| **Xiang Shen Wan** 香参丸<br>Aucklandia & Sophora flavescens Pill | Zhong Fu Tang Gong Xuan Liang Fang | mu xiang, ku shen, gan cao |
| **Xiang Su San** 香苏散<br>Cyperus & Perilla Leaf Powder | He Ji Ju Fang | xiang fu, zi su ye, chen pi, zhi gan cao |
| **Xiao Ban Xia Tang** 小半夏汤<br>Minor Pinellia Decoction | Jin Gui Yao Lüe | zhi ban xia, sheng jiang |
| **Xiao Chai Hu Tang** 小柴胡汤<br>Minor Bupleurum Decoction | Shang Han Lun | chai hu, huang qin, zhi ban xia, ren shen (or dang shen), gan cao, sheng jiang, da zao |
| **Xiao Cheng Qi Tang** 小承气汤<br>Minor Order the Qi Decoction | Shang Han Lun | da huang, hou po, zhi shi |
| **Xiao Feng San** 消风散<br>Eliminate Wind Powder | Wai Ke Zheng Zong | jing jie, fang feng, dang gui, sheng di huang, ku shen, cang zhu, chan tui, hei zhi ma, niu bang zi, zhi mu, shi gao, mu tong, gan cao |
| **Xiao Huo Luo Dan** 小活络丹<br>Minor Activate the Collaterals Special Pill | He Ji Ju Fang | zhi chuan wu, zhi cao wu, di long, zhi tian nan xing, ru xiang, mo yao |
| **Xiao Ji Yin Zi** 小蓟饮子<br>Small Thistle Drink | Ji Sheng Fang | sheng di huang, xiao ji, hua shi, mu tong, chao pu huang, ou jie, dan zhu ye, dang gui, shan zhi zi, zhi gan cao |
| **Xiao Jian Zhong Tang** 小建中汤<br>Minor Construct the Middle Decoction | Shang Han Lun | gui zhi, bai shao, sheng jiang, da zao, gan cao, yi tang |
| **Xiao Luo Wan** 消瘰丸<br>Reduce Scrophula Pill | Yi Xue Xin Wu | xuan shen, duan mu li, zhe bei mu |
| **Xiao Qing Long Tang** 小青龙汤<br>Minor Blue Green Dragon Decoction | Shang Han Lun | ma huang, gui zhi, bai shao, zhi ban xia, gan jiang, wu wei zi, xi xin, zhi gan cao |
| **Xiao Ru Tang†** 消乳汤<br>Disperse Breast [Lumps] Decoction | Yi Xue Zhong Zhong Can Xi Lu | zhi mu, lian qiao, jin yin hua, ru xiang, mo yao, dan shen, quan gua lou, chuan shan jia (now wang bu liu xiang) |
| **Xiao Xian Xiong Tang** 小陷胸汤<br>Minor D. [for Pathogens] Stuck in the Chest | Shang Han Lun | huang lian, zhi ban xia, quan gua lou |
| **Xiao Yao San** 逍遥散<br>Rambling Powder | He Ji Ju Fang | chai hu, dang gui, chao bai shao, chao bai zhu, fu ling, zhi gan cao, bo he, pao jiang |
| **Xiao Ying Tang** 消瘿汤<br>Eliminate Goitre Decoction | Zhong Yao Lin Chuang Shou Ce | huang yao zi, hai zao, kun bu, mu li, tu bei mu (土贝母 Bolbostematis Rhizoma; can use zhe bei mu) |
| **Xie Bai San** 泻白散<br>Drain the White Powder | Xiao Er Yao Zheng Zhi Jue | sang bai pi, di gu pi, gan cao, geng mi (rice) |
| **Xie Huang San** 泻黄散<br>Drain the Yellow Powder | Xiao Er Yao Zheng Zhi Jue | huo xiang, shan zhi zi, fang feng, shi gao, gan cao |
| **Xie Xin Tang** 泻心汤<br>Drain the Heart Decoction | Jin Gui Yao Lüe | da huang, huang lian, huang qin |
| **Xin Yi San** 辛夷散<br>Magnolia Flower Powder | Ji Sheng Fang | xin yi hua, bai zhi, xi xin, mu tong, chuan xiong, fang feng, gao ben, sheng ma, qiang huo, gan cao |
| **Xing Jun San†** 行军散<br>Marching Powder | Huo Luan Lun | niu huang, zhen zhu, bing pian, mang xiao, gold leaf, she xiang, peng sha, xiong huang |
| **Xing Pi Wan** 醒脾散<br>Awaken the Spleen Powder | Pu Ji Ben Shi Fang | tian ma, quan xie, fang feng, ren shen (or dang shen), bai zhu, hou po, rou gui, liu huang |
| **Xing Su San** 杏苏散<br>Apricot Seed & Perilla Powder | Wen Bing Tiao Bian | xing ren, zi su ye, zhi ban xia, fu ling, qian hu, jie geng, zhi ke, ju hong (or chen pi), gan cao, sheng jiang, da zao |
| **Xu Duan Wan** 续断丸<br>Dipsacus Pill | Pu Ji Ben Shi Fang | xu duan, du zhong, wu jia pi, yi yi ren, fang feng, huai niu xi, mu gua, bi xie, bai zhu, qiang huo, sheng di huang |
| **Xu Sui Zi Wan** 续随子丸<br>Caper Spurge Seed Pill | Yi Xue Fa Ming | qian jin zi, ren shen, mu xiang, han fang ji, chi fu ling, bing lang, hai jin sha, chao ting li zi, sang bai pi |
| **Xu Sui Zi Wan†** 续随子丸<br>Caper Spurge Seed Pill | Sheng Ji Zong Lu | qian jin zi, qing dai, qing fen |
| **Xuan Bi Tang** 宣痹汤<br>Disband Painful Obstruction Decoction | Wen Bing Tiao Bian | han fang ji, xing ren, hua shi, lian qiao, shan zhi zi, zhi ban xia, can sha, yi yi ren, chi xiao dou |
| **Xuan Du Fa Biao Tang** 宣毒发表汤<br>Dissipate Toxin & Release the Exterior Dec. | Yi Zong Jin Jian | sheng ma, ge gen, xing ren, lian qiao, niu bang zi, qian hu, fang feng, mu tong, zhu ye, jie geng, jing jie, zhi ke, bo he, gan cao |
| **Xuan Du San** 宣毒散<br>Dissipate Toxin Powder | Zheng Zhi Zhun Sheng | feng fang, cao wu, tian nan xing, chi xiao dou, bai fan, vinegar |
| **Xuan Fu Dai Zhe Tang** 旋复代赭汤<br>Inula & Hematite Decoction | Shang Han Lun | xuan fu hua, dai zhe shi, zhi ban xia, ren shen (or dang shen), sheng jiang, zhi gan cao, da zao |

| Formula | Source text | Ingredients |
|---|---|---|
| **Xuan Fu Hua Tang** 旋复花汤<br>Inula Decoction | Ji Sheng Fang | xuan fu hua, zhi ban xia, ju hong, gan jiang, bing lang, ren shen, bai zhu, zhi gan cao |
| **Xuan Qi San** 宣气散<br>Disband Qi Powder | Dan Xi Xin Fa | dong kui zi, shan zhi zi, hua shi, mu tong, gan cao shao, deng xin cao |
| **Xuan Shen Gan Jie Tang** 玄参甘桔汤<br>Scrophularia, Licorice & Platycodon Dec. | Zhong Yao Cheng Yao Zhi Ji Shou Ce | xuan shen, gan cao, jie geng, mai dong |
| **Xuan Yu Tong Jing Tang** 宣郁通经汤<br>Dissipate Constraint & Promotes Menses Dec. | Fu Qing Zhu Nu Ke | yu jin, chai hu, dang gui, bai shao, mu dan pi, shan zhi zi, huang qin, xiang fu, bai jie zi |
| **Xue Fu Zhu Yu Tang** 血府逐瘀汤<br>Disperse Stasis from the Mansion of Blood D. | Yi Lin Gai Cuo | dang gui, sheng di, chi shao, chuan xiong, tao ren, hong hua, chuan niu xi, chai hu, zhi ke, jie geng, gan cao |
| **Xue Jie San** 血竭散<br>Daemonorops Powder | Sheng Ji Zong Lu | xue jie, ru xiang, mo yao |
| **Yang He Tang** 阳和汤<br>Harmonious Yang Decoction | Wai Ke Zheng Zhi Quan Sheng Ji | shu di huang, bai jie zi, lu jiao jiao, rou gui, pao jiang, ma huang, gan cao |
| **Yang Qi Shi Wan** 阳起石丸<br>Actinolite Pill | He Ji Ju Fang | duan yang qi shi, gan jiang, wu zhu yu, shu di huang, huai niu xi, bai zhu |
| **Yang Qi Shi Wan** 阳起石丸<br>Actinolite Pill | Fu Ke Yu Chi | duan yang qi shi, tu si zi, lu rong, jiu cai zi, shi hu, chen xiang, rou cong rong, fu pen zi, sang ji sheng, wu wei zi, zhi fu zi |
| **Yang Ti Gen San** 羊蹄根散<br>Rumex Powder | Yi Zong Jin Jian | yang ti gen, bai fan |
| **Yang Xin Tang** 养心汤<br>Nourish the Heart Decoction | Zheng Zhi Zhun Sheng | ren shen (or dang shen), zhi huang qi, dang gui, chuan xiong, chao suan zao ren, chao bai zi ren, fu ling, fu shen, wu wei zi, zhi ban xia, yuan zhi, gan cao, rou gui |
| **Yang Yin Qing Fei Tang** 养阴清肺汤<br>Nourish Yin & Clear the Lungs Decoction | Chong Lou Yu Yao | sheng di huang, mai dong, xuan shen, bai shao, chuan bei mu, gan cao, mu dan pi, bo he |
| **Yang Zang Tang**† 养脏汤<br>Nourish the Organs Decoction | He Ji Ju Fang | rou dou kou, ren shen (or dang shen), bai zhu, rou gui, mu xiang, wei he zi, dang gui, zhi gan cao, zhi ying su ke |
| **Yi Fu San**† 一服散<br>One Dose Powder | Shi Yi De Xiao Fang | wu mei, zhi ban xia, e jiao, xing ren, zi su ye, gan cao, sheng jiang, zhi ying su ke |
| **Yi Guan Jian** 一贯煎<br>Linking Decoction | Xu Ming Yi Lei An | bei sha shen, mai dong, sheng di huang, gou qi zi, dang gui, chuan lian zi |
| **Yi Huang Tang** 易黄汤<br>Benefit the Yellow Decoction | Fu Qing Zhu Nu Ke | huang bai, qian shi, bai guo, chao shan yao, che qian zi |
| **Yi Mu Sheng Jin Dan** 益母生金丹<br>Motherwort Special Pill to Produce Gold | Yi Xue Xin Wu | yi mu cao, chong wei zi, dang gui, shu di huang, bai shao, chuan xiong, dan shen, bai zhu, xiang fu |
| **Yi Pi Bing** 益脾饼<br>Augment the Spleen Cake | Yi Xue Zhong Zhong Can Xi Lu | bai zhu, gan jiang, ji nei jin, da zao, wheat flour |
| **Yi Qi Cong Ming Tang** 益气聪明汤<br>Augment the Qi & Improve Vision Decoction | Zheng Zhi Zhun Sheng | huang qi, ren shen (or dang shen), ge gen, man jing zi, bai shao, huang bai, sheng ma, zhi gan cao |
| **Yi Wei Tang** 益胃汤<br>Augment the Stomach Decoction | Wen Bing Tiao Bian | nan sha shen, mai dong, yu zhu, sheng di huang, yi tang |
| **Yi Yi Fu Zi Bai Jiang San** 薏苡附子败酱散<br>Coix, Aconite & Patrinia Powder | Jin Gui Yao Lüe | yi yi ren, zhi fu zi, bai jiang cao |
| **Yi Yi Ren Tang** 薏苡仁汤<br>Coix Decoction | Ming Yi Zhi Zhang | yi yi ren, cang zhu, ma huang, dang gui, gui zhi, bai shao, zhi gan cao |
| **Yi Zhi San** 益智散<br>Alpinia Powder | Zheng Zhi Zhun Sheng | yi zhi ren, sha ren, ren shen (or dang shen), bai zhu, huang qi, fu ling, huo xiang, dang gui, zhi fu zi, ding xiang, hou po, gao liang jiang, chuan xiong, chen pi, rou gui, sheng jiang, da zao |
| **Yin Chen Hao Tang** 茵陈蒿汤<br>Virgate Wormwood Decoction | Shang Han Lun | yin chen hao, shan zhi zi, da huang |
| **Yin Chen Si Ni Tang** 茵陈四逆汤<br>Virgate Wormwood D. for Frigid Extremities | Zhang Shi Yi Tong | yin chen hao, zhi fu zi, gan jiang, gan cao |
| **Yin Chen Wu Ling San** 茵陈五苓散<br>Virgate Wormwood & Five Ingredient Powder | Jin Gui Yao Lüe | yin chen hao, fu ling, zhu ling, ze xie, bai zhu, gui zhi |
| **Yin Chen Zhu Fu Tang** 茵陈术附汤<br>Virgate Wormwood, Atractylodes & Aconite D. | Yi Xue Xin Wu | yin chen hao, bai zhu, gan jiang, zhi fu zi, rou gui, zhi gan cao |
| **Yin Qiao San** 银翘散<br>Lonicera & Forsythia Powder | Wen Bing Tiao Bian | jin yin hua, lian qiao, bo he, jie geng, niu bang zi, jing jie, zhu ye, lu gen, dan dou chi, gan cao |
| **You Gui Wan** 右归丸<br>Restore the Right [Kidney] Pill | Jing Yue Quan Shu | shu di huang, shan zhu yu, shan yao, gou qi zi, du zhong, tu si zi, zhi fu zi, rou gui, dang gui, lu jiao jiao |
| **Yu Dai Wan** 愈带丸<br>Cure Discharge Pill | Shang Hai Shi Yao Pi Bian Zhun | chun pi, bai shao, gao liang jiang tan, huang bai tan |
| **Yu Guan Wan** 玉关丸<br>Jade Gate Pill | Jing Yue Quan Shu | wu bei zi, he zi, wu wei zi, bai fan |
| **Yu Li Ren Tang** 郁李仁汤<br>Bush Cherry Seed Decoction | Sheng Ji Zong Lu | yu li ren, sang bai pi, chi xiao dou, chen pi, zi su ye, bai mao gen |

| Formula | Source text | Ingredients |
|---|---|---|
| **Yu Nu Jian** 玉女煎<br>Jade Woman Decoction | Jing Yue Quan Shu | shi gao, shu di huang, mai dong, zhi mu, huai niu xi |
| **Yu Ping Feng San** 玉屏风散<br>Jade Wind Screen Powder | Dan Xi Xin Fa | huang qi, bai zhu, fang feng |
| **Yu Quan Wan** 玉泉丸<br>Jade Spring Pill | Za Bing Yuan Liu Xi Zhu | ge gen, tian hua fen, mai dong, ren shen, fu ling, wu mei, huang qi, zhi huang qi, gan cao |
| **Yu Ye Tang** 玉液汤<br>Jade Fluid Decoction | Yi Xue Zhong Zhong Can Xi Lu | shan yao, huang qi, zhi mu, ji nei jin, wu wei zi, tian hua fen, ge gen |
| **Yu Zhen San** 玉真散<br>True Jade Powder | Wai Ke Zheng Zong | zhi tian nan xing, zhi bai fu zi, bai zhi, tian ma, qiang huo |
| **Yue Bi Jia Zhu Tang** 越婢加术汤<br>Maidservant from Yue's D. plus Atractylodes | Jin Gui Yao Lüe | ma huang, shi gao, sheng jiang, bai zhu, gan cao, da zao |
| **Yue Hua Wan**† 月华丸<br>Moonlight Pill | Yi Xue Xin Wu | sheng di huang, shu di huang, tian dong, mai dong, nan sha shen, bai he, chuan bei mu, shan yao, fu ling, e jiao, san qi, ju hua, sang ye, ta gan (獭肝 otter liver) |
| **Yue Ju Wan** 越鞠丸<br>Escape Restraint Pill | Dan Xi Xin Fa | xiang fu, chuan xiong, cang zhu, shan zhi zi, shen qu |
| **Yun Nan Bai Yao** 云南白药<br>Yunnan White Medicine | Prepared medicine | san qi, other ingredients proprietary secret |
| **Zai Zao San** 再造散<br>Renewal Power | Shang Han Liu Shu | huang qi, ren shen (or dang shen), gui zhi, gan cao, zhi fu zi, xi xin, qiang huo, fang feng, chuan xiong, bai shao, pao jiang, da zao |
| **Zan Yu Dan** 赞育丹<br>Special Pill to Aid Fertility | Jing Yue Quan Shu | shu di huang, bai zhu, dang gui, gou qi zi, du zhong, xian ling pi, xian mao, ba ji tian, shan zhu yu, rou cong rong, jiu cai zi, she chuang zi, zhi fu zi, rou gui |
| **Zao Jia Wan** 皂荚丸<br>Gleditsia Fruit Pill | Jin Gui Yao Lüe | zao jia, feng mi, da zao |
| **Ze Lan Tang** 泽兰汤<br>Bugleweed Decoction | Zhong Yi Fu Ke Jing Yan Fang Xuan | ze lan, hong hua, xiang fu, dang gui, xu duan, bai zi ren, chi shao, huai niu xi, yan hu suo |
| **Ze Xie Tang** 泽泻汤<br>Alisma Decoction | Jin Gui Yao Lüe | ze xie, chao bai zhu |
| **Zeng Ye Cheng Qi Tang** 增液承气汤<br>Increase Fluids & Order the Qi Decoction | Wen Bing Tiao Bian | sheng di huang, xuan shen, mai dong, da huang, mang xiao |
| **Zeng Ye Tang** 增液汤<br>Increase Fluids Decoction | Wen Bing Tiao Bian | sheng di huang, xuan shen, mai dong |
| **Zhen Gan Xi Feng Tang** 镇肝熄风汤<br>Sedate the Liver & Extinguish Wind Dec. | Yi Xue Zhong Zhong Can Xi Lu | huai niu xi, dai zhe shi, long gu, mu li, gui ban, bai shao, xuan shen, tian dong, chuan lian zi, mai ya, yin chen hao, gan cao |
| **Zhen Ling Dan**† 震灵丹<br>Astonishingly Effective Special Pill | He Ji Ju Fang | chi shi zhi, yu yu liang, zi shi ying, dai zhe shi, wu ling zhi, ru xiang, mo yao, zhu sha |
| **Zhen Ni Tang** 镇逆汤<br>Suppress Rebellion Decoction | Yi Xue Zhong Zhong Can Xi Lu | dai zhe shi, bai shao, long dan cao, zhi ban xia, ren shen (or dang shen), qing dai, sheng jiang, wu zhu yu |
| **Zhen Wu Tang** 真武汤<br>True Warrior Decoction | Shang Han Lun | zhi fu zi, bai zhu, fu ling, bai shao, sheng jiang |
| **Zhen Yuan Yin** 贞元饮<br>Original & Faithful Drink | Jing Yue Quan Shu | shu di huang, dang gui, zhi gan cao |
| **Zhen Zhu Mu Wan** 珍珠母丸<br>Mother of Pearl Pill | Pu Ji Ben Shi Fang | zhen zhu mu, dang gui, shu di huang, ren shen, suan zao ren, bai zi ren, fu shen, chen xiang, shui niu jiao, long chi |
| **Zhen Zhu San** 真珠散<br>True Pearl Powder | Zheng Zhi Zhun Sheng | zhen zhu, qing xiang zi, huang qin, ren shen (or dang shen), ju hua, shi jue ming, chuan xiong, zhi gan cao |
| **Zheng Gu Tang Yao** 正骨烫药<br>Repair Bones Decoction | Zhong Yi Shang Ke Jiang Yi | tou gu cao, gu sui bu, xu duan, mo yao, ru xiang, qiang huo, hong hua, bai zhi, fang feng, mu gua, hua jiao |
| **Zhi Bai Di Huang Wan** 知柏地黄丸<br>Anemarrhena, Phellodendron & Rehmannia Pill | Jing Yue Quan Shu | zhi mu, huang bai, shu di huang, shan zhu yu, shan yao, mu dan pi, fu ling, ze xie |
| **Zhi Bao Dan**† 至宝丹<br>Greatest Treasure Special Pill | He Ji Ju Fang | hu po, bing pian, niu huang, an xi xiang, gold leaf, silver leaf, xi jiao (now shui niu jiao), dai mao, zhu sha, xiong huang, she xiang |
| **Zhi Gan Cao Tang** 炙甘草汤<br>Prepared Licorice Decoction | Shang Han Lun | zhi gan cao, ren shen (or dang shen), sheng di huang, e jiao, gui zhi, mai dong, huo ma ren, sheng jiang, da zao |
| **Zhi Jing San** 止痉散<br>Stop Spasm Powder | Liu Xing Xing Yi Xing Nao Yan Zhong Yi Zhi Liao Fa | quan xie, wu gong |
| **Zhi Shi Dao Zhi Wan** 枳实导滞丸<br>Unripe Orange Pill to Guide Out Stagnation | Nei Wai Shang Bian Huo Lun | zhi shi, da huang, shen qu, fu ling, huang qin, huang lian, bai zhu, ze xie |

| Formula | Source text | Ingredients |
|---|---|---|
| **Zhi Shi Xiao Pi Wan** 枳实消痞丸<br>Unripe Orange Pill to Reduce Distension | Lan Shi Mi Cang | zhi shi, gan jiang, huang lian, hou po, mai ya, fu ling, bai zhu, ban xia qu, ren shen, zhi gan cao |
| **Zhi Shi Xie Bai Gui Zhi Tang** 枳实薤白桂枝汤<br>Unripe Orange, Chive & Cinnamon D. | Jin Gui Yao Lüe | zhi shi, xie bai, gui zhi, quan gua lou, hou po |
| **Zhi Sou San** 止嗽散<br>Stop Cough Powder | Yi Xue Xin Wu | bai bu, bai qian, zi wan, jie geng, chen pi, jing jie, gan cao |
| **Zhi Zhu Wan** 枳术丸<br>Unripe Orange & Atractylodes Pill | Pi Wei Lun | zhi shi, bai zhu |
| **Zhi Zi Bai Pi Tang** 栀子柏皮汤<br>Gardenia & Phellodendron Decoction | Shang Han Lun | shang zhi zi, huang bai, zhi gan cao |
| **Zhi Zi Chi Tang** 栀子豉汤<br>Gardenia & Prepared Soybean Decoction | Shang Han Lun | shan zhi zi, dan dou chi |
| **Zhong Ru Bu Fei Tang** 钟乳补肺汤<br>Stalactite Decoction to Supplement Lungs | He Ji Ju Fang | zhong ru shi, sang bai pi, mai dong, zi shi ying, ren shen (or dang shen), wu wei zi, kuan dong hua, rou gui, zi wan |
| **Zhong Ru Wan** 钟乳丸<br>Stalactite Pill | Zhang Shi Yi Tong | zhong ru shi, xing ren, ma huang, gan cao, feng mi |
| **Zhong Ru Tang** 钟乳汤<br>Stalactite Decoction | Jing Yan Fang | zhong ru shi, tian hua fen, lou lu, tong cao |
| **Zhou Che Wan**† 舟车丸<br>Vessel & Vehicle Pill | Jing Yue Quan Shu | qian niu zi, gan sui, cu yuan hua, cu hong da ji, da huang, qing pi, chen pi, mu xiang, bing lang, qing fen |
| **Zhu Gen San** 苎根散<br>Boehmeria Powder | Sheng Ji Zong Lu | zhu ma gen, ren shen (or dang shen), hai ge qiao, bai e 白垩 (chalk) |
| **Zhu Gen Tang** 苎根汤<br>Boehmeria Decoction | Xiao Pin Fang | zhu ma gen, dang gui, bai shao, sheng di huang, e jiao, gan cao |
| **Zhu Huang San** 珠黄散<br>Pearl & Cattle Gallstone Powder | Shang Hai Shi Yao Pi Bian Zhun | zhen zhu, niu huang |
| **Zhu Jing Wan** 驻景丸<br>Preserve Vistas Pill | Zheng Zhi Zhun Sheng | tu si zi, shu di huang, che qian zi, gou qi zi |
| **Zhu Li Da Tan Wan** 竹沥达痰丸<br>Bamboo Sap Pill to Thrust Out Phlegm | Shen Shi Zun Sheng Shu | zhu li, sheng jiang, zhi ban xia, chen pi, bai zhu, da huang, mang xiao, huang qin, qing meng shi, chen xiang, ren shen, fu ling, zhi gan cao |
| **Zhu Li Hua Tan Wan** 竹沥化痰丸<br>Bamboo Sap Pill to Transform Phlegm | Wan Bing Hui Chun | zhu li, dan nan xing, zhi ban xia, zhi shi, chen pi, bai zhu, cang zhu, tao ren, hong hua, xing ren, bai jie zi, cu hong da ji, cu yuan hua, gan sui, huang bai, jiu da huang |
| **Zhu Ling Tang** 猪苓汤<br>Polyporus Decoction | Shang Han Lun | zhu ling, fu ling, ze xie, hua shi, e jiao |
| **Zhu Ye Liu Bang Tang** 竹叶柳蒡汤<br>Phyllostachys, Tamarisk & Burdock Seed D. | Xian Xing Zhai Yi Xue Guang Bi Ji | zhu ye, xi he liu (西河柳 Tamaricis Cacumen), chan tui, niu bang zi, ge gen, xuan shen, mai dong, zhi mu, jing jie, bo he, gan cao |
| **Zhu Ye Shi Gao Tang** 竹叶石膏汤<br>Phyllostachys & Gypsum Decoction | Shang Han Lun | zhu ye, shi gao, ren shen, mai dong, zhi ban xia, gan cao, rice |
| **Zi Cao Xiao Du Yin** 紫草消毒饮<br>Lithospermum Drink to Eliminate Toxin | Zhang Shi Yi Tong | zi cao, lian qiao, niu bang zi, jing jie, shan dou gen, gan cao |
| **Zi Cao You** 紫草油<br>Lithospermum Oil | Zhong Yi Wai Ke Xue | zi cao, bai zhi, ren dong teng, bing pian, |
| **Zi Jin Ding**† 紫金锭<br>Purple & Gold Tablet | Wan Shi Ni Zhuan Pian Yu Xin Shu | shan ci gu, wu bei zi, qian jin zi, hong da ji, she xiang (now ren gong she xiang), xiong huang, zhu sha |
| **Zi Ling Wan** 紫灵丸<br>Purple Ganoderma Pill | Sheng Ji Zong Lu | ling zhi, bai zi ren, zhi shi, ba ji tian, fu ling, ren shen, sheng di huang, mai dong, wu wei zi, zhi ban xia, mu dan pi, zhi fu zi, yuan zhi, ze xie, dong gua zi |
| **Zi Ran Tong San** 自然铜散<br>Pyrite Powder | Zhang Shi Yi Tong | duan zi ran tong, ru xiang, mo yao, dang gui, qiang huo, gu sui bu |
| **Zi Shi Ying Wan** 紫石英丸<br>Fluorite Pill | Sheng Ji Zong Lu | zi shi ying, lu rong, yu yu liang, dang gui, chuan xiong, zhi ke, ai ye, e jiao zhu, chi shao, gui zhi, bai zhi, mu xiang, ce bai ye, hai piao xiao |
| **Zi Wan Tang** 紫菀汤<br>Aster Decoction | Yi Fang Ji Jie | zi wan, zhi mu, chuan bei mu, e jiao zhu, jie geng, ren shen (or dang shen), fu ling, wu wei zi, gan cao |
| **Zi Xue Dan**† 紫雪丹<br>Purple Snow Special Pill | He Ji Ju Fang | shi gao, han shui shi, hua shi, ci shi, chen xiang, xuan shen, sheng ma, ding xiang, mang xiao, zhi gan cao, xi jiao (now shui niu jiao), ling yang jiao, qing mu xiang, she xiang, zhu sha, po xiao |
| **Zi Xue Tang** 滋血汤<br>Enrich the Blood Decoction | San Yin Ji Yi Bing Zheng Fang Lun | chi shao, mu dan pi, dang gui, chuan xiong, ma bian cao, jing jie, zhi ke, rou gui |
| **Zuo Gui Wan** 左归丸<br>Restore the Left [Kidney] Pill | Jing Yue Quan Shu | shu di huang, shan yao, gou qi zi, shan zhu yu, huai niu xi, tu si zi, lu jiao jiao, gui ban jiao |
| **Zuo Jin Wan** 左金丸<br>Left Metal Pill | Dan Xi Xin Fa | jiang huang lian, yan wu zhu yu |

**Abscess** (*yōng* 痈; *jū* 疽) An abscess is an intense localized collection of toxic heat that destroys tissue and creates pus. Abscesses can occur on the skin or affect the internal organs. In Chinese medicine the term includes not only encapsulated suppurative lesions, but also localized areas of redness, swelling and suppuration. There are two types of abscess, yang and yin. Yang abscesses are acute, raised, hot, painful and can change rapidly. Any discharge is thick, colored and malodorous. Yin abscesses (also described as yin sores) are chronic, flat, not especially painful and not noticeably warmer than the surrounding skin. They may ooze a thin, watery inoffensive material. A Chinese medically defined yang abscess may be diagnosed biomedically as acne, boils and carbuncles, but also cellulitis, erysipelas and mastitis, as well as severe respiratory infections, pelvic inflammatory disease and so on. Yin sores may be diagnosed as chronic localized infections, chronic abscess or chronic osteomyelitis. Also known as a welling abscess or flat abscess (Wiseman 1998).

**Accumulation disorder** (*gān jí* 疳积) Accumulation disorder is a disorder of children, previously associated with various forms of malnutrition and the development of the characteristic pot belly with scrawny limbs, sallow complexion and so on. Also known as childhood nutritional impairment (Bensky 2009) and gan accumulation (Wiseman 1998). The modern clinical definition has been expanded to include a variety of symptoms associated with overloading of the immature childhood digestive system with excessive or inappropriate foods, resulting in a blockage to the qi dynamic, and the generation of phlegm and heat. Children typically present with round firm abdomens, abdominal pain, mucus problems, irritability, and digestive and behavioral problems.

**Aids discharge of pus** (*pái nóng* 排脓) Encourages suppurative sores to form a head and rupture.

**Aids Gallbladder function** (*lì dǎn* 利胆) Improves secretion of bile, and the movement of qi through the Liver Gallbladder organ system.

**Aids Kidney in grasping qi** (*nà qì* 纳气) Treats wheezing and asthma of a chronic Kidney deficiency type.

**Alleviates dysuria** (*tōng lín* 通淋) Treats lin syndrome of various types.

**Alleviates food stagnation** (*xiāo shí* 消食) Improves digestion and transit of food through the Stomach and Intestines.

**Alleviates hyperacidity** (*zhǐ suān* 止酸)

**Alleviates jaundice** (*tuì huáng* 退黄)

**Alleviates spasm** (*jiě jìng* 解痉) A treatment method that relieves muscle spasm and rigidity, as well as tremors and convulsions. Also known as resolves tetany (Wiseman 1998) and releases spasms (Bensky 2009).

**Alleviates toxicity** (*jiě dú* 解毒) Mitigates the unwanted or toxic effects of some herbs, and alleviates food poisoning.

**Alleviates wheezing** (*píng chuǎn* 平喘) Treats wheezing mostly associated with excess patterns. See also Aids Kidney in grasping qi.

**Ascites** Fluid accumulation in the abdominal cavity, usually as the result of yang deficiency or blockage of the Triple Burner by damp heat or blood stasis. Generally synonymous with drum-like abdominal distension (*gǔ zhàng* 鼓胀).

**Astringes bleeding** (*shōu liǎn zhǐ xuè* 收敛止血) Stops bleeding by contracting vessels and tissues. Can be used for all types of bleeding, except blood stasis.

**Astringes fluid leakage** (*gù sè* 固涩) Stops fluid leakage (sweat, urine, vaginal) by toning and contracting tissues.

**Astringes the Lungs** (*liǎn fèi* 敛肺) Restrains leakage of Lung qi to stop cough from deficiency.

**Augments essence and blood** (*yì jīng xuè* 益精血) Although jing cannot be replaced, its consumption can be slowed by the use of dense substances with a 'meaty' richness. These substances also promote the generation of blood via their action on jing and hence, the marrow.

**Augments the Kidneys** (*yì shèn* 益肾) Augmenting the Kidneys refers to a mild yin nourishing action not as strong or potentially cloying as tonifying, and without the greasy richness of the major yin tonic herbs.

**Bai he disease** (*bǎi hé bìng* 百合病) An ancient disorder first described in the Essentials from the Golden Cabinet (*Jin Gui Yao Lüe*), characterized primarily by emotional and mental symptoms. The patient is taciturn, sleepy but is unable to sleep, desires to walk but is too weak, wants to eat but cannot tolerate the smell of food, has poor temperature regulation and is easily cold or overheated, is restless and mutters to themselves. May be diagnosed as depression or other psychological disorder. Also known as Lilium syndrome (Maciocia 2008) and Lily bulb disorder (Bensky 2004).

**Benefits hearing** (*cōng ěr* 聪耳) Treats tinnitus and hearing loss from various causes.

**Binds the Intestines** (*sè cháng* 涩肠) Harnesses the gathering and contracting nature of astringency to tone and tighten intestinal tissues to stop chronic diarrhea and alleviate prolapse.

**Breaks up blood stasis** (*pò xuè zhú yū* 破血逐瘀) The most powerful blood stasis dispersing action, and one that carries significant potential to damage normal qi and blood. Not suitable for prolonged use.

**Breaks up stagnant qi** (*pò qì* 破气) The most powerful of the qi mobilizing actions, with potential to damage normal qi. For relatively severe qi stagnation anywhere in the body. Excellent for quickly and powerfully mobilizing qi, but not suitable for long term use.

**Brightens the eyes** (*míng mù* 明目) A generic term describing herbs that improve a variety of visual parameters, including weakness and loss of vision, obstruction by cataracts or nebulae, and infection.

**Buerger's disease** A condition of the extremities characterized by impaired blood circulation, necrosis, with eventual tissue death and ulceration. Usually attributed to blood stasis as a result of damp heat or phlegm collecting in the channels, or depletion of yin from ingestion of heating and drying substances (especially tobacco). Similar to gangrene (*tuō jū* 脱疽), which is also known as sloughing flat abscess (Wiseman 1998) and sloughing ulcer (Bensky 2009).

**Calcining** (*duàn* 煅) Involves heating of a substance, usually a mineral or shell, to a high temperature to cause loss of moisture or decomposition of the calcium carbonate fraction to calcium oxide. The process increases astringency and facilitates pulverization, and extraction of active components when decocted.

**Calms a restless fetus** (*ān tāi* 安胎) The term restless fetus implies a threatened miscarriage, so herbs that calm fetal restlessness can assist in alleviating abdominal pain and bleeding during pregnancy.

**Calms the Liver** (*píng gān* 平肝) Reduces the Livers' tendency to excessive exuberance, qi constraint and ascendant yang. A mild to moderate effect on pacifying ascendant yang, usually facilitated by herbs that soften the Liver, replenish yin or in some way restore the normal free flow of Liver qi. See also Pacifies ascendant yang.

**Calms and sedates the *shen*** (*ān shén zhèn jīng* 安神镇静) Usually minerals that heavily weigh down and sedate an unstable or manic *shen* that is disturbed by heat, phlegm or ascendant yang.

**Calms the *shen*** (*ān shén* 安神) Usually nourishing herbs that tonify yin and blood to provide a firm foundation for, and thus assist in anchoring, the *shen*.

**Cervical lymphadenitis** (*luǒ lì* 瘰疬) Traditionally this term refers to tuberculosis of the cervical lymph nodes, also known as scrofula or the Kings evil in previous times. Cervical lymphadenitis is used here because the herbs used to treat *luǒ lì* can also be applied effectively for the more commonly seen inflammation, swelling and nodulation of lymph nodes from causes other than tuberculosis.

**Checks malarial disorder** (*jié nüè* 截疟) *see* Malarial disorder

**Clears damp heat** (*qīng rè zào shī* 清热燥湿; *qīng shī rè* 清湿热)

**Clears deficient heat** (*tuì xū rè* 退虚热) Alleviates heat generated by deficiency of yin or blood.

**Clears Heart fire** (*xiè xīn huŏ* 泻心火) A method of treating strong heat in the Heart generated by qi constraint, pent up emotion or heat transferred from the Liver via the *sheng* cycle.

**Clears heat** (*qīng rè* 清热) A generic terms for cooling herbs.

**Clears Stomach heat/fire** (*qīng wèi rè* 清胃热)

**Clears the nose and sinuses** (*tōng bí qiào* 通鼻窍; *tōng qiào* 通窍) Treats nasal congestion and accumulation of phlegm or phlegm heat in the sinuses.

**Clears toxic heat** (*qīng rè jiě dú* 清热解毒) Herbs designated as toxic heat clearing may do one or all of: **1.** treat suppurative sores and other festering lesions; **2.** alleviate systemic 'toxicity' (illnesses presenting with high fever, malaise, disturbances of consciousness, skin rashes and so on); **3.** alleviate and repair the damage done by burns and scalds, usually applied topically; **4.** treat erythematous skin disorders.

**Closed disorder** (*bì zhèng* 闭证) Loss of consciousness with increased muscle tone – clenched jaw and fists, clonic spasm of the extremities – as a result of wind stroke, fever or syncope. Can be associated with heat or cold pathology. Also known as impediment pattern (Wiseman 1998) and closed type stroke (Bensky 2009). See also Flaccid collapse.

**Common cold** (*găn mào* 感冒) The various manifestations of the common cold. In Chinese medicine a variety of different pathogens can cause common cold, but they are characteristically mild and self limiting, in contrast to warm diseases, which may appear initially to be similar, but tend to be more severe and persistent.

**Cools the blood** (*liáng xuè* 凉血) Clears heat from the blood resulting from both heat excess and yin deficiency conditions.

**Cools the Heart** (*qīng xīn* 清心) A method of treating heat in the Heart generated by yin deficiency. See also Clears Heart fire.

**Cools the Liver** (*qīng gān* 清肝) Treats heat and fire generated by constrained qi or heat introduced through the diet.

**Cools the Lungs** (*qīng fèi* 清肺; *qīng xiè fèi rè* 清泄肺热) Treats heat or phlegm heat patterns of the Lungs.

**Diabetes** (*xiāo kě* 消渴) Refers to disorders characterized by excessive thirst, hunger and urination. May be diagnosed as diabetes mellitus, or rarely, diabetes insipidus. Also known as wasting and thirsting disorder (Bensky 2009) and dispersion–thirst (Wiseman 1998).

**Diffuse fluid retention syndrome** (*yì yǐn* 溢饮) A condition characterized by edema of the limbs accompanied by chills, myalgia, absence of sweating. Also known as flooding thin mucus (Bensky 2009) and spillage rheum (Wiseman 1998).

**Diffuses the Lungs** (*xuān fèi* 宣肺) Promotes the aspect of Lung function that distributes fluids and qi towards the exterior and surface of the body.

**Directs blood and fire down** (*yǐn xuè yǐn huŏ xià xíng* 引血引火下行) A method used to pull heat and ascendant yang away from the head and towards the lower body; used for upper body bleeding, headache, dizziness and so on.

**Directs qi downward** (*xià qì* 下气; *jiàng qì* 降气) Causes qi to move downwards in the body. Used in the treatment of bloating and constipation, and when natural descent of qi is blocked causing cough, wheezing, bloating, nausea and vomiting.

**Dispels cold** (*sàn hán* 散寒) A method of eliminating cold from the exterior of the body. Utilizes pungency and warmth to eject superficial cold on the surface or in the channels. Used in the treatment of wind cold common cold patterns and cold type bi syndrome.

**Dispels summerheat** (*jiě shŭ* 解暑)

**Dispels wind** (*qū fēng* 祛风) Eliminating or extinguishing wind from the surface and smooth muscles with acrid mild herbs.

**Dispels wind cold** (*sàn fēng hán* 散风寒) Eliminating wind and cold from the surface layers with acrid warm herbs.

**Dispels wind damp** (*qū fēng shī* 祛风湿; *sàn fēng shī* 散风湿)

**Dispels wind heat** (*shū sàn fēng rè* 疏散风热; *xuān sàn fēng rè* 宣散风热) A method of eliminating wind and heat from the surface layers with acrid cool herbs.

**Dispels wind phlegm** (*qū huà fēng tán* 祛化风痰) A method of treating the effects of wind phlegm, such as the sudden onset of vertigo, headaches, disturbance of consciousness and hemiplegia.

**Disperses blood stasis** (*sàn yū* 散瘀; *qū yū* 祛瘀) The middle level of blood activation and stasis removal, with strength in between regulating blood (*huó xuè* 活血) and breaking up blood stasis (*pò xuè* 破血). A moderately strong blood stasis dispersing effect, with the possibility of side effects and dispersal of normal qi and blood if overused.

**Disperses cold** (*sàn hán wēn zhōng* 散寒温中) A method of warming and counteracting internal cold in the chest, abdomen and uterus. The same Chinese character is used for dispels cold, above, but the area of influence and mode of action is different.

**Disperses phlegm** (*xiāo tán* 消痰) A method to break up phlegm accumulation in the extremities and joints, and in nodules.

**Dissipates masses** (*sàn jié* 散结) Treats localized accumulations of phlegm and/or blood stasis.

**Dissolves stones** (*pái shí* 排石) The characters actually mean eject stones, but in fact the treatment of stones is a slow process that gradually whittles them away until they can be discharged by natural physiological processes.

**Domain** (*guī jīng* 归经) The area of influence of a herb, which includes the organ system and channel pathway, its related tissues and sense organs.

**Drains fluid from Lungs** (*xiè fèi* 泻肺) A powerful method of driving fluids downwards and out through the Bladder, used in the treatment of severe wheezing, pulmonary edema and orthopnea.

**Drains Kidney fire** (*qīng shèn huŏ* 清肾火) A method of clearing a type of Kidney heat (ministerial fire) that gives rise to premature ejaculation and involuntary seminal emission.

**Dredges the Liver** (*shū gān* 疏肝) Restores the normal free flow of Liver qi. Alleviates qi constraint. Herbs that dredge the Liver have a specific effect on qi constraint resulting from pent up emotion.

**Dries damp** (*zào shī* 燥湿) Utilizes pungency to dry dampness in situ. The strongest drying herbs are considered 'parching' (cang zhu in particular), an effect that carries a likelihood of damage to fluids and yin. See also transforms damp.

**Drives out phlegm** (*zhú tán* 逐痰) A method of eliminating phlegm that utilizes the 'big exit', i.e. the bowel, resulting in swift discharge. Used for severe or emergency situations with phlegm in the upper body affecting the Heart (as in mania) or the head (a type of wind stroke) that must be quickly driven down and out.

**Dysenteric disorder** (*lì jí* 痢疾) A disorder characterized by urgent diarrhea with mucus and/or pus and/or blood. May be associated with infections such as amebic or bacterial dysentery, or with inflammatory conditions such as ulcerative colitis and Crohn's disease.

**Dysuria** (*lín zhèng* 淋证) Also known as painful urination syndrome, this group of disorders is characterized by pain or discomfort around urination.

**Eases the throat** (*lì hóu* 利喉) This term has a broad meaning, and includes treating sore throat, and alleviating hoarseness and loss of voice.

**Eruptive disease** (*shā qì* 痧气) Acute seasonal infectious disorders occurring in late summer, characterized by violent abdominal pain, vomiting, diarrhea and skin rash. Caused by virulent summerheat pathogens. May be diagnosed biomedically as measles and scarlet fever.

**Erysipelas** (*dān dú* 丹毒; *huŏ dú* 火毒) A condition characterized by acute onset of redness, swelling, heat and pain of the skin. The lesion enlarges rapidly and has a sharply demarcated raised edge.

Accompanied by fever, chills, nausea, vomiting and general illness. This may occur anywhere, but most often seen on the face and extremities. Usually attributed to a collection of intense wind or damp toxic heat invading the blood. Also known as cinnabar toxin (Wiseman 1998) and fire toxin (Bensky 2009). See also Abscess, and Clears toxic heat.

**Essence** (*jīng* 精) In broad terms the template inherited from both parents that determines ones constitutional vitality; in narrow terms sperm. The quantity of inherited essence is fixed at birth and cannot be replaced, but its use (it is consumed by living) can be slowed.

**Excess fluid in the hypochondrium and epigastrium** (*zhī yǐn* 支饮) One of the thin mucus disorders, in which pathological fluids accumulate in the Lungs causing wheezing and orthopnea. Also known as prodding thin mucus (Bensky 2009) and propping rheum (Wiseman 1998).

**Expels phlegm** (*qū tán* 祛痰) Encourage expectoration of phlegm from the Lungs.

**Exterior releasing** (*fā hàn jiě biǎo* 发汗解表) These acrid dispersing herbs dispel pathogens from the surface layers by opening the pores and encouraging sweating.

**Extinguishes wind** (*xī fēng* 息风) Alleviates the manifestations of internally generated wind – tics, tremors, spasms, involuntary movements and convulsions.

**Fèi láo** (肺劳) A chronic wasting disease of the Lungs, characterized by cough, hemoptysis, sweating and weakness. Includes biomedical disorders such as tuberculosis, but also may be associated with other chronic consumptive respiratory illnesses. Also known as Lung taxation (Wiseman 1998) and Lung consumption disorder (Bensky 2009).

**Fèi láo** (肺痨) Tuberculosis.

**Fetal restlessness** (*tāi dòng bù ān* 胎动不安) This term describes problems during pregnancy, including abdominal and lumbar pain, a heavy or bearing down sensation and/or vaginal bleeding. It is a euphemism for threatened miscarriage. Also known as stirring fetus (Wiseman 1998).

**Flaccid collapse** (*tuō zhèng* 脱证) Loss of consciousness with decreased muscle tone – incontinence of bladder and bowels, sagging jaw, flaccid limbs and profuse sweating – as a result of severe collapse of yang. Known as desertion pattern (Wiseman 1998) and abandoned pattern (Bensky 2009). Similar to shock. See also Closed disorder.

**Fortifies the exterior** (*gù biǎo* 固表) Improves the ability of the pores to stay closed and protects against invasion by an external pathogen.

**Generates fluids** (*shēng jīn* 生津)

**Genital pain** (*shàn qì* 疝气) A group of disorders characterized by pain and swelling of the external genitals and lower abdomen, usually associated with cold or constrained qi affecting the Liver channel. Mostly affecting men, with the commonest manifestation being various types of hernia, and testicular swelling and pain. Diagnosed biomedically as hydrocele or varicocele, testicular torsion, epididymitis, orchitis, inguinal or inguinolabial hernia. Also known as bulging disorders (Bensky 2009) and mounting (Wiseman 1998).

**Harmonizes *shào yáng*** (*hé jiě shào yáng* 和解少阳) To vent pathogens from the *shào yáng* level.

**Harmonizes the middle** (*hé zhōng* 和中) Treats indigestion by activating the qi dynamic, balancing the Liver and Spleen/Stomach and promoting the correct movement of middle burner qi.

**Harmonizes the Stomach** (*hé wèi* 和胃) Directs Stomach qi downwards to treat nausea, vomiting, reflux and hiccups.

**Hydrothorax** see *xuán yǐn* 悬饮

**Indefinable epigastric discomfort** (*cáo zá* 嘈杂) An uncomfortable sense of hunger and emptiness in the pit of the stomach without wanting to eat. Also given as clamoring stomach (Wiseman 1998).

**Induces vomiting** (*yǒng tù* 涌吐) Utilizes the emetic method to quickly eject pathogens, mostly phlegm, from the interior.

**Intestinal abscess** (*cháng yōng* 肠痈) An enclosed space occupying lesion within the abdomen usually, but not always, involving the intestines. There may be suppuration, in which case there is fever and focal abdominal pain. Also known as Intestinal welling abscess (Wiseman 1998). May be diagnosed biomedically as appendicitis, diverticulitis, diverticulosis or mesenteric adenitis.

**Intestinal wind** (*cháng fēng* 肠风) Bleeding of fresh red blood from the bowel. Usually associated with hemorrhoids.

**Invigorates blood** (*huó xuè* 活血) The gentlest form of blood mobilizing, suitable for mild blood stasis and prolonged use, with few, if any of the negative effects the stronger blood moving or breaking herbs may produce.

**Itchy damp rash** (*shī zhěn* 湿疹) Pruritic rashes with wet or weeping lesions. May be diagnosed as certain types of eczema such as pompholyx.

**Itchy wind rash** (*fēng zhěn* 风疹) Typically acute and extremely pruritic rashes on skin that is dry. May be diagnosed as various types of allergy, urticaria or dermatitis.

**Kills parasites** (*shā chóng* 杀虫) A broad term for herbs that treat intestinal, blood and skin parasites, worms, fungi, insects and other travellers.

**Leg qi** (*jiǎo qì* 脚气) A condition of the legs characterized by edema, cramping and numbness, attributed to external damp or damp heat invading the local network vessels. Can be associated with prolonged contact with water (i.e. in paddy field workers) or with an inadequate diet. Occasionally diagnosed as the vitamin $B_1$ deficiency disorder beriberi, but may be associated with other biomedical diseases.

**Lung abscess** (*fèi yōng* 肺痈) A Lung abscess, in Chinese medical terms, is a disorder characterized by fever, cough and chest pain with purulent, malodorous and blood streaked sputum. It may be diagnosed biomedically as an actual abscess (rare), but also includes severe lung infections such as pneumonia and bronchiectasis.

**Malarial disorder** (*nüè bìng* 疟病) Disorders characterized by a distinctive fever pattern, in which the fever alternates with chills. Includes not only true (plasmodium) malaria, but also other conditions with the characteristic fever pattern.

**Miscarriage, threatened** *see* Fetal restlessness

**Moistens dryness** (*rùn zào* 润燥) A generic term for herbs that lubricate surfaces that need to remain moist to function efficiently – for example, the Lungs, Stomach and Intestines.

**Moistens the intestines** (*rùn cháng* 润肠) Specifically treat constipation from dryness, due either to fluid damage by heat or lack of lubrication from blood deficiency.

**Moistens the Lungs** (*rùn fèi* 润肺) Specifically treat cough, respiratory problems and skin conditions from dryness, yin deficiency or fluid damage following a heat condition.

**Moves qi** (*xíng qì* 行气) A moderately strong and general effect on mobilizing qi anywhere in the body, used to alleviate qi stagnation. Strength is in between regulating qi and breaking up qi.

**Muscle weakness and atrophy** (*wěi zhèng* 痿证) A group of disorders characterized by acute or progressive muscular weakness and loss of motor function, with or without gradual atrophy. Mostly affects the lower body and legs. Also known as atrophy disorder (Bensky 2009) and wilting patterns (Wiseman 1998).

**Nasosinusitis** (*bí yuān* 鼻渊) A condition characterized by acute or chronic nasal and sinus congestion, with persistent mucus secretion, swelling of the mucous membranes or low grade infection in the sinuses. Also known as deep source nasal congestion in Wiseman (1998) and Bensky (2009).

**Nodules and masses** (*jié* 结, *tán jié* 痰结) These are superficial lumps affecting the subcutaneous tissues, breast, neck, groin and axilla. They are predominantly associated with phlegm and may be diagnosed biomedically as lipomata, ganglia, fibrocystic breast disease, benign thyroid nodules and chronic lymphatic swellings. These lumps are distinct from abdominal masses, which are predominantly associated with blood stasis.

**Nourishes the Heart** (*yǎng xīn* 养心) Applied to *shen* calming herbs, it implies an ability to help build and secure Heart blood and yin, and thus forms a good foundation for stabilizing the *shen*.

**Nourishes yin** (*zī yīn* 滋阴) A form of tonification, utilizing herbs with a particular gelatinous quality, moisture content or sweet sour flavour, that lubricate and moisten dry surfaces, augment the yin without being overly cloying, and clear mild to moderate deficient heat. Applies primarily to the shallow yin of the Lungs and Stomach, but may also be applied to the Liver and Heart.

**Opens orifices** (*tōng qiào* 通窍, *kāi qiào* 开窍) This term has two meanings: **1.** Restores consciousness, using piercingly fragrant and acrid substances to break through and disperse phlegm, or other pathogenic blockage, of the Heart and senses (as found on page 50); **2.** Opening up of blocked or congested senses, mostly the nose or ear.

**Opens the bowels** (*tōng biàn* 通便) Promotes bowel movement.

**Pacifies ascendant yang** (*qián yáng* 潜阳) A method of forcefully weighing down and restraining ascendant yang, mostly using minerals, shells and horns. May simply put a lid on rising yang, or also replenish yin in order to restore the balance naturally. See also Calms the Liver.

**Painful obstruction** (*bì zhèng* 痹证) Arthritic and musculoskeletal pain, stiffness and numbness.

**Phlegm damp** (*tán shī* 痰湿) Phlegm damp is a thin mucoid secretion resulting from poor fluid metabolism, weak Spleen function or a phlegm inducing diet. The term is used here to specifically refer to phlegm damp congesting the Lungs and/or digestive tract, in contrast to the phlegm that congeals into nodules and lumps or clouds the Heart and *shen*, and the phlegm complicated by heat (below). The consistency of the phlegm damp can range from thin and watery, to a more glutinous opaque or white substance.

**Phlegm heat** (*tán rè* 痰热) There are three broad types of phlegm heat disorder: **1.** Thick viscid colored sputum in the Lungs causing cough and wheezing; **2.** Mental disorders, mania, seizures and loss of consciousness from phlegm heat disrupting the Heart and *shen*; **3.** Encapsulated masses such as hot thyroid nodules, inflamed lymph nodes, breast lumps and other inflammatory swellings.

**Pleural effusion** (*xuán yǐn* 悬饮) A condition characterized by accumulation of pathological fluids in the pleural cavity resulting in chest oppression and pain, shortness of breath and cough. Xuan yin is associated with pleural effusion as a result of conditions such as pleurisy. Also known as suspended thin mucus (Bensky 2009), and suspended rheum (Wiseman 1998).

**Promotes fluid metabolism** This term describes the unique function of prepared aconite root (zhi fu zi 制附子) in supporting the transforming fire of the Kidneys, which in turn supports the other organs of fluid transformation, the Spleen, Lungs and Heart.

**Promotes healing** (*shēng jī* 生肌, *liàn chuāng* 敛疮) The literal translation of the first term is 'generates flesh', but the implication is one of assisting in the healing of all tissues that have been damaged by heat, infection or trauma. The second means to 'contain or close open sores'. Herbs that promote healing are applied topically to the affected lesion.

**Promotes healing of bones** (*xù gǔ* 续骨; *jiē gǔ* 接骨) Usually herbs that invigorate blood, stimulate the Kidneys to lay down new bone, or both. Used for poor or impaired healing of fractures and breaks.

**Promotes lactation** (*tōng rǔ* 通乳) Encourages flow of milk in situations where the flow is blocked by heat or stasis. Not a technique suited for insufficient lactation from blood deficiency, which requires blood tonification.

**Promotes menstruation** (*tōng jīng* 通经) Encourages menstruation, especially in situations where flow is obstructed by blood stasis, phlegm or cold. Not a technique suited for amenorrhea or scanty menses from blood deficiency, which requires blood tonification.

**Promotes sweating** (*fā hàn* 发汗) The diaphoretic method used for expelling pathogens from the surface.

**Promotes urination** (*lì niào* 利尿; *lì shuǐ* 利水) Herbs that promote urination are diuretics and, depending on the context, they reduce edema, alleviate dysuria or jaundice.

**Purges fluids** (*lì niào zhú shuǐ* 利尿逐水) A powerful ejection of fluids through the bladder by strong diuresis, and in some cases via the bowel as well. Used for severe edema, fluid accumulation in enclosed spaces (such as the pleura) and ascites.

**Purges the Intestines** (*xiè xià* 泻下) A method of forcefully expelling the contents of the Intestines by stimulating strong peristalsis, usually with bitter cold herbs.

**Qi dynamic** (*qì jī* 气机) The pivot of qi movement through the digestive system, and a significant contributor to qi distribution through the whole body, the qi dynamic is the dynamo created by the ascent of Spleen qi and the descent of Stomach qi.

**Qi constraint** (*qì yù* 气郁) Impediment to the free flow of qi as a result of Liver dysfunction, usually as the result of emotional factors or alteration of natural cycles (shift work etc).

**Qi stagnation** (*qì zhì* 气滞) Obstructed or impaired movement of qi anywhere in the body, commonly affecting the Spleen, Stomach and digestive system, for reasons not necessarily associated with emotion or Liver dysfunction.

**Raises yang and sinking qi** (*shēng jǔ yáng qì* 升举阳气) The technique of encouraging the normal ascent of Spleen qi, thus counteracting the pull of gravity on lax tissues, by utilizing herbs that promote the elevation of qi and the normal flow of yang (which should rise).

**Rebellion** (*nì* 逆) The pathological movement of qi in the opposite direction to its natural flow. Applied in this text to the Stomach and Lungs, whose qi should descend, but when blocked or in some way disturbed, rebels upwards to cause cough and wheezing, or nausea, vomiting, hiccups and reflux.

**Reduces lactation** (*huí rǔ* 回乳) Used to reduce milk production when weaning or when abnormal from heat or other pathology.

**Reduces visual opacity** (*tuì yì* 退翳) Treats cataracts, nebulae, and clouding of the superficial tissues of the eye.

**Regulates menstruation** (*tiáo jīng* 调经) Herbs that encourage the establishment of a regular and pain free menstrual cycle by regulating qi, nourishing blood and tonifying the Kidneys and Liver.

**Regulates qi** (*lǐ qì* 理气) Mobilizes stagnant or sluggish qi anywhere in the body, but most commonly the digestive system and qi dynamic. This is a gentler qi mobilizing action than moving qi or breaking up stagnant qi, and so is better for long term application with fewer negative effects. See also dredges the Liver.

**Releases the exterior** (*jiě biǎo* 解表) Herbs that release the exterior dispel pathogens trapped in the skin, and do so by opening the pores to enable the escape of the pathogen. Some actively promote sweating as well as an extra impetus to expel a pathogen (diaphoretics), while others simply free the surface. Can be used for cold, heat and damp surface pathogens.

**Releases the muscle layer** (*jiě jī* 解肌) Dispels pathogens trapped beneath the skin. Usually the pathogen is wind which can get through the surface more quickly than cold. Because the skin is not blocked, there is mild sweating. The mechanism of elimination involves restoring the balance of nutritive and defensive qi, and promoting normal qi movement through the muscle layer. This gently nudges the pathogen outwards. Also known as resolving the flesh (Wiseman 1998).

**Restless organs** (*zàng zào* 脏燥) A psychological and emotional disorder characterized by irrational behavior, emotional lability, hypersensitivity, depression, agitation and sudden loss of speech or motor control. Often associated with menopause or hysteria. Also known as restless organ syndrome (Bensky 2009) and visceral agitation (Wiseman 1998).

**Restores collapsing yang** (*huí yáng* 回阳) Used as an emergency treatment to prevent dissipation of yang and death. Collapsing yang is akin to shock.

**Restores consciousness** (*kāi qiào* 开窍) Revives from partial or total loss of consciousness, using piercingly fragrant and acrid substances, usually in prepared medicine form.

**Restrains urine** (*suō niào* 缩尿) Reduces urinary volume when excessive or frequent, usually by improving Kidney function or applying astringency.

**Secures essence** (*gù jīng* 固精) Prevents leakage or involuntary discharge of semen or urine. See also Sperm – involuntary loss of.

**Separates turbid and pure** (*fēn qīng qù zhuó* 分清去浊) Assists the Kidneys in segregating the impure portion of fluids, i.e those waste fluids destined for excretion, from the pure portion that will be recycled. Failure of separation results in cloudy urine and turbid vaginal discharge.

**Softens hardness** (*ruǎn jiān* 软坚) The method of gradually breaking down and resolving phlegm nodules and masses with salty substances.

**Softens the Liver** (*ruǎn gān* 软肝) Tonifying of Liver blood and yin to increase the Livers' suppleness and pliability, and to counteract its tendency to become stiff and unyielding.

**Sperm – involuntary loss of** (*yí jīng* 遗精) Traditionally this term refers to involuntary seminal emission during sleep – wet dreams – a condition considered undesirable and even pathological in Chinese medicine. Usually caused by Kidney weakness or heat of some type, the concept has been expanded to include inability to prevent or delay ejaculation during intercourse. Also known as spermatorrhea (Bensky 2009), and seminal emission (Wiseman 1998).

**Stabilizes the Kidneys** (*gù shèn* 固肾) Improves the Kidneys control of the 'lower yin', to prevent leakage of urine, sperm and other fluids from the lower burner.

**Stifling sensation in the chest** (*xiong men* 胸闷) A sense of fullness, constriction or tightness in the chest, often described by patients as difficulty in getting a deep breath. A symptom of qi constraint or phlegm accumulation.

**Stops bleeding** (*zhǐ xuè* 止血)

**Stops cough** (*zhǐ ké* 止咳)

**Stops diarrhea** (*zhǐ xiè* 止泻)

**Stops dysentery** *zhǐ lì* 止痢)

**Stops hiccup** (*zhǐ è* 止呃)

**Stops itch** (*zhǐ yǎng* 止痒)

**Stops leukorrhea** (*zhǐ dài* 止带)

**Stops pain** (*zhǐ tòng* 止痛; *dìng tòng* 定痛)

**Stops spasm** (*zhǐ jìng* 止痉; *jiě jìng* 解痉) The character *jìng* 痉 can refer to a range of conditions from simple smooth or skeletal muscle spasm (esophagus, intestines in irritable bowel, hypertonicity following stroke, spastic diplegia), through rhythmic spasms like tremor or convulsions, to the opisthotonic spasm of tetanus.

**Stops tremor** (*zhǐ jīng* 止惊; *zhèn jīng* 镇惊; *dìng jīng* 定惊) The character *jīng* 惊, can refer to a feeling of anxiety, agitation or disquiet, but more commonly in the context of the herbs that have this function, refers to tremors, fearful shaking or even convulsions, especially in children.

**Stops sweating** (*zhǐ hàn* 止汗; *liǎn hàn* 敛汗)

**Stops thirst** (*zhǐ kě* 止渴)

**Stops vomiting** (*zhǐ ǒu* 止呕)

**Strengthens sinew and bone** (*qiáng jīn jiàn gǔ* 强筋健骨) Treats atrophy and weakness, atrophy conditions in general (*wei* syndrome), bi syndromes, back pain from Kidney and Liver deficiency, and some types of pain and tissue damage from trauma.

**Strengthens the Spleen** (*jiàn pí* 健脾)

**Sudden turmoil disorder** (*huò luàn* 霍乱) An acute disorder characterized by sudden onset of vomiting and diarrhea.

**Tonifies blood** (*bǔ xuè* 补血, *yǎng xuè* 养血)

**Tonifies essence** (*bǔ jīng* 补精; *bǔ yì jīng xuè* 补益精血; also often combined with *yì suǐ* 益髓 augmenting the marrow) Although essence cannot be replaced, its consumption can be slowed by the use of tonic herbs with a particular richness and density. The act of tonifying essence also has a generative effect on the blood. *See also* Augmenting essence and blood.

**Tonifies Kidney yang** (*bǔ shèn yáng* 补肾阳) Strengthens and warms the yang functions of the Kidneys.

**Tonifies Kidney yin** (*bǔ shèn yin* 补肾阴) Strengthens and replenishes the yin components of the Kidneys.

**Tonifies Liver and Kidney** (*bǔ shèn gān* 补肾肝) strengthens the yang and yin components and overall function of the Liver and Kidneys. Herbs with this function can be used for patterns of yang deficiency with some component of yin deficiency, as long as there is no significant heat. *See also* Warms the Kidneys.

**Tonifies Liver yin** (*bǔ gān yin* 补肝阴) Strengthens and replenishes the yin components of the Liver.

**Tonifies Lung and Kidney** (*bǔ fèi shèn* 补肺肾) Strengthens respiratory function in the treatment of chronic Lung disease.

**Tonifies Lung qi** (*bǔ fèi qì* 补肺气) Specifically strengthens respiratory and defensive qi function.

**Tonifies Lung yin** (*bǔ fèi yin* 补肺阴)

**Tonifies qi** (*bǔ qì* 补气; *bǔ pí yì fèi* 补脾益肺) Strengthens Spleen and Lungs function to enhance manufacture of qi in general.

**Tonifies qi and blood** (*bǔ qì xuè* 补气血)

**Tonifies Spleen yang** (*bǔ pí yáng* 补脾阳; *wēn pí yáng* 温脾阳)

**Tonifies Stomach yin** (*yǎng wèi* 养胃) Enhances the moisture lining of the Stomach, to both lubricate and cool the Stomach.

**Tonifies the Kidneys** (*bǔ shèn* 补肾; *zī shèn* 滋肾) Strengthens and replenishes both the yin and yang aspects of Kidney function.

**Tonifies source qi** (*bǔ yuán qì* 补元气)

**Thin mucus disorders** (*tán yin* 痰饮) Generally refers to a group of conditions (see also *xuán yin*, *zhi yin* and *yi yin*) characterized by localized accumulation of fluid in a body cavity and/or the extremities. Specifically, *tán yin* refers to accumulation of pathological fluids in the Stomach and Intestines. Thin mucus disorders are clinically indistinguishable from phlegm damp accumulation, and the same principles of treatment apply.

**Transforms damp** (*huà shī* 化湿) Improves the Spleen's function of metabolizing dampness and prevents more damp from being formed. Some utilize a piercing fragrance (huo xiang [p.16] for example, of the aromatic group) that breaks up and disperses damp allowing it to be more easily transformed. *See also* Dries damp.

**Transforms maculae** (*huà bān* 化斑) Treats macular or purpuric skin rashes, usually due to heat, that sometimes accompany high fever.

**Transforms phlegm** (*huà tán* 化痰) Transforming phlegm means improving the Spleen's ability to metabolise fluids, to get rid of the phlegm that is already present, and to prevent more from being formed. *See also* Expels phlegm.

**Transforms phlegm heat** (*huà tán rè* 化痰热) Treats phlegm heat disorders. These substances usually have some degree of sweetness or saltiness which moistens and softens hot phlegm. They are not as acrid and drying as cold phlegm transforming herbs and so do not aggravate the heated phlegm's already pronounced stickiness.

**Treats accumulation disorder** (*qīng gān rè* 清疳热; *chú gān rè* 除疳热) *See* Accumulation disorder

**Treats suppurative sores** (*xiāo yōng* 消痈; *liáo chuāng* 疗疮) Treats festering sores that are due to dampness with varying degrees of heat. *See also* Clears toxic heat.

**True heat, false cold** (*zhēn rè jiǎ hán* 真热假寒) A condition wherein heat is constrained within the trunk, and its presence blocks the distribution of yang qi to the extremities, which feel cold. The condition is characterized by icy cold limbs and a pale face, but the tongue is red, urine concentrated, and the patient restless and irritable.

**Unbinds the chest** (*jié xiōng* 解胸) Treats stifling sensation in the chest, a sense of constriction, stuffiness or tightness in the chest.

**Unblocks channels** (*tōng jīng* 通经) Herbs with an ability to remove obstructions from the channels, used in the treatment of pain and bi syndrome.

**Unblocks chest yang** (*tōng yáng sàn jié* 通阳散结) Stimulate the circulation of qi and blood through the chest, and particularly the Heart. Used in the treatment of chest pain and angina.

**Unblocks collaterals** (*tōng luò* 通络; *huó luò* 活络) Herbs with an ability to drill deeply into the smallest vessels and dislodge blood stasis. For stubborn and chronic pain and painful obstruction patterns.

**Unblocks yang** (*tōng yáng* 通阳) This terms has a broad meaning that includes the stimulation of correct yang movement where the yang is blocked or sluggish (usually in one or more of the upper, middle and lower burners), and activation of the transforming power of yang. The latter is specifically seen in the ability of herbs such as gui zhi (Cinnamoni Ramulus), to activate fluid metabolism and the transformation of phlegm damp and thin fluids.

**Vents from the qi level** (*tòu qì fèn* 透气分) Encourages the outward movement of pathogens from the qi level and muscles to the surface to escape.

**Vents rashes** (*tòu zhěn* 透疹) A method used when a patient, usually a child, is too weak to mount a robust defense and expel a heat pathogen, indicated by a pale or sparse rash in a child who is pale, mildly febrile and persistently malaised. A vigorous rash is considered a sign of robust normal qi, and an indication that the infection has been completely expelled. Also known outthrusts papules (Wiseman 1998).

**Vents the nutritive level** (*tòu yíng fèn* 透营分) Encourages the outward movement of a pathogen from the ying level towards a surface (a yang organ or the surface of the body) from which it can escape.

**Warm diseases** (*wēn bìng* 温病) Conditions characterized by acute and chronic fever, and damage to yin and fluids. May be associated with a variety of pathogens, in particular damp heat and summerheat. Also known as warm pathogen diseases (Bensky 2009) or warm heat disease (Wiseman 1998).

**Warms Kidney yang** (*wēn shèn yáng* 温肾阳; *zhuàng yáng* 壮阳) A strong effect of warming and stimulating Kidney yang. Used for vigorously activating movement of yang and fluid metabolism. Quick to stimulate yang, but less sustained than tonifying.

**Warms channels** (*wēn jīng* 温经) Treats cold accumulation in the channels of the extremities, causing pain and stiffness of joints and muscles.

**Warms the Intestines** (*wēn cháng* 温肠) Treats cold type constipation.

**Warms the Kidneys** (*wēn shèn* 温肾) A mild effect of warming Kidney yang deficiency with acrid warmth. Mostly used for cold type pain of the lower burner and to assist the Kidneys in grasping qi for chronic wheezing. Quick to activate yang, but with a less sustained effect than tonification. See also Warms Kidney yang.

**Warms the Lungs** (*wēn fèi* 温肺) Treats cold conditions of the Lungs.

**Warms the middle burner** (*wēn zhōng* 温中) Supports the yang functions of the Spleen and Stomach.

**Warms the uterus** (*wēn jīng* 温经) The characters used here are the same as those used for warms the channels, but depending on the context, they also literally mean warms the menstrual flow. The implication is that herbs so described treat cold conditions affecting the uterus, specifically menstrual irregularity, dysmenorrhoea, amenorrhea, gynecological masses and infertility.

**Wears away sores** (*gōng dú shí chuāng* 攻毒蚀疮) Literally 'attacks toxin and corrodes sores', a powerful counterirritant effect for especially hard or resistant lesions.

**Wind stroke** (*zhōng fēng* 中风) An acute condition characterized by sudden onset of loss of motor function, paralysis, hemiplegia and possibly impairment of consciousness. Analogous to biomedical conditions such as stroke (cerebrovascular accident) and Bell's palsy.

**Withdrawal mania** (*diān kuáng* 癫狂) A disorder characterized by alternating periods of manic or irrational behavior, and depression. Usually attributed to the oscillating influence of phlegm and phlegm heat on the Heart.

**Yin sores** *See* abscesses.

Main sources used to compile this text

**Herbs**

Bensky D, Clavey S and Stoger E (2004) Chinese Herbal Medicine: Materia Medica, (3rd ed.) Eastland Press, Seattle

Chen J and Chen T (2004) Chinese Medical Herbology and Pharmacology. Art of Medicine Press, City of Industry

*Shi Yong Zhong Yao Xue* 实用中药学 Practical Chinese Herbs (1985) Zhou Feng-Wu (ed.), Shandong Science and Technology Press, Shandong

Xu Li and Wang Wei (2002) Chinese Materia Medica; Combinations and Applications. Donica Publishing

*Zhong Yao Xue* 中药学 Chinese Herbs (2000) Gao Xue-Min et al., Peoples Medical Publishing House, Beijing

*Zhong Yao Xue* 中药学 Chinese Herbs (1997) Yan Zheng-Hua (ed.), Peoples Medical Publishing House, Beijing

**Formulae**

*Fang Ji Xue* 方剂学 Chinese Herbal Formulae (2002); Li Fei (ed.), Peoples Medical Publishing House, Beijing

Maclean W (2016) The Clinical Manual of Chinese Herbal Patent Medicines, (3rd ed.) Pangolin Press, Sydney

*Shi Yong Fang Ji Xue* 实用方剂学 Practical Chinese Herbal Formulae (1989) Zhou Feng-Wu (ed.), Shandong Science and Technology Press, Shandong

*Zui Xin Fang Ji Shou Ce* 最新方剂手册 Handbook of the Latest Prescriptions (1998) Fan Wei-Hong (ed.), Central Plains Publishing, Henan

**Other cited references**

Eastland Press Draft Glossary for Chinese Medicine (2009)

Maciocia G (2008) The Practice of Chinese Medicine, 2nd ed. Churchill Livingstone, Edinburgh

Wiseman N, Feng Ye (1998) A Practical Dictionary of Chinese Medicine) 2nd ed., Paradigm Publications, Brookline, MA

Original source of prescriptions noted in the text

*Bai Ling Fu Ke* 百灵妇科 (Bai Ling's Gynecology), Han Bai-Ling 1983 Heilongjiang Publishing, Heilongjiang

*Bao Ming Ji* 保命集 (Collection for Maintenance of Life), Zhang Bi-Zhuan, Yuan dynasty

*Bao Ying Cuo Yao* 保婴撮要 (Outline of Infant Care) Xue Kai, Ming dynasty

*Bei Jing Shi Zhong Yao Cheng Fang Xuan Ji* 北京市中药成方选集 (Chinese Prepared Medicines from the Beijing Municipality)

*Ben Cao Gang Mu* 本草纲目 (The Great Materia Medica), Li Shi-Zhen 1596

*Ben Cao Hui Yan* 本草汇言 (Treasury of Words on the Materia Medica), Ni Zhu-Mo 1624

*Ben Cao Yan Yi* 本草衍义 (Extension of the Materia Medica), Kou Zong-Shi 1116

*Bian Zheng Lu* 辨证录 (Records of Differentiation of Symptoms), Chen Shi-Dou 1687

*Bu Yao Xiu Zhen Xiao Er Fang Lun* 补要袖珍小儿方论 (Supplement to the Pocket Sized Discussion of Formulas for Children) Zhuang Ying-Qi, Late Ming dynasty

*Cheng Fang Bian Du* 成方碥读 (Convenient Reader of Established Formulas), Yu Gen-Chu 1776

*Chong Ding Tong Su Shang Han Lun* 重订通俗伤寒伦 (Revised Popular Guide to the Discussion of Cold Induced Disorders), Zhang Bing-Cheng 1904

*Chong Lou Yu Yao* 重楼玉钥 (Jade Key to Layered Stories), Zheng Mei-Jian 1838

*Chuan Xin Shi Yong Fang* 传信适用方 (Transmitted Trustworthy and Suitable Formulas), Wu Yan-Kui 1180

*Ci Shi Nan Zhi* 此事难知 (Hard Won Knowledge), Wang Hao-Gu 1308

*Dan Xi Xin Fa* 丹溪心法 (Teachings of Zhu Dan-Xi), Zhu Dan-Xi 1481

*Dan Xi Xin Fa Fu Yu* 丹溪心法附余 (Additions to the Teachings of Zhu Dan-Xi), Fang Guang-Lei 1536

*Dong Yuan Shi Xiao Fang* 东垣试效方 (Effective Formulas from Li Dong-Yuan's Practice), Li Dong-Yuan 1266

*Dou Zhen Shi Yi Xin Fa* 痘疹世医新法 (Teachings of Generations of Physicians about Pox), Wan Quan 1568

*Fu Ke Yu Chi* 妇科玉尺 (Jade Rule Gynecology) Shen Jin-Ao, Qing dynasty

*Fu Qing Zhu Nu Ke* 傅青主女科 (Women's Diseases According to Fu Qing-Zhu), Fu Qing-Zhu 1827

*Fu Ren Liang Fang* 妇人良方 (Fine Formulas for Women), Chen Zi-Ming 1237

*Gu Jin Yi Jian* 古今医鉴 (Medical Reflections Ancient and Modern), Gong Xin 1589

*Han Shi Yi Tong* 韩氏医通 (Comprehensive Medicine According to Master Han), Han Mao 1522

*He Ji Ju Fang* 和剂局方 (Imperial Grace Formulary of the Tai Ping Era), Imperial Medical Department 1107-1110

*Hong Shi Ji Yan Fang* 洪氏集验方 (Master Hong's Experiential Formulae), Hong Zun 1170

*Huo Luan Lun* 霍乱论 (Discussion of Sudden Turmoil Disorders), Wan Shi-Xiong 1862

*Ji Feng Pu Ji Fang* 鸡峰普济方 (Ji-Feng's Formulas of Universal Benefit), Zhang Ji-Feng 1133

*Ji Lin Di Si Lin Chuang Xue Yuan Gu Ke Jing Yan Fang* 吉林第四临床学院骨科经验方 (Experiential Formulas of the Jilin Fourth Clinical Teaching Hospital Orthopedic Department), Jilin 1974

*Ji Sheng Fang* 济生方 (Formulas to Aid the Living), Yan Yong-He 1253

*Ji Shi Yang Sheng Ji* 济世养生集 (Collected Writings on Preserving Health of Benefit to the World), Mao Shi-Hong 1791

*Jiao Zhu Fu Ren Liang Fang* 校注妇人良方 (Revised Fine Formulas for Women), Chen Zi-Ming 16th Cent.

*Jin Gui Yao Lüe* 金匮要略 (Essentials from the Golden Cabinet), Zhang Zhong-Jing 210

*Jing Xiu Tang Yao Shuo* 敬修堂要说 (Medicinal Teachings from the Respectfully Decorated Hall), Qian Shu-Tian, Late 18th Cent.

*Jing Yan Fang* 经验方 (Experiential Formulae) These are prescriptions derived from modern works, and are usually the experience of physicians in various hospital across China.

*Jing Yue Quan Shu* 景岳全书 (The Complete Works of Jing Yue), Zhang Jing-Yue 1624

*Lan Shi Mi Cang* 兰室秘藏 (Secrets from the Orchid Chamber), Li Dong-Yuan 1336

*Lei Yun Shang Song Feng Tang Fang* 雷允上诵芬堂方 (Formulas from Lei Yu-Shang's Pharmacy) Lei Yu-Shang 18th Cent.

*Lei Zheng Huo Ren Shu* 类证活人书 (Book to Safeguard Life Arranged According to Pattern), Zhu Gong 1108

*Lei Zheng Zhi Cai* 类证治裁 (Tailored Treatments According to Pattern), Lin Pei-Qin 1839

*Liang Fang Ji Ye* 良方集腋 (Small Collection of Fine Formulas), Xie Yuan-Qing 1842

*Liu Xing Xing Yi Xing Nao Yan Zhong Yi Zhi Liao Fa* 流行性乙性脑炎中医治疗法 (Chinese Medical Treatment for Epidemic Encephalitis B), Hebei Provincial Health Workers Association 1955

*Ma Ke Huo Ren Quan Shu* 麻科活人全书 (Complete Book on Rashes to Safeguard Life) Xie Yu Qiong-En 1748

*Ma Zhen Quan Shu* 麻疹全书 (Complete Treatise on Measles), Hua Shou (att.) Yuan dynasty

*Ming Yi Zhi Zhang* 明医指掌 (Displays of Enlightened Physicians), Huang Fu-Zhong, Ming dynasty

*Nan Yang Huo Ren Shu* 南阳活人书 (The Nanyang Book to Safeguard Life), Zhu Gong 1111

*Nei Ke Zhai Yao* 内科摘要 (Summary of Internal Medicine), Yu Ying-Tai 19th Cent.

*Nei Wai Shang Bian Huo Lun* 内外伤辨惑论 (Clarifying Doubts about Injury from Internal and External Causes), Li Dong-Yuan 1231

*Pi Wei Lun* 脾胃轮 (Discussion of the Spleen and Stomach), Li Dong-Yuan 1249

*Pu Ji Ben Shi Fang* 普济本事方 (Formulas of Universal Benefit from My Practice), Xu Shi-Wei 1150

*Qi Xiao Liang Fang* 奇效良方 (Remarkably Effective Fine Formulas), Dong Su, Fang Xian 1470

*Qian Jin Yao Fang* 千金要方 (Thousand Ducat Formulas), Sun Si-Miao 652

*Qian Jin Yi Fang* 千金翼方 (Supplement to The Thousand Ducat Formulas), Sun Si-Miao 682

*Qing Dao Tai Xi Yi Yuan Jing Yan Fang* 青岛台西医原经验方 (Experiential Prescriptions from the Qing Dao Taixi Hospital)

*Quan Sheng Zhi Mi Fang* 全生指迷方 (Guiding Formulas for the Whole Life), Sun Ren-Cun, Song dynasty

*Ren Zhai Zhi Zhi* 仁斋直指 (Straight Directions from Ren-Zhai), Yang Shi-Ying 1264

*Ru Men Shi Qin* 儒门事亲 (Confucians' Duties to their Parents) Zhang Cong-Zheng 1228

*Rui Zhu Tang Jing Yan Fang* 瑞竹堂经验方 (Experiential Formulas from the Auspicious Bamboo Hall), Sha-Tu Mu-Su 1326

*San Yin Ji Yi Bing Zheng Fang Lun* 三因极一病症方论 (Discussion of Illnesses, Patterns and Formulas Related to the Unification of the Three Etiologies), Chen Yan 1174

*Shan Xi Sheng Zhong Yi Yan Fang Mi Fang Hui Ji* 山西省中医验方秘方汇集 (Collection of Experiential and Secret Formulas from Shanxi Province), Shanxi Provincial Health Bureau 1956

*Shang Hai Shi Yao Pi Bian Zhun* 上海市药品标准 (Shanghai Municipal Medicine Standards) 1974

*Shang Hai Shu Guang Yi Yuan Jing Yan Fang* 上海曙光医原经验方 (Experiential Prescriptions from the Shanghai Shuguang Hospital) 1950's

*Shang Han Huo Ren Shu Kuo* 伤寒活人书括 (Book to Safeguard Life on Cold Induced Disorders), Li Zhi-Xian 1564

*Shang Han Liu Shu* 伤寒六书 (Six Texts on Cold Induced Disorders), Tao Hua 1445

*Shang Han Lun* 伤寒论 (Discussion of Cold Induced Disorders), Zhang Zhong-Jing 210

*She Sheng Mi Pou* 摄生秘剖 (Secret Investigations into Obtaining Health), Hong Ji 1638

*She Sheng Zhong Miao Fang* 摄生众妙方 (Marvelous Formulas for the Health of the Multitudes), Zhang Shi-Che 1550

*Shen Shi Yao Han* 审视瑶函 (Scrutiny of the Precious Jade Case), Fu Yun-Ke 1644

*Shen Shi Zun Sheng Shu* 沈氏尊生书 (Master Shen's Book for Revering Life), Shen Jin-Ao 1773

*Sheng Ji Zong Lu* 圣济总录 (Comprehensive Recording of the Sages Benefits) Tai Yi Medical College 1111-1117

*Shi Bing Lun* 时病论 (Discussion of Seasonal Diseases), Lei Feng 1882

*Shi Bu Zhai Yi Shu* 世补斋医书 (Medical Texts from the Bettering the World Studio), Lu Jiu-Zhi 1884

*Shi Fang Ge Kuo* 时方歌括 (Compendium of Songs on Modern Formulas), Chen Nian-Zi 1801

*Shi Re Tiao Bian* 湿热条辨 (Systematic Differentiation of Damp Heat), Xue Sheng-Bai, Qing dynasty

*Shi Yao Shen Shu* 十药神书 (Miraculous Book of Ten Remedies), Ge Qian-Sun 1348

*Shi Yi De Xiao Fang* 世医得效方 (Effective Formulae from Generations of Physicians), Wei Yi-Lin 1345

*Shi Zhai Bai Yi Yuan Fang* 是斋百一选方 (Selected Formulas from the Praiseworthy Studio), Wang Qiu 1196

*Shou Shi Bao Yuan* 寿世保元 (Protecting the Source for Long Life), Gong Ting-Xian 1615

*Su Wen Bing Ji Qi Yi Bao Ming Ji* 素问病机气宜保命集 (Collection of Writings on the Mechanism of Illness, Suitability of Qi and the Safeguarding of Life as Discussed in the Basic Questions), Zhang Yuan Su 1186

*Tai Ping Sheng Hui Fang* 太平圣惠方 (Formulas from Benevolent Sages Compiled during the Taiping Era), Wang Hui-Yin et al 992

*Ti Ren Hui Bian* 体仁汇编 (Compilation of Materials of Benevolence for the Body), Peng Yong-Guang 1549

*Tong Su Shang Han Lun* 通俗伤寒论 (Popular Guide to the Discussion of Cold Induced Disorders), Yu Gen-Chu 1776

*Wai Ke Da Cheng* 外科大成 (Great Compendium of External medicine), Qi Kun 1665

*Wai Ke Zheng Zhi Quan Sheng Ji* 外科证治全生集 (Complete Collection of Patterns and Treatments in External Medicine), Wang Wei-De 1740

*Wai Ke Zheng Zong* 外科正宗 (True Lineage of External Medicine), Chen Shi-Gong 1617

*Wai Tai Mi Yao* 外台秘要 (Arcane Essentials from the Imperial Library), Wang Tao 752

*Wan Bing Hui Chun* 万病回春 (Return to Spring from the Myriad Diseases), Gong Ting-Xian 1587

*Wan Shi Mi Zhuan Pian Yu Xin Shu* 万氏秘传片玉心书 (Wan Family's Secret Commentaries on the Pure Hearted Jade Book), Li Zi-Yin, Qing dynasty

*Wei Sheng Bao Jian* 卫生宝鉴 (Precious Mirror of Health), Luo Tian-Yi, Yuan dynasty, 13th Cent.

*Wen Bing Quan Shu* 温病全书 (Complete Book of Warm Diseases)

*Wen Bing Tiao Bian* 温病条辨 (Systematic Differentiation of Warm Diseases), Wu Ju-Tong, 1798

*Wen Re Feng Yuan* 温热逢原 (Encountering the Source of Warm-Heat Pathogen Diseases), Liu Bao-Yi, late Qing dynasty

*Wen Re Jing Wei* 温热经纬 (Warp and Woof of Warm Febrile Diseases), Wang Meng-Ying 1852

*Wen Re Lun* 温热论 (Discussion of Warm Heat Pathogen Disorders), Ye Tian-Shi 1766

*Wen Yi Lun* 温疫论 (Discussion of Epidemic Warm Disease), Wu You-Ke 1642

*Xian Shou Li Shang Xu Duan Mi Fang* 仙授理伤续断秘方 (Secret Formulas to Manage Trauma and Reconnect Fractures Received from an Immortal, Daoist priest Lin, 846

*Xian Xing Zhai Yi Xue Guang Bi Ji* 先醒斋医学广笔记 (Wide Ranging Medical Notes from the First Awakened Studio), Miao Xi-Hong 1613

*Xiao Er Dou Zhen Fang Lun* 小儿痘疹方论 (Discussion of Formulas for Pediatric Pox Rashes) Chen Wen-Zhong 13th Cent.

*Xiao Er Yao Zheng Zhi Jue* 小儿药证直诀 (Craft of Medical Treatments for Childhood Disease Patterns), Qian Yi 1119

*Xiao Pin Fang* 小品方 (Formulas with Short Articles), Chen Yan-Zhi 14th Cent.

*Xin Fang* 新方 (New Formulae) These are new prescriptions derived from modern works, and are usually the experience of physicians in various hospital across China.

*Xu Ming Yi Lei An* 续名医类案 (Continuation of Famous Physicians Cases Organized by Categories), Wei Zhi-Xiu 1770

*Xuan Ming Fang Lun* 宣明方论 (Clear and Open Discussion of Formulas), Liu Wan-Su 1172

*Yan Fang Xin Bian* 验方新编 (New Compilation of Experiential Formulas), Bao Xiang-Ao 1846

*Yang Ke Xin De Ji* 疡科心得集 (Collected Experience on Treating Sores), Gao Bin-Jun 1806

*Yang Shi Jia Zang Fang* 杨氏家藏方 (Collected Formulas of the Yang Family), Yang Tan 1178

*Yang Yi Da Quan* 疡医大全 (Comprehensive Treatment of Skin Sores), Gu Shi-Cheng 1760

*Ye Tian Shi Nu Ke Zhen Zhi Mi Fang* 叶天士女科诊治秘方 (Secrets Formulas for the Treatment of Gynecological Disorders from Ye Tian-Shi), Ye Tian-Shi, 18th Cent.

*Yi Chun Sheng Yi* 医醇賸义 (The Refined in Medicine Remembered) Fei Bo-Xiong 1863

*Yi Fang Ji Jie* 医方集解 (Analytic Collection of Medical Formulas), Wang Ang 1682

*Yi Fang Kao* 医方考 (Investigations of Medical Formulas), Wu Kun 1584

*Yi Ji Bao Jian* 医级宝鉴 (Precious Mirror for Advancement of Medicine), Dong Xi-Yuan 1777

*Yi Lin Gai Cuo* 医林改错 (Corrections of Errors among Physicians), Wang Qing-Ren 1830

*Yi Men Fa Lu* 医门法律 (Precepts for Physicians), Yu Chang 1658

*Yi Xue Fa Ming* 医学发明 (Medical Innovations), Li Dong-Yuan 13th Cent.

*Yi Xue Ru Men* 医学入门 (Introduction to Medicine), Li Chan 1575

*Yi Xue Tong Zhi* 医学统旨 (Systematic Instructions on Medicine) Ye Wen-Ling 1534

*Yi Xue Xin Wu* 医学心悟 (Medical Revelations), Cheng Guo-Peng 1732

*Yi Xue Zheng Chuan* 医学正传 (True Lineage of Medicine), Yu Tian-Min 1515

*Yi Xue Zhong Zhong Can Xi Lu* 医学衷中参西录 (Records of Heart Felt Experience in Medicine with Reference to the West) Zhang Xi-Chun 1918-1934

*Yi Yuan* 医原 (Origin of Medicine), Shi Shou-Tang 1861

*Yi Zhen Yi De* 疫疹一得 (Achievements Regarding Epidemic Rashes), Yu Shi-Yu 1794

*Yi Zong Bi Du* 医宗必读 (Required Reading from the Masters of Medicine), Li Zhong-Zi 1637

*Yi Zong Jin Jian* 医宗金鉴 (The Golden Mirror of Medicine), Wu Qian 1742

*Yong Lei Qian Fang* 永类钤方 (Everlasting Categorization of Inscribed Formulas), Li Zhong-Nan 1331

*You You Xin Shu* 幼幼新书 (New Treatise on Children), Liu Fang, Song dynasty

*Yu Ying Jia Mi Fang* 育婴家秘方 (Secret Formulas for Infants), Wan Mi-Zhai 1549

*Za Bing Yuan Liu Xi Zhu* 杂病源流犀烛 (Wondrous Lantern for Peering into the Origin and Development of Miscellaneous Diseases), Shen Jin-Ao 1773

*Zeng Bu Wan Bing Hui Chun* 增补万病回春 (Supplement to the Return to Spring from the Myriad Diseases)

*Zhang Shi Yi Tong* 张氏医通 (Comprehensive Medicine According to Master Zhang), Zhang Lu 1695

*Zheng Ti Lei Yao* 正体类要 (Catalogued Essentials for Correcting the Body), Bi Li-Zhai 1529

*Zheng Yin Mai Zhi* 症因脉治 (Symptoms, Cause, Pulse and Treatment), Qin Zhi-Zhen 1706

*Zheng Zhi Zhun Sheng* 证治准绳 (Standards of Patterns and Treatment), Wang Ken-Tang 1602

*Zhong Fu Tang Gong Xuan Liang Fang* 种福堂公选良方 (Effective Prescriptions from Hall of Cultivating Happiness), Ye Gui 1894

*Zhong Guo Yao Dian* 中国药典 (Chinese Pharmacopoeia)

*Zhong Guo Yao Wu Da Quan* 中国药物大全 (Complete Book of Chinese Medicinals)

*Zhong Guo Yi Xue Da Ci Dian* 中国医学大辞典 (Encyclopedia of Chinese Medicine)

*Zhong Guo Zhong Yao Cheng Yao Chu Fang Ji* 中国中药成药处方集 (Formulary of Chinese Prepared Medicines)

*Zhong Xi Yi Jie He Zhi Liao Ji Fu Zheng* 中西医结合治疗急腹症 (Combined Chinese and Western Medical Treatment of the Acute Abdomen)

*Zhong Yao Cheng Yao Zhi Ji Shou Ce* 中药成药制剂手册 (Handbook of Chinese Herbal Prepared Medicines)

*Zhong Yao Zhi Shi Shou Ce* 中药知识手册 (Handbook of Chinese Herbal Knowledge)

*Zhong Yi Fu Ke Jing Yan Fang Xuan* 中医妇科经验方选 (Anthology of Experiential Herbal Formulas for Gynecological Conditions)

*Zhong Yi Nei Ke Jiang Yi* 中医内科讲义 (Teaching Notes on Chinese Internal Medicine)

*Zhong Yi Zhi Ji Shou Ce* 中医制剂手册 (Handbook of Chinese Medicinal Pharmaceutics), Chinese Academy of Medical Sciences 1974

*Zhong Yi Nei Ke Za Bing Zheng Zhi Xin Yi* 中医内科杂病证治新义 (New Treatments for Miscellaneous Internal Diseases), Hu Guang-Ci 1958

*Zhong Yi Pi Fu Bing Xue Jian Bian* 中医皮肤病学简编 (Concise Chinese Medical Dermatology)

*Zhong Yi Shang Ke Jiang Yi* 中医伤科讲义 (Teaching Notes on Chinese Medical Traumatology)

*Zhong Zang Jing* 中藏经 (Treasury Classic), attributed to Hua Tuo, 4th Cent.

*Zhou Hou Bei Ji Fang* 肘后备急方 (Emergency Formulas to Keep up Ones Sleeve), Ge Hong 3rd Cent.

Major references are in bold

Due to the physical limitations of the table format, index entries do not always correlate exactly to those found in the tables. Cross referencing between indications and functions may be necessary in some cases to find the precise herb.

# HERB INDEX
Pin Yin – Pharmaceutical cross reference